TECHNOLOGY-BASED HEALTH PROMOTION

To my cherished husband, Pablo, with sincere
acknowledgment of your unwavering support. (SB)

To all those who have taught me—parents, teachers, husband, children, friends—with
unending gratitude and my hope of passing on some of the great gifts you gave me. (MM)

TECHNOLOGY-BASED HEALTH PROMOTION

SHEANA BULL
University of Colorado, Denver

with contributions by
MARY MCFARLANE
Centers for Disease Control and Prevention

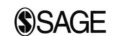

Los Angeles | London | New Delhi
Singapore | Washington DC

For information:

SAGE Publications, Inc.
2455 Teller Road
Thousand Oaks,
  California 91320
E-mail: order@sagepub.com

SAGE Publications India Pvt. Ltd.
B 1/I 1 Mohan Cooperative
  Industrial Area
Mathura Road, New Delhi 110 044
India

SAGE Publications Ltd.
1 Oliver's Yard
55 City Road
London EC1Y 1SP
United Kingdom

SAGE Publications
  Asia-Pacific Pte. Ltd.
33 Pekin Street #02-01
Far East Square
Singapore 048763

Printed in the United States of America.

Library of Congress Cataloging-in-Publication Data

Bull, Sheana.
  Technology-based health promotion / Sheana Bull; with contributions by Mary McFarlane.
      p.; cm.
  Includes bibliographical references and indexes.
  ISBN 978-1-4129-7060-0 (pbk.: alk. paper)
    1. Medical informatics. 2. Health promotion. I. McFarlane, Mary. II. Title.
  [DNLM: 1. Health Promotion—trends. 2. Cellular Phone—trends. 3. Medical Informatics
  Applications. 4. Program Evaluation—trends. WA 590]

R858.B85 2011
362.10285—dc22   2010032451

This book is printed on acid-free paper.

10   11   12   13   14   10   9   8   7   6   5   4   3   2   1

Acquisitions Editor:	Vicki Knight
Associate Editor:	Lauren Habib
Production Editor:	Karen Wiley
Copy Editor:	Melinda Masson
Typesetter:	C&M Digitals (P) Ltd.
Proofreader:	Wendy Jo Dymond
Indexer:	Gloria Tierney
Cover Designer:	Edgar Abarca
Permissions Editor:	Adele Hutchison

Brief Contents

Detailed Contents

Preface

We live in an era with a constantly evolving and ever-expanding landscape of opportunities to communicate and interact with others using technology. Public health, health science, and social science professionals run the risk of being perceived as behind the times if they cannot incorporate technological tools in the promotion of health and prevention of disease.

This book was written to orient health professionals to the enormous potential that exists in using technology for health promotion and disease prevention. At the same time, it is intended as a caution against an uncritical consideration of technology. We should carefully consider ways to maximize technology for health promotion without sacrificing the critical and effective traditional strategies that we know can be effective to help people choose and sustain healthy behaviors. The book was written because of the perception that there is a gap in textbook material for students in the health sciences; they have very good textbooks on how to design and implement program evaluation. Students can also access good textbooks on how to design and implement effective health promotion programs. However, there is little available to students in one textbook that focuses on ways to

    (a) consider innovations using technology in health promotion;
    (b) critically examine ethical considerations related to use of technology in health promotion;
    (c) learn both the best practices and the challenges associated with developing, implementing, and evaluating technology-based health programs, with special consideration for how to do this for diverse audiences; and
    (d) be exposed to case studies of technology-based programs using computer kiosks, the Internet, and mobile phones.

In Chapter 1, students and readers are introduced to a history of the use of technology for health promotion, as well as technology-based strategies and programs that have been developed related to numerous health outcomes. Chapter 2 offers an important consideration of ethics and their relationship to technology; just because we *can* do something technologically doesn't mean we *should*. The considerations for this chapter allow the reader to explore some unique issues that arise when using technology for health promotion. Chapter 3 focuses on how to develop a technology-based health promotion program, and focuses specifically on program development that is appropriate for diverse target audiences, disease conditions, and settings. In Chapter 4, the reader is introduced to issues and challenges that are specific to technology-based program implementation such as collection and management of data from large samples and using technology to communicate and follow up with program participants. Chapter 5 explores unique issues related to program evaluation using technology, including such important topics as making sure participants are who they say they are and harnessing the potential for sophisticated analyses given our opportunities to collect data from large samples via technology.

Chapters 6 through 8 offer detailed case studies of technology-based health promotion using computer kiosks, the Internet, and mobile phones. These programs were designed to address heart disease, HIV, diabetes, and smoking and offer the reader a detailed description of program elements and technology-based features.

In the Epilogue, the reader can consider the future of technology-based health promotion and the challenge related to being flexible enough to adopt new innovations as they emerge (such as using social networking sites for health promotion) while simultaneously taking the time to evaluate if we are reaching who we need to with messages and effective approaches to promote health.

In each chapter the reader will find a resource section, which identifies additional reading and websites to explore. Readers can go to www.sagepub.com/bull for regular updates to these resource lists. In addition, professors who assign this book for their undergraduate or graduate classes can access slide sets and notes that accompany the material presented in each chapter. Students and professors have exercises in most chapters that are designed for a more in-depth exploration of the material presented in each chapter.

ACKNOWLEDGMENTS

There are numerous people who have contributed to this book, and we owe them our sincere thanks and acknowledgment. First, many thanks to Erin Wright and Nora Lee, our research assistants, who helped edit, review tables, compile references, and track down permissions.

We gratefully recognize the effort and work contributed by the many reviewers of this manuscript, and the constructive comments they offered to improve this work, including Eric G. Benotsch, Virginia Commonwealth University; David Daniel Bogumil, California State University, Northridge; Karen L. Carlson, The University of New Mexico; William R. Carpenter, University of North Carolina at Chapel Hill; S. Alan Fann, Emory University School of Medicine; Maria Gilson Sistrom, Oregon Health & Sciences University; Chanda Nicole Holsey, San Diego State University, Graduate School of Public Health; Jeffrey B. Kingree, Clemson University; Francesca M. Maresca, Rutgers University; Sheila M. Patterson, Cleveland State University; Roberta P. Pawlak, Edgewood College; Ralph Renger, University of Arizona; John G. Ryan, University of Miami Miller School of Medicine; Laurie Selz-Campbell, University of North Carolina at Chapel Hill; Manoj Sharma, University of Cincinnati; Jiunn-Jye (JJ) Sheu, University of Florida; Julie K. Suzuki-Crumly, University of Alabama at Birmingham; and Ken W. Watkins, University of South Carolina.

Thank you also to all of the manuscript contributors—Anne Bowen, Russ Glasgow, Beau Gratzer, Deb Levine, Marguerita Lightfoot, Simon Rosser, Joel Selanikio and EpiSurveyor, and

HSAGlobal. Your innovations and creative ideas offer wonderful examples for others interested in technology-based health promotion. We gratefully acknowledge Dr. John Douglas from the Centers for Disease Control and Prevention; Drs. Willo Pequegnat and Susannah Allison from the National Institute of Mental Health (NIMH); Dr. Patrice Desvigne-Nickens from the National Heart, Lung, and Blood Institute (NHLBI); and Dr. Jeanette Hosseini from the National Institute of Nursing Research (NINR) for their support as project officers and program directors.

    We acknowledge the help and inspiration of longtime collaborators and colleagues, Dr. Kees Rietmeijer, Dr. Rachel Kachur, and Mr. Stephan Adelson. Finally, the information offered here was generated in part with support from the following federally sponsored research grants: R01 MH63690 and MH63690S, R21 MH083318, HL079208, and R01NR010492.

About the Authors

Sheana Bull, PhD, MPH, is trained in public health and sociology and works as an associate professor with appointments in the Department of Community and Behavioral Health at the Colorado School of Public Health and in the Department of Health and Behavioral Sciences, both at the University of Colorado Denver. She has been researching the use of technology for health promotion for over a decade and has developed and tested numerous technology-based interventions to facilitate prevention of sexually transmitted infections, including HIV, and to promote improvements in physical activity and nutrition. Her work includes collaborations with researchers and public health experts in Colorado, Wyoming, California, Pennsylvania, Virginia, Kentucky, and Texas, and she is involved in technology-based research for HIV prevention in Uganda, East Africa. She has published over four dozen research articles related to public health and is nationally and internationally recognized as a leader and innovator in the field of technology-based health promotion.

Mary McFarlane, PhD, was trained as a quantitative psychologist at the University of North Carolina at Chapel Hill. Since 1996, she has held positions in the Division of STD Prevention at the U.S. Centers for Disease Control and Prevention in Atlanta, Georgia. She originally served as a research behavioral scientist and is now the prevention partnerships coordinator, working to ensure that the field of public health continues to engage with partners in innovation, technology, communication, policy, and health promotion. She is widely published in the field of STD prevention and technology-based disease control and prevention, and continues to investigate new technologies and innovations for the advancement of public health.

PART I ⊞

Orientation to Technology-Based Health Promotion

1 ▪▪▪

A Primer on Technology-Based Health Promotion

CHAPTER OVERVIEW

This chapter introduces readers to the use of computers, the Internet, mobile phones, and mobile devices in health promotion. We offer specific examples from a growing body of literature that illustrate *how these modalities are unique and different from traditional health promotion efforts.* We also offer examples from the literature that illustrate the challenges we face with technology-based health promotion. This dynamic field has offered us several programs that we can highlight as current "best practices," and we will describe these as well. In this section, we will also consider the role of theory in technology-based health promotion, offering a conceptual framework to link the unique aspects of this field to health promotion generally. Finally, we consider emerging trends in technology-based health promotion. After reading this chapter, the reader should be able to (a) summarize unique elements of technology-based health promotion; (b) identify current "best practices" in computer, Internet, mobile phone, and mobile devices to promote health; (c) describe limitations to technology-based health promotion; (d) identify theoretical concepts that should be considered in development and implementation of technology-based health promotion efforts; and (e) describe emerging trends in the field.

WHAT IS UNIQUE AND BENEFICIAL ABOUT TECHNOLOGY-BASED HEALTH PROMOTION?

Efforts to promote health are obviously not new. We emphasize that our role in this textbook is not to describe health promotion generally but rather to consider what is *unique* and *different* that technology can add to our efforts to promote health. In this segment we consider these unique features of technology-based health promotion by reviewing selected publications that exemplify this point. Text Box 1.1 identifies the key unique elements of technology-based health promotion we describe in this chapter, and the Appendix (p. 236) offers a brief review of selected technology-based health promotion programs that exemplify the points we make in this chapter.

Reaching Larger Numbers With Health Promotion Programs—Including Disadvantaged and Marginalized Groups

One of the most significant contributions technology-based health promotion programs offer is *reach*. The Internet offers unprecedented opportunities to reach large numbers of people with health promotion programs. With the advent of the Internet (aka the World Wide Web) and browsers designed to search webpages, health promotion entered a new era. The Pew Internet & American Life Project reported that in 2000, there were 52 million Americans who had gone online seeking health information; that number had risen by 2002 to 73 million and by 2006 to 113 million (Fox & Rainie, 2000; Horrigan, 2004; Pew Internet & American Life Project, 2006).

Whereas computers could be used effectively by health care providers to promote health in clinic settings, individuals could now be proactive in seeking health information, and could do so in the privacy of their own homes, on their own time. Programs can now be delivered to people outside traditional clinic, educational, and social service settings, and therefore, they may have the potential to reach people who do not have access to any of these settings.

There remains evidence of a digital divide; that is, poor persons and persons living in resource-poor settings do not have equal access to the equipment used for technology-based health promotion or the levels of bandwidth required to deliver high-quality and graphic-rich content. This suggests that technology-based programs may actually be problematic in that they could bias the delivery of programs to those with computer access and high-speed Internet access. We further discuss this particular limitation of technology-based health promotion in the section on "bias and the ongoing digital divide" below. Of note, however, is recent evidence of a reverse digital divide—wherein lower-income populations and those residing in resource-poor settings are among the fastest-growing consumers of mobile phones, airtime minutes, and text messaging (Cellular-News, 2006). When we consider reach with technology-based health promotion, it is certainly valuable to consider the possibility of even greater penetration and reach into potentially higher-risk groups using mobile phones. Chapter 8 focuses specifically on case studies of health promotion using mobile phones.

Why is reach in health promotion of such critical importance? Consider the classic argument of public health impact. Our health promotion programs are often evaluated to determine if they work—or whether they have *efficacy*. Public health researchers are also concerned about other factors, including whether they can work for a large and diverse number of people—that is, whether they are *effective*. Ultimately, if programs have a high degree of efficacy but they work for only a small number and/or select group of people, they

TEXT BOX 1.1

What is *unique* about technology-based health promotion?

Unique element	*Why technology-based programs differ from traditional health promotion*	*Examples of this element from technology-based health promotion*	*Examples of this element from traditional health promotion*
Reach	• Technology-based programs have the potential to reach many more people than could be served in traditional programs. • People aren't required to travel to a site to participate and can access it outside traditional educational or social service settings.	(Gustafson et al., 2002)	Providers work to adapt their programs to make them more appealing to target audiences at elevated risk—for example, Latinos facing high morbidity related to diabetes (Eakin, Bull, Glasgow, & Mason, 2002).
Standardized information	• Technology-based programs' content is delivered in exactly the same way each time to every user. • Technology-based programs aren't dependent on the personality or charisma of one individual to deliver content.	(Siek, Khan, & Ross, 2009)	Project RESPECT, a two-session counseling program with demonstrated efficacy for reduction in STD (sexually transmitted disease) risk behavior and related STD infection, is designed to be delivered by staff trained in client-centered counseling. The program will differ depending on the quality of the training and the individual skills of the staff members (Kamb et al., 1998).
Tailoring	• Technology-based programs can take specific information offered by a user and generate responses, using preprogrammed algorithms that are crafted for the individual.	The Wyoming Rural AIDS Prevention Project involved a multisession interactive Internet program for men who have sex with men to address issues related to HIV prevention. Users could choose to role-play situations related to HIV risk that was most salient and relevant to them, and	The Safe in the City video project, while demonstrating efficacy, was designed to target specific risk groups but did not tailor information. Rather, persons watching the video saw information specific to topics such as condom negotiation, skills in condom use, and disclosure of STD infection to

Unique element	Why technology-based programs differ from traditional health promotion	Examples of this element from technology-based health promotion	Examples of this element from traditional health promotion
	• Traditional health promotion programs can do this as well—consider, for example, the counselor who tailors recommendations to an individual—but such efforts cannot be widely standardized or replicated.	they could avoid role plays related to situations that were not relevant (Bowen, Horvath, & Williams, 2007).	partners. Viewers could not choose a particular segment they wished to watch (Warner et al., 2008).
Interactivity with computerized device	• Technology-based programs allow for users to get instant feedback and interact with a computer. While traditional programs allow for interaction with other people, technology-based programs allow for interaction with computers and people simultaneously.	While successful traditional programs utilize interactivity to deliver content, computers can use such attractive features as video games, multiplayer games, and large-scale contents. For the younger generation dubbed "technology natives," this can be of particular appeal (Crutzen, Oenema, Brug, & de Vries, 2008).	Evidence suggests that dynamic, engaging material is critical to facilitate efficacy in health promotion. Traditional programs rely on real-world interactivity with other group members, games, and stimulating discussion (Ramirez et al., 1995; Veazie et al., 2005).
Privacy	• Programs with sensitive information or information about health that individuals may not wish to disclose to anyone else can be delivered using technology. • Evidence shows that participants may be more willing to disclose sensitive information when interacting with a machine.	Studies intended to deliver sensitive information are effective in reducing symptoms of depression while maintaining participant privacy (Christensen & Griffiths, 2002).	Group-level interventions where participants meet weekly to cover health promotion content have been shown to have efficacy for health promotion. However, everyone in the group is privy to information about other participants in the group. This can affect levels and intensity of participation, especially if programs rely on disclosure of personal or sensitive information (Eakin, Glasgow, & Riley, 2000).

(Continued)

(Continued)

Unique element	Why technology-based programs differ from traditional health promotion	Examples of this element from technology-based health promotion	Examples of this element from traditional health promotion
Autonomy	• Participants in technology-based programs can have the option of choosing program elements that are relevant and appealing to them. Traditional programs may often require users to complete elements in a particular sequence. • Technology-based programs are "always on," allowing access at any time of day or on any day of the week that is convenient to the user.	(Levine, Madsen, Barar, Wright, & Bull, 2009)	Delivery of programs with proven efficacy require participants to attend sessions that are delivered on a specific day of the week and at a specific time of day (Diclemente et al., 2004).
Portability	• Technology-based programs can be ubiquitous and portable if available on a laptop or mobile phone.	Recent innovations in the delivery of health promotion programs using mobile phones—for example, the STOMP smoking cessation program described in more detail in Chapter 8—can be accessed anytime and anywhere a person can use a mobile phone (Rodgers et al., 2005).	Traditional smoking cessation programs with counseling, while demonstrated as effective, still require users to attend sessions in person at a physical location.
Potentially lower program costs	• If technology-based programs reach greater numbers of people, can be standardized, and can be delivered at any time in diverse locations, we have the potential to lower the program costs associated with delivering health promotion.	This pilot study of an Internet-based weight loss program was more cost-effective than other information delivery channels (Booth, Nowson, & Matters, 2008).	(Glasgow, Klesges, Dzewaltowski, Estabrooks, & Vogt, 2006; Linke, Murray, Butler, & Wallace, 2007).

References

Booth, A. O., Nowson, C. A., & Matters, H. (2008). Evaluation of an interactive, Internet-based weight loss program: A pilot study. *Health Education Research, 23*, 371–381.

Bowen, A., Horvath, K., & Williams, M. (2007). A randomized controlled trial of Internet-delivered HIV prevention targeting rural MSM. *Health Education Research, 22*, 120–127.

Christensen, H., & Griffiths, K. M. (2002). The prevention of depression using the Internet. *Medical Journal of Australia, 177*(Suppl.), 122–125.

Crutzen, R., de Nooijer, J., Brouwer, W., Oenema, A., Brug, J., & de Vries, N. K. (2008). Internet-delivered interventions aimed at adolescents: A Delphi study on dissemination and exposure. *Health Education Research, 23*, 427–439.

Diclemente, R. J., Wingood, G. M., Harrington, K. F., Lang, D. L., Davies, S. L., Hook, E. W., III, et al. (2004). Efficacy of an HIV prevention intervention for African American adolescent girls: A randomized controlled trial. *JAMA, 292*, 171–179.

Eakin, E. G., Bull, S. S., Glasgow, R. E., & Mason, M. (2002). Reaching those most in need: A review of diabetes self-management interventions in disadvantaged populations. *Diabetes / Metab Research and Reviews, 18*, 26–35.

Eakin, E. G., Glasgow, R. E., & Riley, K. M. (2000). Review of primary care-based physical activity intervention studies: Effectiveness and implications for practice and future research. *Journal of Family Practice, 49*, 158–168.

Glasgow, R. E., Klesges, L. M., Dzewaltowski, D. A., Estabrooks, P. A., & Vogt, T. M. (2006). Evaluating the impact of health promotion programs: Using the RE-AIM framework to form summary measures for decision making involving complex issues. *Health Education Research, 21*, 688–694.

Gustafson, D. H., Hawkins, R. P., Boberg, E. W., McTavish, F., Owens, B., Wise, M., et al. (2002). CHESS: 10 years of research and development in consumer health informatics for broad populations, including the underserved. *International Journal of Medical Informatics, 65*, 169–177.

Kamb, M. L., Fishbein, M., Douglas, J. M., Jr., Rhodes, F., Rogers, J., Bolan, G., et al. (1998). Efficacy of risk-reduction counseling to prevent human immunodeficiency virus and sexually transmitted diseases: A randomized controlled trial. Project RESPECT Study Group. *JAMA 280,* 1161–1167.

Levine, D., Madsen, A., Barar, R., Wight, E., & Bull, S. (2009). *Asynchronous focus groups on MySpace: Creating cultural and environmental relevance for hard-to-reach populations.* Unpublished manuscript.

Linke, S., Murray, E., Butler, C., & Wallace, P. (2007). Internet-based interactive health intervention for the promotion of sensible drinking: Patterns of use and potential impact on members of the general public. *Journal of Medical Internet Research, 9,* e10.

Ramirez, A. G., McAlister, A., Gallion, K. J., Ramirez, V., Garza, I. R., Stamm, K., et al. (1995). Community level cancer control in a Texas barrio: Part I. Theoretical basis, implementation, and process evaluation. *Journal of the National Cancer Institute Monographs,* 117–122.

Rodgers, A., Corbett, T., Bramley, D., Riddell, T., Wills, M., Lin, R. B., et al. (2005). Do u smoke after txt? Results of a randomised trial of smoking cessation using mobile phone text messaging. *Tobacco Control, 14,* 255–261.

Siek, K., Khan, D., & Ross, S. (2009). A usability inspection of medication management in three personal health applications. *Proceedings of Human Computer Interaction International, 1,* 129–138.

Veazie, M. A., Galloway, J. M., Matson-Koffman, D., Labarthe, D. R., Brownstein, J. N., Emr, M., et al. (2005). Taking the initiative: Implementing the American Heart Association Guide for Improving Cardiovascular Health at the Community Level: Healthy People 2010 Heart Disease and Stroke Partnership Community Guideline Implementation and Best Practices Workgroup. *Circulation, 112,* 2538–2554.

Warner, L., Klausner, J. D., Reitemeijer, C., Malotte, C. K., O'Donnell, L., Margolis, A. D., et al. (2008). Effect of a brief video intervention on incident infection among patients attending sexually transmitted disease clinics. *PLoSMed, 5,* 919–927.

will have less impact. Programs that may have relatively lower efficacy but whose effects can be realized by larger and more diverse groups of people will have greater impact overall. This impact is of critical importance, because without it, we cannot hope to affect reductions in morbidity and mortality and improve health.

Several researchers have paid close attention to public health impact. Thyrian and Ulrich (2007) argue that a program that can produce an effect on a specific behavioral outcome such as smoking will not necessarily have a substantial impact on smoking prevalence in the population or subsequently on smoking-related morbidity unless it can be designed to reach many people and unless those people can remain engaged with the program over time. Other researchers emphasize the same—unless we can reach large proportions of the audience targeted for a health promotion endeavor, they argue, our program will have limited impact regardless of efficacy (Glasgow, Klesges, Dzewaltowski, Estabrooks, & Vogt, 2006; Klesges, Estabrooks, Dzewaltowski, Bull, & Glasgow, 2007). Glasgow and colleagues take this argument further—they also consider that reach to individuals is indeed critical for program impact, but in addition, they consider that in order to achieve improvements in reach we need to make programs easy for organizations and communities to adopt and to implement. It isn't enough to reach large proportions of a target audience; in order to sustain program effects over time, you must ensure that organizations coming in contact with a target audience can easily adopt and implement a program (Glasgow, Lichtenstein, & Marcus, 2003).

How exactly would this be relevant for a technology-based health promotion program? Using technology in health promotion certainly has potential for reaching many more individuals than may otherwise participate in traditional face-to-face programs in clinics, schools, and community settings. Using technology could also be appealing for organizations in that technology-based programs (such as a CD-ROM or Internet program) may require fewer human resources to implement than other programs (e.g., a six-session group counseling program for weight loss may require personnel time and clinic space; a similar CD-ROM program only would require a computer and perhaps a short amount of staff time to introduce and orient a patient or participant to the program).

Thus, while it is of course important that our programs show positive effects, it is only by disseminating these effects widely that we will achieve our goals of health promotion and disease prevention. The importance of program *reach* cannot be overstated (Glasgow, McKay, Piette, & Reynolds, 2001). Consider the following references for a more detailed exploration of public health impact (Dzewaltowski et al., 2010; Klesges et al., 2007; Thyrian & Ulrich, 2007); included in these resources are specific calculations for quantifying the impact of a program.

Standardizing Information

Another advantage offered by technology-based health promotion is that of standardization in program delivery. By offering health promotion via computers, early innovators in this area were able to demonstrate fidelity and standardization as key advantages in the use of technology. Because program content is delivered in the exact same way each time, it removes reliance on individuals for health promotion whose skills and demeanor may be unique and difficult to duplicate (Prochaska, DiClemente, Velicer, & Rossi, 1993; Strecher et al., 1994; Taylor, Houston-Miller, Killen, & DeBusk, 1990).

Tailoring Information

In addition to standardization, another important element of technology-based programs is tailoring. The emergence of computer software and "expert systems" allows for the production and dissemination of individually tailored print material (Bental, Cawsey, & Jones, 1999; Campbell, Peterkin, Abbott, & Rogers, 1997; Campbell et al., 1994; de Vries & Brug, 1999; Kreuter & Strecher, 1996; Lipkus, Lyna, & Rimer, 1999; Marcus et al., 1998; Rakowski et al., 1998; Rimer et al., 1999; Rimer & Glassman, 1998; Skinner, Siegfried, Kegler, & Strecher, 1993; Skinner, Strecher, & Hospers, 1994). This body of research has shown that tailoring increases the "self-relevance" of print material for subjects; that such material is more likely to be read, comprehended, and remembered; and that it can produce significant behavior change (Kreuter, Farrell, Olevitch, & Brennan, 2000; Strecher, 1999) across a wide variety of behavioral outcomes (e.g., smoking cessation, diet and nutrition, cancer screening). This algorithm-driven tailoring is a key element that blends the traditional mass media or even targeted media campaign with an individual-level intervention that can be delivered to large numbers of people. We can create libraries of branching content that allows for multiple situations and circumstances that can be unique and may not be taken into account in a traditional program.

Interactivity and Social Media

Computer-based programs allow for users to explore interactively and discover different outcomes or options either through interacting via different branches throughout the program or through interaction with other program users via social media.

Interactivity with different branches or scenarios is a key feature of computer games, and these elements have often been available historically through computer-based health promotion. More recently, a review of interactive games in computer-based health promotion has shown that the absorption allowed by the interaction appears to increase user attention and engagement (Baranowski, Buday, Thompson, & Baranowski, 2008). While evaluations from traditional health promotion efforts have demonstrated the critical importance of using engaging and interactive techniques to deliver their program content, the difference we underscore here may be most relevant for the younger, or "technology-native," user, who will appreciate the ability to interact with components such as video games designed to send a health promotion message online.

Another facet of interactivity is through connection with other users via social media. The advent of social media elements on the Internet has allowed users to interact with each other online through such activities as web logging or "blogging," threaded discussion groups, online chatting, instant messaging, and text messaging on the telephone. Pew Internet & American Life reports that over 70% of teens and young adults (up to age 29) engage in social media and social networking sites (Carter-Sykes, 2010). Thus, while we have relatively little data to date on the efficacy of using these social media tools for health promotion, we anticipate that the growing popularity of devices online and on cell phones and other mobile devices such as tablet computers and the iPad™ (Apple, 2010), a mobile device bigger than a phone intended to link users to the Internet, e-mail, photos, and music, will create many opportunities for health promotion programs to rely on user-generated interaction to introduce, process, and reinforce messages about health, health behavior, and health outcomes.

Privacy

In a landmark study of audio computer-assisted self-interview (ACASI), Turner and colleagues (1998) found that more sensitive behaviors are revealed to computers than to in-person interviewers or to paper-and-pencil surveys. While this work is more specific to research on health than health promotion per se, the advantages for health promotion are evident. When asking persons to complete health promotion programs for sensitive or stigmatized issues, such as mental health, sexuality, eating disorders, and/or substance use, there may be an advantage to the privacy afforded to the individual who interacts with a computer instead of an individual or a group. In a recent qualitative assessment of youth opinions regarding the value of using computers to convey information on sexuality in Uganda, for example, participants indicated a high level of interest in the approach, stating,

> I think this program is better. It is more private; when you ask about some sensitive things, you feel shy and when these people come to school, when you have personal problems, you can not ask because you are many, you just feel shy. But when you go to this program you get to know your problem and you discuss it and you find the solution without being interrupted by any one. (Bull, Biringi, Nambembezi, Kiwanuka, & Ybarra, 2010)

Autonomy

Prior to the Internet, computer-based health promotion programs were unidirectional; that is, they were created by the care provider based on assumptions regarding patient needs in clinic settings. While these assumptions were likely to be data driven, the Internet offered users a new opportunity in autonomy by allowing them to pose questions about health and peruse multiple sites to find answers to these questions.

Individuals could seek information from multiple sources and compare and contrast information they found. Pew Internet & American Life reports that the typical health information seeker during the early days of the Internet sought information on prescription drugs, approaches for weight loss, and specific diseases (Fox & Rainie, 2000). Over time, reports have consistently shown that online health information seekers (a) want updated and current information, (b) need to trust the information source, and (c) don't typically find information on commercial sites selling products credible. Finding ways to communicate information to the widest possible audience involved ensuring that the information was readable, captured the viewer's attention, and was accurate, up-to-date, and credible. Initially, the Internet seemed to represent a perfect medium for communicating health information, and whole medical encyclopedias appeared online (ADAM, WebMD, etc).

With the advent of social networking sites and other user-driven features online (discussed in more detail in this chapter, in the section on emerging and evolving trends) users can contribute to site content through posting a web log (called blogging), participating in threaded discussions, or offering testimonials.

Portability

In the early part of the 21st century we began seeing additional technology-based health promotion opportunities arise to join computers and the Internet. The proliferation of mobile phones—extending in many cases in some developing country settings to users who had never before had a phone because the landline infrastructure was not developed—has offered additional new opportunities beyond computers and the Internet for health promotion. The critical aspects of the mobile phone that can enhance health promotion include (a) portability and accessibility and (b) increased access by disadvantaged groups.

The mobile phone has the advantage of being able to fit into a pocket or purse, and evidence is growing that phones are ubiquitous. Recent data from the Pew Internet & American Life Project show that over 60% of U.S. adults are connected through a mobile device (Horrigan, 2008).

A mobile phone is much more affordable than a computer. Web-enabled phones that can receive or send data are also more affordable than computers, although the costs of such features are often subsidized in the United States by having users sign up for user contracts that will incur stiff penalties if broken.

In 2010 we have also seen the emergence of other portable devices such as the iPad™, which allows users access to the Internet through a device with a larger screen—because this device is still relatively new, we know little about the advantages and accessibility of the product but anticipate it will offer portability and may improve access to the Internet and continue to make computing ubiquitous. The initial price of this device is $500—much more expensive than a phone, but less expensive than a laptop computer. We anticipate that many of the advantages of portability may be realized through this type of device.

As mentioned above, we face a digital divide in access to technology and, by extension, to technology-based health promotion. Much has been written about this disparity in access to the Internet and high-speed broadband or cable access among high-income and more often White populations in the United States compared to lower-income and minority groups (Bernhardt, 2000; Chang et al., 2004; Gustafson et al., 2005; Jackson et al., 2008). Even though there is evidence that the digital divide is shrinking, there is also evidence that it persists. Data on mobile phone usage have shown in multiple settings—both domestic and international—that the digital divide is substantially less for mobile phone users, and other sources show that minority users are trendsetters for phone purchase and use of minutes and data via phones (Jackson et al., 2008; Lenhart & Horrigan, 2003; Lorence, Park, & Fox, 2006).

Potentially Lower Program Costs

If the advantages of technology-based health promotion cited here are realized, we have the potential to lower program costs related to the delivery of health promotion. Specifically, reaching larger numbers of people means lower costs per person for program delivery; standardized information delivery means fewer costs expended for training staff; tailoring information can save time in reducing exposure to superfluous information; and increasing access through ubiquitous computing may allow for fewer resources devoted to brick-and-mortar program elements. In addition, because the computer program offers additional reach, it is possible that more people could access and utilize a computer-based health promotion program than could interact with staff in traditional programs (Booth, Nowson, & Matters, 2008; Brendryen & Kraft, 2008; Bull, Gaglio, McKay, & Glasgow, 2005; Cassell, Jackson, & Cheuvront, 1998; Feil, Glasgow, Boles, & McKay, 2000; Formica, Kabbara, Clark, & McAlindon, 2004; Glasgow et al., 2007; Rainie, Horrigan, Wellman, & Boase, 2006).

WHAT ARE CHALLENGES WE FACE WITH TECHNOLOGY-BASED HEALTH PROMOTION?

While technology-based health promotion has the potential to achieve the benefits outlined here, it is important to consider the challenges we currently face in realizing this potential. Without careful consideration of these challenges and potential limitations, we may fail to identify important factors that can reduce the overall benefit and impact that our efforts in technology-based health promotion achieve. The issues considered in this section are summarized in Text Box 1.2.

Sampling and Generalizability

While technology-based work certainly does have the opportunity of reaching many more people than face-to-face programs, it is imperative that we carefully consider the methods in which we reach our audiences.

Sampling and generalizability are not issues that are unique to technology-based health promotion. However, it is important to examine some specific considerations when recruiting exclusively in a virtual environment. While the Internet offers the unprecedented reach to populations described above, appropriate sampling in this medium is challenging. Given daily additions and deletions of websites, we do not have the ability to define a sampling frame of all Internet sites, or even all sites of a particular type online. We may have better luck within a site, where we could sample users of the site—although the same challenge presents itself when users join and stop using sites. One approach to this problem from a research perspective has been employed by Harris Interactive (2010), which utilizes a panel method for sampling. This, however, is specific to research. A panel approach to sampling could be used to pretest program ideas and pilot-test program elements.

It is essential to realize that not all information discovered in online venues can be generalized to the real world, or even to the rest of the Internet. One early example involved "gift giving" and "bug chasing," the processes by which an individual intentionally infects another with HIV or seeks infection from an HIV-positive person. The *gift giver* is a term

TEXT BOX 1.2
What challenges do we face with technology-based health promotion?

Challenge	Specific challenges technology-based programs face in this area
Sampling and generalizability	• While it is easy to accrue large samples for programs that are delivered online, it isn't easy to select them systematically online. • Strategies such as banner advertising yield participation rates of <.01, making it impossible to generalize findings to the larger audience using the Internet.
Identification of users and confidentiality	• People may engage in deception to participate in Internet- or phone-based programs. • While confidentiality and privacy are likely more secure online than in face-to-face programs, users may distrust programs, and program planners may face challenges in establishing credibility.
Attention span and competing priorities online and with mobile devices	• Because of the volume of information that technology users must process, multitasking has become commonplace. Evidence shows that multitasking is on the increase (Carrier, Cheever, Rosen, Benitez, & Chang, 2009) but also that it actually reduces the ability to absorb or comprehend material. • The growing volume of information and activities available online means health promoters must compete for participant attention with often better-financed games, videos, and so on online.
Bias and ongoing digital divide	• Evidence remains that persons with less income have less access to the Internet and use it less often, suggesting programs relying on the Internet to deliver content will be biased. • While Internet users tend to be more affluent, lower-income communities are among the fastest-growing consumers of mobile phone technology.
Technological obsolescence	• Technology-based health promotion that relies on lengthy development and evaluation periods may find some or all elements of the program obsolete by the time it is implemented and evaluated.

References

Carrier, L. M., Cheever, M.A., Rosen, L. D., Benitez, S., Chang, J. (2009). Multitasking across generations: Multitasking choices and difficulty ratings in three generations of Americans. *Computers in Human Behavior, 25*(2), 483–489.

given to someone infected with HIV who makes it known that he or she is willing to infect another individual. The *bug chaser* is the name given to the individual intentionally seeking an HIV-infected partner for sex to increase his or her own chances of infection. This is a behavior that can occur in non-Internet venues, but one can easily imagine that the Internet can magnify the potential for partnerships to form and infection to be spread rapidly. As a research topic, this attracted some attention and concern, and even some media activity; however, in general, the phenomenon of bug chasing and gift giving has not been shown to be widespread (Grov & Parsons, 2006). Many countercultural websites are fascinating and bizarre (examples such as proanorexia websites, violence-oriented sites, and sites promoting self-destructive activities abound); however, users of these sites are either very few or nonexistent, and the online phenomenon does not always translate to real-life behavior. Thus, observing the web to learn about health promotion activities can be misleading, which implies that we must exercise caution in generalizing from observational studies to the population as a whole.

While observational studies clearly have their place, they should be substantiated by further research that indicates the size, scope, and impact of the issue being studied.

Another concern with generalizability arises with the use of banner advertising for recruitment, be it for surveillance or program activities. Our own experience, for example, shows that persons clicking on banner advertisements represent only .01% of those exposed to the banner, and those who continue the program after clicking on the ad are only a fraction of those clicking (Bull, Vallejos, & Ortiz, 2008). Such low "click through" rates, as they are named, illustrate the impossibility of generalizing any program findings to a larger audience. We will cover specific strategies for sampling and recruitment to address these challenges in Chapter 4.

These sampling concerns are related to the concern of validity. If we cannot generalize our findings based on representative samples, how valid will our programs be, particularly across diverse technology users? We submit that the issue of validity for technology-based programs isn't unique to technology per se: Rather, it remains one of concern for any health promotion program. We advocate attention to validity for programs whether they are technology based or based in other settings. What technology-based programs do afford that other programs may not is a platform to more easily test our validity across groups because of the ease inherent in contacting and interacting with groups that technology affords. Therefore, processes of development and testing programs can include plans for adaptation and validity testing for diverse technology-based audiences.

Identification of Users and Confidentiality

When recruiting for any technology-based program using virtual approaches, the identification of users and participant privacy can be a challenge. Similarly, when delivering program content using technology, it isn't always possible to know if the person you intend to expose to your content is the person who receives and views it. This issue is only exacerbated in Internet and mobile phone programs when enrollment and program activities are divorced from direct face-to-face staff contact. Persons enrolling on the Internet may lie about program eligibility criteria, and they may attempt to enroll multiple times (especially if there is an incentive). Persons using mobile phones may not be the exclusive users of a phone, or their phone could be used or answered by a friend or family member. Many of the problems inherent with self-reported data are exacerbated by the Internet. While anonymity and accessibility can provide an environment of honest and open communication, it can also allow respondents to falsify data, misunderstand questions, or otherwise provide inaccurate responses. Online survey data can be maliciously or accidentally falsified, and there is no in-person support if respondents have questions or concerns. Privacy concerns online are paramount, and no one wants to report sensitive behaviors to a system that can be "hacked" by online vandals. Similarly, it is difficult to imagine reporting illegal behaviors to a government behavioral surveillance system. This is a factor in in-person interviewing as well, but an in-person interviewer has the opportunity to answer questions and address concerns from the respondent. Online, the respondent must trust that the person on the other end of the survey is beneficent and intends to keep the data confidential. We will further discuss issues of user identification and verification in Chapter 4, and of user privacy in Chapter 2.

Attention Span and Competing for Attention Online and With Mobile Devices

Attention spans are an increasing concern with technology-based health promotion. Surveys are often long and occasionally tedious, and Internet and mobile phone users are accustomed to brief interactions; thus, a long survey may appear even longer when conducted using technology. When in a face-to-face interview, the respondent and the interviewer may develop a rapport that allows the survey to feel more like a friendly interaction. Using technology, however, the sterile nature of the site may contribute to boredom, wandering attention, and high dropout or noncompletion rates.

An additional concern is the competition for attention in the virtual world. New websites are regularly added to the Internet, and there is an ever increasing volume of data transmitted via e-mail as well. This suggests that we have challenges in creating and disseminating content for health promotion using technology that will effectively compete with the other content that is constantly being sent to technology users. We will have to strategize about how to gain and hold participant attention in an environment that is increasingly crowded, likely with content that is more appealing, entertaining, and personally relevant for users.

Bias and Ongoing Digital Divide

There is an inherent bias in technology-based health promotion, because such programs are only available to people who have access to the appropriate technology. In some populations of interest, this strikes a major blow to the ability to generalize the survey results to the larger population. It is a well-established fact that health issues of persons with low socioeconomic status are very different from those of wealthier, educated, employed, insured citizens. The likelihood of owning a computer or mobile device with Internet access may be similarly related to socioeconomic status. Thus, surveying health problems via Internet questionnaires may result in a biased sample of mostly wealthy, educated persons and an inaccurate portrayal of the health conditions of the poor. As mentioned above, however, mobile phones may someday fill this "digital divide" by ensuring access for people who lack the means to purchase a full computer system. At present, a desktop or laptop computer with reasonably fast Internet access costs, at a minimum, several hundred dollars. A mobile phone, on the other hand, costs far less and may provide many of the same communication and information features found on laptops. Thus, online behavioral surveillance and other Internet-based health promotion efforts will likely need to be adapted to the more compact, mobile medium.

There is evidence that information offered on the web about health is frequently delivered at a very high level of literacy—that is, greater than a ninth-grade reading level (Bull, Leeman-Castillo, Ortiz, & Gutierrez-Raghunath, 2008). With ample evidence that persons with lower literacy skills and limited English proficiency also suffer disproportionately from negative health outcomes, it is imperative that we do more to ameliorate this situation.

The fact that technologies haven't been widely used for health promotion with less literate, less educated, or non-English-speaking groups is ironic, given the potential for technology to overcome these challenges with audio, video, cartoons, and other interactive but more accessible content. There are some exceptions to this finding to date, however; research is currently being done with Latinos in the Denver metropolitan area to use computer algorithms to offer feedback on physical activity, nutrition, and smoking in an effort to promote healthy behaviors (Bull, et al., 2008).

Data have consistently shown lags in access to and use of technology among poor people, minorities (inasmuch as these groups are overrepresented among the poor), and elderly (King et al., in press). While new assessments of this digital divide show that these lags are diminishing, they do remain. It is important that health promoters recognize the existence of the digital divide and try to assess how large it actually is for the population they wish to engage with technology-based health promotion. Failure to do so can bias samples to overrepresent higher-income and better-resourced groups, and limit generalizability of findings to those groups that may not have as great a need for intervention. Program planners need to consider whether they want to conduct technology-based health promotion because it is the most appropriate modality to use, or because it is convenient and easy for them.

Even when barriers to access and literacy have been addressed, there may be cultural considerations to conducting technology-based health promotion with specific groups. In preparation for a pilot study of a computer kiosk to promote heart-healthy behaviors for Latinos, researchers learned that there were assumptions within the Latino populations they hoped to reach that use of the Internet and computers was anathema to many within their community, and, recognizing that, they made substantial effort to create a program that was culturally relevant and engaging for Latinos specifically (Padilla et al., 2010). More on making programs culturally relevant is discussed in Chapter 3 in the section on best practices in technology-based program development.

Technological Obsolescence

One of the biggest hurdles in technology-based health promotion is obsolescence. Health promotion program planning, implementation, and evaluation have accepted standards of rigor. With rapid evolution of technology, however, we may no longer have the luxury of time to be able to investigate if a technology-based innovation works. If we take several years to design programs, make them culturally appropriate for the audience, accrue samples, and follow them for long periods of time, we may show efficacy for an innovation that is obsolete. One example of our own learning in this area was for an intervention to promote HIV prevention among youth, using primarily static design elements with some tailored feedback, but no interactivity between users. By the time 4 years had passed between obtaining research funding and completing the randomized trial testing the efficacy of our online intervention, the era of social media was upon us with its attendant blogs, threaded discussion, and user-generated commentary, making our own intervention potentially obsolete (Bull, Pratte, Whitesell, Rietmeijer, & McFarlane, 2009).

While evaluation of health promotion efforts is known for attention to detail and rigorous methodologies, the rapid evolution of the Internet and other technologies is proving to set up a tension that has important implications for our work. We need to keep pace with the rapid evolution in technology with similar agility in our research methods. As researchers began to document patterns of web usage and behaviors and to test out the efficacy of providing information online, using algorithms to give feedback and communicating in a bidirectional manner using e-mail, the Internet world was moving into a new era altogether—the so-called "Web 2.0" world of social media and social networking. This is an era that moves beyond uni- and bidirectional communication into a much stronger emphasis on social networking and an explosion of information sharing.

Should we relax our standards, then, to allow for more rapid assessment and evaluation? It may not be necessary to do so. We do need to investigate approaches that can prepare us to rapidly implement our research so that findings are relevant. In Chapter 2 of this book, researchers and program planners can learn strategies for priming their institutional review boards (IRBs), and other internal ethics committees so that when technology-based research and program evaluation opportunities arise they can knowledgably review protocols and quickly approve them. In Chapters 3 through 5, we touch on issues that will allow health promoters to increase their capacity to collect, manage, and analyze high-quality data quickly, both on computers and on mobile phones. In Chapter 8, we go into more detail on the promise of social media and social networking sites and how we might capitalize on them for health promotion. In each chapter we identify new horizons for technology-based health promotion—that is, what we foresee in the coming years that we can prepare to utilize to our advantage for remaining leaders in the assessment of development, testing, and translating technology-based health promotion to reach the highest audience for the greatest impact.

In general, the Internet and mobile phones have become well integrated into the fabric of modern life. However, interventions on health behaviors seemingly have not kept pace with this fast-moving technology. It seems that as soon as we learn to use and evaluate the use of current technology, it is already outdated. As we write this, new innovations in ubiquitous computing are in development. Technologies will allow users to monitor their own biological outcomes, such as sugar levels for diabetics or biobehavioral cues (galvanic skin response, increased heart rate) for addicts who begin to experience withdrawal or craving symptoms. When the monitors detect a problem, they can send a digital signal to a remote counselor or health provider, and the user can receive a phone call or text message offering support or assistance. This level of tailored health intervention is within reach, but we do not yet grasp its full potential.

THE ROLE OF THEORY IN
TECHNOLOGY-BASED HEALTH PROMOTION

The discussion above outlining both promises and limitations of technology-based health promotion offers information about elements that can be critical for inclusion in a conceptual framework hypothesizing processes through which technology-based health promotion operates.

Reviews of technology-based health promotion reveal that there has not been systematic attention to the role of theory in technology-based interventions. The types of interventions that have been employed remain largely focused on offering individuals opportunities to make behavior changes. These interventions have the opportunity to employ well-known individual-level theoretical perspectives related to behavior change such as the health belief model (Rosenstock, 1974) and the theory of planned behavior (Azjen, 1991). In addition, they offer options for including an understanding of how individuals interact with others whom they consider important, through application of social cognitive theory (Bandura, 1986) and diffusion of innovations (Rogers, 1995). Indeed, there is evidence from nontechnology interventions that when these theoretical perspectives are appropriately applied to interventions, they contribute substantially to intervention content and are considered invaluable for promotion of healthy behaviors (Albarracin, Fishbein, Johnson, & Muellerleile, 2001; Albarracin et al., 2005).

We know of at least two technology-based interventions shown in the Appendix that paid explicit attention to applications of individual-level health behavior change theories, and these are two interventions with positive results, the D-Net trial and the LUCHAR (Latinos Using Cardio Health Action to Reduce Risk) pilot study (Bull et al., 2008; Glasgow, Boles, McKay, Feil, & Barrera , 2003).

Within the broader field of public health, there certainly has been attention to theories of social interaction, culture, and environment and their varied influence on health. For example, researchers have explored the relationship between social stigma and health (Benzies & Allen, 2001; Centers for Disease Control and Prevention, 2000; Crooks, 2001; Fortenberry et al., 2002), the role of culture in health (Caldwell, Caldwell, Caldwell, & Pieris, 1998; Chin, 2000; Duffy, 2005; Fisher & Ball, 2002), the influence of social networks on health outcomes (Christakis & Fowler, 2007), and the concept of structural violence that perpetuates limitations in access to care and suggestions of individual responsibility for health outcomes even in the face of marginalization, poverty, and environmental degradation (Farmer, 1999; Farmer, Connors, & Simmons, 1996). However, we do not regularly see these theories explicitly applied to health interventions in general, and they have not been applied to technology-based health promotion in particular. As technology-based health promotion has evolved, the integration of relevant theories into programs that can offer conceptual frameworks to guide program development and explain program success or limitation has been notably lacking.

As mentioned above, we know from extensive research in health promotion that interventions at the individual level focused on specific concepts that precede behavior change have been shown to be effective (Albarracin et al., 2005; Courneya, Estabrooks, & Nigg, 1997; Courneya, Nigg, & Estabrooks, 1998; Wallace, Buckworth, Kirby, & Sherman, 2000).

This constellation of constructs includes such things as behavioral beliefs and decisional balance, or the idea that performing a behavior will offer more benefits than drawbacks when compared to not performing a behavior. Norms, or the beliefs about what important others do and think, also influence behavior—it is important to think that a group of peers would approve of a behavior, for example (Azjen, 1985). Self-efficacy, or the belief that one can perform a challenging behavior, even under difficult circumstances, is also important (Bandura, 1986). Finally, forming specific intentions to perform a behavior increases the likelihood of doing so (Azjen, 1985).

All of these individual-level constructs can be impacted through exposure to technology-based programs. Several that are described in detail later in the book have utilized these concepts in their program design (see Chapters 6–8 for case studies).

As will be discussed in greater detail below, one element of technology that recently emerged that has already impacted the landscape of technology in general and technology-based health promotion in particular is that of social networking online, also called Web 2.0. Web 2.0 allows users to interact not only with a machine but also with other computer users via the Internet. The proliferation of Web 2.0 features such as threaded discussions and posting opinions via web logs (called blogs) has opened up substantial interest in the role of social networks in health and health promotion. Researchers have recently demonstrated the importance that social networks in real life have for such important health issues as obesity and smoking (Christakis & Fowler, 2007).

Of particular interest, therefore, within technology-based health promotion, is the theoretical perspective of social networks, both real world and virtual. What is possible to study, but is essentially an unexplored area, is the influence that virtual social networks have on health outcomes and how they can be harnessed in health promotion efforts.

In addition to social networks, the theoretical perspective of social support may be particularly helpful to consider in the Web 2.0 era (Beal, Ausiello, J., & Perrin, 2001; Boutin-Foster, 2005). Investigators can take the opportunity to consider how having social support via social networking sites can enhance or detract from health outcomes. They can explore how user-generated content may increase ownership or identification with health concerns or responses to health concerns.

Given the potential critical importance that reach will have for increasing the impact of technology-based health promotion, we also have a need to make explicit theory-based approaches for increasing and facilitating exposure to and engagement with technology-based health promotion by users.

Finally, technology-based research allows for consideration of completely new theoretical ideas. For example, what is different about the interaction with technology that occurs simultaneously with human interaction? How does the technology mediate or moderate effects of an intervention that includes social networks and social support? We have unprecedented opportunity to intervene in social networks online, and to research networks and technology use among mobile phone users. What new theoretical contributions about the interaction between people moderated by machines will emerge?

Figure 1.1 offers one depiction of how all of these theoretical perspectives come together for technology-based work. Individual-level concepts such as beliefs, norms, and self-efficacy are

Figure 1.1   Theoretical elements to consider in technology-based
                health promotion

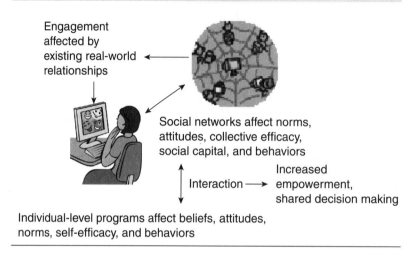

Engagement
affected by
existing real-world
relationships

Social networks affect norms,
attitudes, collective efficacy,
social capital, and behaviors

Interaction ⟶ Increased
empowerment,
shared decision making

Individual-level programs affect beliefs, attitudes,
norms, self-efficacy, and behaviors

depicted below the picture of a computer user. The user has the potential to interact with others in a real or virtual social network, as depicted in the center of the figure. It is of importance to consider the role that persons within these networks may play in helping individuals get exposed to online materials, and whether exposure to technology-based health promotion is indeed mediated by others within networks. In addition, concepts such as collective efficacy and consciousness raising within networks and the social capital of groups as they interact with technology are also areas for study.

WHAT ARE THE CURRENT AND BEST PRACTICES IN TECHNOLOGY-BASED HEALTH PROMOTION?

Hybrid Programs—Using Technology to Enhance or Supplement Health Promotion

Observational Studies Using Technology

Health promoters have been using computers, the Internet, and mobile phones to test and refine approaches for health promotion for several decades. The Appendix (p. 235) offers descriptions of selected health promotion efforts that are technology based. This Appendix is intended to be illustrative of key uses for these modalities that are instructive. Given the rapid evolution of the field, we do not anticipate that this table will be exhaustive; rather, we hope that it can serve as a resource to illustrate approaches that represent the types of technology-based health promotion described here.

Observational studies related to health that have been done using technology illustrate the utility of taking the time to understand the environment in which you plan to implement your project. By doing observational work you can better understand the ways that users interact with the technology of interest and how they engage with others using the technology. You can use observational data to design and structure your program and to consider the extent to which the information gleaned can be generalized to the population at large. We will cover processes for observational studies and other formative program development for technology-based health promotion in more detail in Chapter 3.

In one early, observational study (Bull & McFarlane, 2000), we conducted a restricted form of participant observation in multiple online venues that existed for the purpose of facilitating sexual contact between users. We observed individuals seeking sexual contact, finding potential partners in chat rooms, and moving to "private" chat or other, nonpublic communication venues. We looked for information that might indicate that online sex-seeking is common, that the sex facilitated is anonymous and unprotected by condoms, and that seeking sex online could increase a person's risk for sexually transmitted infections (including HIV, the virus that causes AIDS). This observational study was a key element in program development, allowing us to better understand how and when people used the Internet—these data could then be used for more effective program development to intervene and address sexual risk behavior online.

The main purpose of an observational study such as the one described above is discovery, leading to formative work in preparation for a health promotion program. In this example, the researchers tried to understand the process by which users engage in online activity. Components of online activity that interest health promoters include health-seeking behaviors as well as risk-seeking behaviors. How do users look for information? What type of format is especially appealing? What makes some information credible and other information blatantly untrustworthy? What attracts people online? What makes them think and feel and learn in ways that will enhance their personal and public health? Watching the way users interact with information, with online experts, and with other users is an excellent method of discovering new directions for health promotion activities.

Technology-based health promotion is not limited to health promotion for the individual. Technology can be used at the observational level to determine how well providers or organizations are meeting standards for health promotion and care delivery. In an observational study, we reviewed and coded features of 87 publicly available diabetes websites hosted by governmental, health plan, commercial, pharmaceutical, and not-for-profit organizations. We assessed whether each website was using online opportunities in the areas of interactivity, theory-based interventions, social support, and evidence-based care. The majority of sites provided information, essentially using an electronic newspaper or pamphlet format. Few sites offered interactive assessments, social support, or problem-solving assistance, although there were some significant differences in these characteristics across the types of site. The authors concluded that current diabetes websites fall short of their potential to help consumers, and made specific suggestions for ways to improve the helpfulness and interactivity of these resources (Bull et al., 2005).

Technology to Facilitate Surveillance

Surveillance work offers an opportunity to assess the scope of a health promotion issue. For example, we may learn in observational studies that thousands of users read websites about hypnosis for smoking cessation. But how many people actually undergo hypnosis and quit smoking? People most likely read about a wide variety of treatments for whatever condition they may be experiencing, and they gather information from other (offline) sources as well. To understand the full range of health-seeking behaviors, it is useful to conduct surveillance surveys. The aim of these surveys is to comprehensively study a set of health behaviors or conditions in a quantitative, structured way. For health promoters, the appeal of a technology-based survey—whether it is delivered at a computer kiosk, online, or through a mobile device—is obvious: The automated, user-entered data process streamlines data collection and eliminates the need for cumbersome paper-and-pencil surveys and time-consuming data entry. If entered data are illogical or out of range, the survey software can prompt respondents to check their answers for accuracy. Technology-based surveys can be completed in a fairly short time frame and can circumvent the need to train interviewers. Additionally, survey respondents can be presented with different versions of the survey, depending on their answers to previous questions. This type of survey is called an adaptive questionnaire, because later questions are adapted to accommodate information provided in earlier questions.

Those using the Internet for surveys have the added advantage of being able to reach many more respondents in a very short time. Further benefits of Internet-based surveillance surveys include the ability to surmount the twin obstacles of geography and population mobility. For example, in a study of survivors of childhood cancer (Cantrell & Lupinacci, 2008), participants were geographically scattered and represented a relatively small proportion of the population. Using the Internet, the challenges of finding cancer survivors among the general population could be reduced, although in this particular study, the authors were unsuccessful in recruiting a large number of participants. Similarly, populations of diabetics, people living with HIV, or people with cancer, alcoholism, or mental illness can be found online and offered the opportunity to participate in a survey.

Ultimately, survey data collected using technology can inform program development, which will be discussed in more detail in Chapter 3; it can also be used to assess program effects, which will be discussed in more detail in Chapter 5.

Examples from the review shown in the Appendix illustrate how behavioral surveillance online can facilitate understanding of the scope of a public health concern and opportunities for health promotion intervention. In the study on behavioral risk factors among men who have sex with men (MSM) in China, Zhang, Bi, Hiller, and Lv (2008) showed that collecting data from MSM online versus collecting data from community venues resulted in different behavioral risk profiles. For example, MSM online reported fewer female partners and were more likely to identify as homosexual compared to MSM in community venues. The authors of this study concluded that online interventions for HIV prevention in this group could more readily focus on topics of homosexuality and could concentrate on promotion of condom use with male partners.

Also in China, Sun et al. (2007) used an online behavioral surveillance system to understand the spread of health behaviors in remote areas as well as in densely populated urban centers. The Chinese behavioral surveillance system for HIV-related behaviors, piloted in 2004, involves drug users, female sex workers, men who have sex with men, STD clinic clients, long-distance truckers, and students. Because China is a vast nation with a low HIV prevalence and many remote areas, behavioral surveillance can be of great use in predicting the future directions of HIV incidence.

An online behavioral surveillance of problem drinkers (Lieberman & Huang, 2008) illustrated that over 1,000 users of an alcohol evaluation website were less likely to recognize their drinking as problematic compared to persons seeking treatment face-to-face. In addition, users in the online sample were less likely to take steps to change their drinking behaviors, although they shared a similar level of concern about the effects of their drinking when compared to those seeking treatment. This work illustrates the opportunity to develop online interventions for problem drinking that may be more focused on recognition of pathology and skills building for change.

Technology Used to Enhance or Extend Health Promotion Efforts

There is growing interest in the use of technologies to extend or enhance health promotion efforts that happen in clinics or schools or other settings. Consider, for example, the simple approach to enhance care delivery offered when persons can communicate via e-mail with a nutritionist. This approach was one of the early efforts shown to have efficacy for weight loss (Tate, Wing, & Winett, 2001). Persons enrolled in a nutrition education program could send messages and communicate via e-mail with a counselor at regular intervals. They could also engage in "ask the expert" opportunities to post questions and have them responded to via e-mail or in a more public forum (such as a threaded discussion board). There are relatively few published studies examining the use of technology to extend clinical services, and this could be a ripe area for program development (Glasgow, Bull, Piette, & Steiner, 2004; Marrero et al., 1995; Prochaska, Zabinski, Calfas, Sallis, & Patrick, 2000). In addition, it is critical that we consider the potential for technology to be utilized for multilevel interventions. There has consistently been a call to address health behaviors not only at the individual level but also at the social, organizational, and environmental levels (Friedman et al., 2007; Piot, Bartos, Larson, Zewdie, & Mane, 2008; Rice, Stein, & Milburn, 2008; Sanders, Lim, & Sohn, 2008; Taylor, 2007). We anticipate that intervening through a care provider using technology could be promising—consider, for example, offering care providers detailed tailored information about patient behaviors through shared electronic records. When a patient inputs his or her daily blood pressure or glucose measures and uploads these to a shared file, the physician could be prompted to make care more tailored and appropriate for him or her (Siek, Khan, & Ross, 2009). Another provider-level intervention that could enhance care and potentially behavioral outcomes is one that could deliver updates in guidelines for care to a provider's mobile device.

Technologies could be used beyond the individual to facilitate behavioral change within families—for example, programs already exist to address childhood obesity through parental education. Low-income parents can attend cooking classes and nutrition education workshops that help them identify strategies for more nutritious shopping and cooking (Swindle, Baker, & Auld, 2007). Technology can be utilized to reinforce and enhance such programs; for example, parents could receive recipes or information on days/times for a farmers' market all via text message.

Stand-Alone Interventions for Infectious and Chronic Illness Prevention

As mentioned above, in the pre-Internet era, health promotion experts looked for effective ways to incorporate health messages into the flow of everyday life, reaching people via radio, television, motion pictures, print media, billboards, and community awareness campaigns. Beginning in the 1970s, they also began to deliver health promotion programs via computer. As the computer and Internet became a mainstream tool, a natural early step involved adapting print, and later audio and video materials, to these technologies. Online, billboards were translated to banner ads, and brochures became webpages. Although these communications were intended to raise awareness, they were limited in the sense that there was only one direction to the message: from the experts to the masses. It rapidly became obvious that providing messages to the public, though necessary, was in no way sufficient for changing the behavior of the public in regard to health. Furthermore, unidirectional messages failed to capitalize on the interactivity and multidirectional communications offered by technology.

Interventions aimed at changing health behavior and related outcomes using technology have been attempted in fields as wide-ranging as mental health (depression and anxiety; Spek et al., 2007), physical activity and exercise (van den Berg, Schoones, & Vliet Vlieland, 2007), weight loss (Weinstein, 2006), diabetes (Kim & Kim, 2008), and smoking cessation (Rodgers et al., 2005). The Appendix (p. 235) describes a number of studies in which researchers have intervened upon various behaviors in an attempt to increase the health of the target groups.

In general, the goal of such interventions is to change the way people behave such that their health improves. Thus, we might try to keep people from smoking, overeating, or engaging in unprotected sex. We might discuss food safety, sunscreen, and physical activity. By engaging in multidirectional discussions, we may provide social support or even therapy using technology.

There are numerous examples of best practices in technology-based intervention for health promotion. In a review of weight-loss programs delivered online, Weinstein (2006) considers the potential impact of Internet programs introduced above. Even if they produce smaller changes in behavior than their offline counterparts, Internet programs have the potential for huge impact simply due to the number of people that can be reached for low cost. Internet interventions, she suggests, should take into account the sociocultural background, literacy, and individual needs of the target audience. But it is exactly these contextual, background variables that are difficult to assess online. Thus, Internet interventions with face-to-face components were posited as having the most potential for success. Mixing the media and modalities becomes more and more important as the Internet becomes more portable, accessible, and ubiquitous.

A very promising example of a combined Internet and mobile phone intervention for persons with diabetes was studied by Kim, Yoo, & Shim (2005). Patients in the intervention (Internet/cell phone) group were significantly able to maintain better control of their baseline hemoglobin.

Although this study only included 51 patients, it does show promise for the type of program that could combine clinic-based and technology-based health promotion.

WHAT ARE EMERGING AND EVOLVING TRENDS IN TECHNOLOGY-BASED HEALTH PROMOTION?

Web 1.0 and Web 2.0 and Social Networking

Early in the Internet era, the primary use of the medium was for sharing information, and this involved primarily moving text-based documents from paper to electronic format and placing them online. The Internet was seen as a mechanism to access information.

As the Internet began to grow in popularity, programmers also realized that in addition to simple text-based information, they could also use algorithms to make information personally relevant for people. Thus, the Internet began to shift from simply a mechanism for unidirectional presentation of information to a more interactive environment. People could give the computer information and receive something specific and tailored in return. With the use of pre-programmed algorithms, programs on the Internet could give people specific feedback. For example, in the field of health, if you typed in your height and weight, a program could calculate your body mass index (BMI); your age and gender would yield information on risk for various diseases. These interactive features could be in the form of quizzes, games, or surveys.

In addition to obtaining information and getting feedback based on algorithms, early research initiatives for health considered the efficacy of using e-mail communication as an intervention strategy. This activity begins to move research on the Internet from increasing information access and interactivity with the machine to interactivity with people—albeit limited to bidirectional interactivity, this human interactivity is a hallmark of the Web 2.0 era that we are in today—and is described below.

The other activity that began in this early period was participation in what were called chat rooms and then bulletin boards—electronic equivalents of the corkboard where people could post information and ask for replies. These are two initial examples of Web 2.0, which ushered in a shift to much more interactive multidirectional communication online.

Figure 1.2 shows a screenshot with an example of the text-based information and algorithms that characterize these early online offerings. This time period online has been dubbed "Web 1.0."

During this time, researchers began to consider both how people used the Internet in ways that might put their health at risk and how they might use the Internet to promote health. The primary attraction of the Internet for research was the ability to instantly reach very large numbers of people. Data collection that previously would take months or years could now be accomplished within weeks or even days.

Figure 1.2   Example of a Web 1.0 site

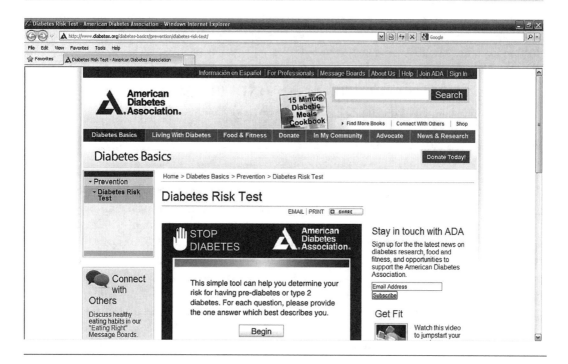

Consider the sample sizes shown in the Appendix. Larger sample sizes also allowed researchers to make better statistical inferences about their findings, and added to the excitement about using the Internet for research. Larger sample sizes alone, however, cannot be the basis for drawing conclusions on inferences from data, and these are specific considerations we will address in Chapter 5.

Web 2.0 is characterized by this multidirectionality. Sites such as MySpace, Facebook, LinkedIn, and others have features that allow people to (a) web log (or blog)—that is, offer online journals on any topic; (b) have threaded discussions or chat sessions; (c) allow people to share testimonials; and (d) in general have "user-driven" content. This user-driven content is characterized by a much more democratic process in placing and posting content. Users will establish policies and self-monitor, but in general there is much greater opportunity for users to give feedback to website designers regarding design and content preferences, and users also want the opportunity to share with each other, cocreating a site and networks of users.

Two of the more famous social networking sites are Facebook and MySpace. Pages on these sites have infinite options for self-expression and can allow the user to post photos, music, video, art, and so on. Social networking sites also allow people to use the sites to promote their product—indeed, MySpace began as a way to promote information about bands. MySpace has been used by bands, politicians, businesses, and other groups and organizations to get information out and share it with others in the MySpace networks. Sharing information becomes easier, since people will list their "friends" (usually people they are close to who also have a page on a given social networking site), and they can easily forward content from one page to the many "friends" they have in their network on that site.

Researchers have begun to utilize MySpace and Facebook in their work. As we will elaborate on further in both Chapters 2 and 8, there is a growing expectation for transparency in evaluations of technology-based health promotion. People can use the Internet to share detailed information, not only in text form but also in digital photos and video. Evaluators of health promotion using technology can consider using social networking sites to create their own profile that they can then post to offer such information about themselves for potential participants. It can lend a sense of credibility to the evaluation endeavor, and also assist in recruitment and retention of participants. Figure 1.3 shows an example of a Facebook page used to explain a program evaluation on that site.

As the Internet continues to evolve, there will likely be a Web 3.0, which, according to early conjecture, may involve access to and transfer of large amounts of data, moving more definitively into a paperless society. There is growing use of what has been termed "cloud computing" (Rosenthal et al., 2010) whereby one can access servers for a limited period essentially renting bandwidth and computational time to run and transfer data. This may be relevant for technology-based health promotion evaluation efforts that seek to gather and analyze large amounts of data simultaneously at lower cost.

Figure 1.3   Explaining program evaluation on a Facebook page

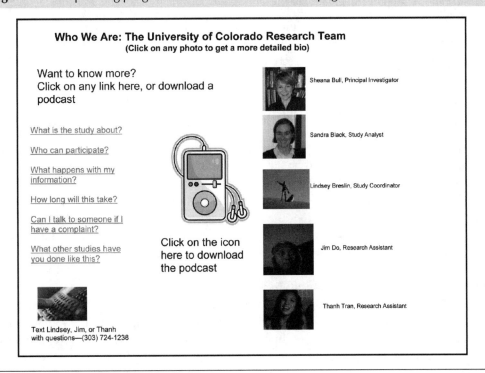

Portability

It is clear that there is increased attention to access to the Internet via mobile phones, and now through other portable devices such as the iPad™, suggesting there will be an emphasis on universal and ubiquitous access to data and information. Ultimately, health promoters will have to consider approaches for conducting their work in this new environment. The emphasis on instant access to information and data suggests we should seek approaches to adapt our methods for rapid implementation of program evaluation, quickly gathering, managing, and analyzing data so that findings can be relevant for the present. Failure to do so may mean our well-controlled and rigorous studies will offer detailed findings on technologies and innovations that are obsolete.

SUMMARY

The use of technology for research in health has proliferated in a decade, and there is promise and potential for continued use of tools such as computers, the Internet, and mobile phones and other portable devices to collect, manage, and analyze data. We can use these technologies (a) to conduct observational studies—for example, to document how, when, and where people engage with a particular modality; (b) to conduct surveillance—to document knowledge, attitudes, and behaviors that are critical for epidemiologic assessment; and (c) to intervene and attempt novel and engaging approaches to improve health outcomes.

We face both opportunities and limitations for health promotion using technologies. Within the field of health promotion, we have tremendous opportunity to use technology to increase the reach of our services and research to the multitudes of people who are connected to computers, the Internet, and mobile phone technologies. In order to capitalize on these opportunities, however, we need to think about smart ways to recruit and engage participants in environments that are increasingly crowded with others vying for users' attention. Expanding the study of social and behavioral science theory to consider ways to capture and maintain attention and subsequently engage individuals in technology-based interventions is a priority. Finding approaches to ensure that we can increase access to technologies is also critical. At the same time, using technologies that diverse populations have already embraced is likely to yield results that are more relevant. We have yet to capitalize on opportunities to go substantially beyond individual-level interventions with technology to integrate technology into institutions to facilitate service delivery; we have yet to see strong examples of health promotion programs that target providers of care or seek institutional, organizational, or societal change rather than individual-level behavior change. Finally, we have a critical need to stay ahead of the curve in technology-oriented research for health. Using traditional time frames for conducting evaluations may only result in findings that are obsolescent by the time they are released. Development of timely, rigorous, and rapid assessment procedures for technology-based program evaluation efforts is of the highest priority.

Emerging trends suggest we have moved from using technology to tailor content and make it attractive to including social networking and ubiquitous computing in our technologies. In the past decade with the proliferation of Internet and mobile phone use, we have also seen a substantial change in the ways that people use technologies, moving from graphic intensive and interactive computer programs to social networking endeavors, where user-driven and -created content is the norm. We are on the cusp of explorations of social networking sites and activities on the Internet and through mobile phones, and this is a promising area for research.

? CONCLUDING QUESTIONS

1. How could traditional research that you are familiar with be improved by using technology-based adaptations and methods for delivering content?

   a. Name three specific benefits you could anticipate from delivering health promotion content using technology.

2. What are some specific drawbacks of using technology to deliver program content for health promotion? Consider a health promotion program you are familiar with in formulating your answer.

3. What new contributions would this work offer in terms of better understanding the theoretical interface between interaction with computers and program content and anticipated behavior change?

4. Identify an example from the literature of at least two health promotion programs that show efficacy in promoting behavior change. Describe the program, what technology was used, and how technology was employed to implement the program.

CHAPTER EXERCISE

Justify the technological adaptation of materials from an existing health promotion program.

1. Consider the Diabetes Prevention Program (DPP). DPP was evaluated in a large research study. The goals of the study were to understand if people with prediabetes could prevent onset of type II diabetes through changes in nutrition and physical activity. The DPP behavioral lifestyle intervention was indeed found to be effective. Detailed findings from this research can be found in the February 7, 2002, issue of the *New England Journal of Medicine.*

2. Review some of the written materials developed for the DPP program at this website: http://www.bsc.gwu.edu/dpp/lifestyle/dpp_part.html.

3. Your task is to do the following:

   a. Write a justification for why an adaptation of program materials is needed and will likely be beneficial. Assume you are writing an executive summary of a grant application in a two- to three-page document.

   b. Consider what advantages the adaptation will offer over and above the program as it is delivered face-to-face. Specify what each advantage will be and why you think achieving this advantage will serve as an improvement over the current program.

   c. Discuss specific limitations that you anticipate to the adaptation for the DPP program to a technology-based content delivery.

   d. Identify specific theoretical constructs that will be useful to evaluate to improve on our understanding of the processes for behavior change in the technological environment.

ADDITIONAL RESOURCES

Additional readings on health promotion programs and interventions delivered using technology:

Books, Articles, and Other Peer Reviewed Literature

Resource	Description
Kroeze, W., Werkman, A., & Brug, J. (2006). A systematic review of randomized trials on the effectiveness of computer-tailored education on physical activity and dietary behaviors. *Annals of Behavioral Medicine, 31*(3), 205–223.	This article describes current knowledge about how effective "expert systems" and tailoring are for influencing physical activity and diet.
Myung, S. K., McDonnell, D. D., Kazinets, G., Seo, H. G., & Moskowitz, J. M. (2009). Effects of web- and computer-based smoking cessation programs: Meta-analysis of randomized controlled trials. *Archives of Internet Medicine, 169*(10), 929–937.	This article describes what we currently know about using computers for smoking cessation.
Neville, L. M., Milat, A. J., & O'Hara, B. (2009). Computer-tailored weight reduction interventions targeting adults: A narrative systematic review. *Health Promotion Journal of Australia, 20*(1), 48–57.	This article describes what we currently know about how effective "expert systems" and tailoring are for promoting weight loss—the work includes more qualitative assessment and program descriptions.
Neville, L. M., O'Hara, B., & Milat, A. (2009). Computer-tailored physical activity behavior change interventions targeting adults: A systematic review. *International Journal of Behavioral Nutrition and Physical Activity, 3*(6), 30.	This article describes current knowledge about effective "expert systems" and tailoring for influencing physical activity.
Noar, S. M., Black, H. G., Pierce, & L. B. (2009). Efficacy of computer technology-based HIV prevention interventions: A meta-analysis. *AIDS, 23*(1), 107–115.	This article looks at multiple computer-based interventions and how effective they are for HIV prevention; the majority are computer programs—two are Internet based.
Portnoy, D. B., Scott-Sheldon, L.A., Johnson, B. T., & Carey, M. P. (2008). Computer-delivered interventions for health promotion and behavioral risk reduction: A meta-analysis of 75 randomized controlled trials, 1988–2007. *Preventive Medicine, 47*(1), 3–16.	This article considers the effectiveness of computer-based programs in general and the evidence of how well they work for influencing multiple behavioral outcomes.

REFERENCES

Albarracin, D., Fishbein, M., Johnson, B. T., & Muellerleile, P. A. (2001). Theories of reasoned action and planned behavior as models of condom use: A meta-analysis. *Psychological Bulletin, 127,* 142–161.

Albarracin, D., Gillette, J. C., Earl, A. N., Glasman, L. R., Durantini, M. R., & Ho, M. H. (2005). A test of major assumptions about behavior change: A comprehensive look at the effects of passive and active HIV-prevention interventions since the beginning of the epidemic. *Psychological Bulletin, 131,* 856–897.

Apple. (2010). *iPad*. Retrieved from http://www.apple.com/ipad/

Azjen, I. (1985). From intentions to actions: A theory of planned behavior. In J. Kuhl & J. Beckman (Eds.), *Action-control: From cognition to behavior* (pp. 11–39). Heidelberg, Germany: Springer.

Azjen, I. (1991). The theory of planned behavior. *Organizational Behavior and Human Decision Processes, 50,* 179–211.

Bandura, A. (1986). *Social foundations of thought and action: A social cognitive theory.* Englewood Cliffs, NJ: Prentice Hall.

Baranowski, T., Buday, R., Thompson, D., & Baranowski, J. (2008). Playing for real: Video games and stories for health-related behavior change. *American Journal of Preventive Medicine, 34,* 74–82.

Beal, A. C., Ausiello, J., & Perrin, J. M. (2001). Social influences on health-risk behaviors among minority middle school students. *Journal of Adolescent Health, 28,* 474–480.

Benzies, K. M., & Allen, M. N. (2001). Symbolic interactionism as a theoretical perspective for multiple method research. *Journal of Advanced Nursing, 33,* 541–547.

Bernhardt, J. M. (2000). Health education and the digital divide: Building bridges and filling chasms. *Health Education Research, 15,* 527–531.

Bental, D. S., Cawsey, A., & Jones, R. (1999). Patient information systems that tailor to the individual. *Patient Education and Counseling, 2,* 171–180.

Booth, A. O., Nowson, C. A., & Matters, H. (2008). Evaluation of an interactive, Internet-based weight loss program: A pilot study. *Health Education Research, 23,* 371–381.

Boutin-Foster, C. (2005). Getting to the heart of social support: A qualitative analysis of the types of instrumental support that are most helpful in motivating cardiac risk factor modification. *Heart Lung, 34,* 22–29.

Brendryen, H., & Kraft, P. (2008). Happy ending: A randomized controlled trial of a digital multi-media smoking cessation intervention. *Addiction, 103,* 478–484.

Bull, S., Biringi, R., Nambembezi, D., Kiwanuka, J., & Ybarra, M. (2010). Cyber-Senga: Ugandan youth preferences for content in an Internet-delivered comprehensive sexuality education program. *East African Journal of Public Health.* Manuscript in preparation.

Bull, S., Gaglio, B., McKay, G., & Glasgow, R. E. (2005). Harnessing the potential of the Internet to promote chronic illness self-management: Diabetes as an example of how well are we doing. *Chronic Illness, 1,* 143–155.

Bull, S., Leeman-Castillo, B., Ortiz, C., & Gutierrez-Raghunath, S. (2008). Latinos Using Cardio Health Actions to Reduce Risk (LUCHAR) Project: Findings from a community-based kiosk intervention to improve nutrition, physical activity, and smoking behavior. Presented at the 136th Meeting of the American Public Health Association.

Bull, S., Pratte, K., Whitesell, N., Rietmeijer, C., & McFarlane, M. (2009). Effects of an Internet-based intervention for HIV prevention: The Youthnet trials. *AIDS and Behavior, 13*(3), 474–487.

Bull, S., Vallejos, D., & Ortiz, C. (2008). Recruitment and retention of youth online for an HIV prevention intervention: Lessons from the Youthnet trial. *AIDS Care, 20,* 887–889.

Bull, S. S., & McFarlane, M. (2000). Soliciting sex on the Internet: What are the risks for sexually transmitted diseases and HIV? *Sexually Transmitted Diseases, 27,* 545–550.

Caldwell, J. C., Caldwell, P., Caldwell, B. K., & Pieris, I. (1998). The construction of adolescence in a changing world: Implications for sexuality, reproduction, and marriage. *Studies in Family Planning, 29,* 137–153.

Campbell, E., Peterkin, D., Abbott, R., & Rogers, J. (1997). Encouraging underscreened women to have cervical cancer screening: The effectiveness of a computer strategy. *Preventive Medicine, 26,* 801–807.

Campbell, M. K., DeVellis, B. M., Strecher, V. J., Ammerman, A. S., DeVellis, R. F., & Sandler, R. S. (1994). Improving dietary behavior: The effectiveness of tailored messages in primary care settings. *American Journal of Public Health, 84,* 783–787.

Cantrell, M. A., & Lupinacci, P. (2008). Methodological issues in online data collection. *Journal of Advanced Nursing, 60,* 544–549.

Carter-Sykes, C. (2010). *Pew Internet & American Life Project.* Retrieved from http://www.pewinternet.org/

Cassell, M. M., Jackson, C., & Cheuvront, B. (1998). Health communication on the Internet: An effective channel for health behavior change? *Journal of Health Communication, 3,* 71–79.

Cellular-News. (2006). *African-Americans and Hispanics dominate cellphone use.* Retrieved from http://www.cellular-news.com/story/15627.php

Centers for Disease Control and Prevention. (2000). *HIV: Related knowledge and stigma. Morbidity and Mortality Weekly Reports, 49,* 1062–1064.

Chang, B. L., Bakken, S., Brown, S. S., Houston, T. K., Kreps, G. L., Kukafka, R., et al. (2004). Bridging the digital divide: Reaching vulnerable populations. *Journal of the American Medical Informatics Association, 11,* 448–457.

Chin, J. L. (2000). A juxtaposition of cultures. *Public Health Reports, 115,* 485–486.

Christakis, N., & Fowler, J. (2007). Change to obesity: The spread of obesity in a large social network over 32 years. *New England Journal of Medicine, 357,* 370–379.

Courneya, K. S., Estabrooks, P. A., & Nigg, C. R. (1997). Predicting change in exercise stage over a three-year period: An application of the theory of planned behavior. *Avante, 3,* 1–13.

Courneya, K. S., Nigg, C. R., & Estabrooks, P. A. (1998). Relationships among the theory of planned behavior, stages of change, and exercise behavior in older persons over a three-year period. *Psychology and Health, 13,* 355–367.

Crooks, D. L. (2001). The importance of symbolic interaction in grounded theory research on women's health. *Health Care for Women International, 22,* 11–27.

de Vries, H., & Brug, J. (1999). Computer-tailored interventions motivating people to adopt health promoting behaviors: Introduction to a new approach. *Patient Education and Counseling, 36,* 99–105.

Duffy, L. (2005). Culture and context of HIV prevention in rural Zimbabwe: The influence of gender inequality. *Journal of Transcultural Nursing, 16,* 23–31.

Dzewaltowski, D., Estabrooks, P., Gaglio, B., Glasgow, R. E., King, D. K., & Klesges, L. (2010). RE-AIM. Retrieved from http://www.re-aim.org/ whoweare/index.html

Farmer, P. (1999). *Infections and inequalities.* Berkeley: University of California Press.

Farmer, P., Connors, M., & Simmons, J. (1996). *Women, poverty, and AIDS: Sex, drugs and structural violence.* Cambridge, MA: Common Courage Press.

Feil, E. G., Glasgow, R. E., Boles, S. M., & McKay, H. G. (2000). Who participates in Internet-based self-management programs? A study among novice computer users in a primary care setting. *Diabetes Educator, 26,* 806–811.

Fisher, P. A., & Ball, T. J. (2002). The Indian Family Wellness project: An application of the tribal participatory research model. *Prevention Science, 3,* 235–240.

Formica, M., Kabbara, K., Clark, R., & McAlindon, T. (2004). Can clinical trials requiring frequent participant contact be conducted over the Internet? Results from an online randomized controlled trial evaluating a topical ointment for herpes labialis. *Journal of Medical Internet Research, 6,* e6.

Fortenberry, J. D., McFarlane, M., Bleakley, A., Bull, S., Fishbein, M., Grimley, D. M., et al. (2002). Relationships of stigma and shame to gonorrhea and HIV screening. *American Journal of Public Health, 92,* 378–381.

Fox, S., & Rainie, L. (2000). *The online health care revolution.* Washington, DC: The Pew Internet & American Life Project. Retrieved from http://www.pewinternet.org/Reports/ 2000/The-Online-Health-Care-Revolution .aspx

Friedman, S. R., Mateu-Gelabert, P., Curtis, R., Maslow, C., Bolyard, M., Sandoval, M., et al. (2007). Social capital or networks, negotiations, and norms? A neighborhood case study. *American Journal of Preventive Medicine, 32,* 160–170.

Glasgow, R., Nelson, C., Kearney, K., Reid, R., Ritzwoller, D., Strecher, V., et al. (2007). Reach, engagement and retention in an Internet-based weight loss program in a multi-site randomized controlled trial. *Journal of Medical Internet Research, 9,* e11.

Glasgow, R. E., Boles, S. M., McKay, H. G., Feil, E. G., & Barrera, M. (2003). The D-Net diabetes self-management program: Long-term implementation, outcomes, and generalization results. *Prevention Medicine, 36,* 410–419.

Glasgow, R. E., Bull, S. S., Piette, J. D., & Steiner, J. F. (2004). Interactive behavior change technology. A partial solution to the competing demands of primary care. *American Journal of Preventive Medicine, 27,* 80–87.

Glasgow, R. E., Klesges, L. M., Dzewaltowski, D. A., Estabrooks, P. A., & Vogt, T. M. (2006). Evaluating the impact of health promotion programs: Using the RE-AIM framework to form summary measures for decision making involving complex issues. *Health Education Research, 21,* 688–694.

Glasgow, R. E., Lichtenstein, E., & Marcus, A. C. (2003). Why don't we see more translation of health promotion research to practice? Rethinking the efficacy-to-effectiveness transition. *American Journal of Public Health, 93,* 1261–1267.

Glasgow, R. E., McKay, H. G., Piette, J. D., & Reynolds, K. D. (2001). The RE-AIM framework for evaluating interventions: What can it tell us about approaches to chronic illness management? *Patient Education and Counseling, 44,* 119–127.

Grov, C., & Parsons, J. (2006). Bug chasing and gift giving: The potential for HIV transmission among barebackers on the Internet. *AIDS Education and Prevention, 18,* 490–503.

Gustafson, D. H., McTavish, F. M., Stengle, W., Ballard, D., Hawkins, R., Shaw, B. R., et al. (2005). Use and impact of eHealth system by low-income women with breast cancer. *Journal of Health Communication, 10*(Suppl. 1), 195–218.

Harris Interactive. (2010). *Home.* Retrieved from http://www.harris interactive.com/

Horrigan, J. (2004). *Pew Internet & American Life Project data memo.* Washington, DC: Pew Internet & American Life Project.

Horrigan, J. (2008). *Mobile access to data and information.* Retrieved from http://www.pewinternet.org/Reports/2008/Mobile-Access-to-Data-and-Information.aspx

Jackson, L. A., Zhao, Y., Kolenic, A., Fitzgerald, H. E., Harold, R., & Von Eye, A. (2008). Race, gender, and information technology use: The new digital divide. *Cyberpsychology & Behavior, 11,* 437–442.

Kim, H. S., Yoo, Y. S., & Shim, H. S. (2005). Effects of an Internet-based intervention on plasma glucose levels in patients with type 2 diabetes. *Journal of Nursing Care Quality, 20.*

Kim, S. I., & Kim, H. S. (2008). Effectiveness of mobile and Internet intervention in patients with obese type 2 diabetes. *International Journal of Medical Informatics, 77,* 399–404.

King, D., Stryker, L., Estabrooks, P., Toobert, D., Bull, S., & Glasgow, R. (in press). Outcomes of a multifaceted physical activity regimen as part of a diabetes self-management intervention. *Annals of Behavioral Medicine.*

Klesges, L., Estabrooks, P., Dzewaltowski, D., Bull, S., & Glasgow, R. E. (2007). Beginning with the application in mind: Designing and planning health behavior change interventions to enhance dissemination. *Annals of Behavioral Medicine, 29,* 6675.

Kreuter, M., Farrell, D., Olevitch, L., & Brennan, L. (2000). *Tailoring health messages: Customizing communication with computer technology.* Mahwah, NJ: Erlbaum.

Kreuter, M. W., & Strecher, V. J. (1996). Do tailored behavior change messages enhance the effectiveness of health risk appraisal? Results from a randomized trial. *Health Education Research, 11,* 97–105.

Leeman-Castillo, B. F., Beaty, B. F., Raghunath, S. F.A. U., Steiner, J., Steiner, J. F., & Bull, S. (2010). LUCHAR: Using computer technology to battle heart disease among Latinos. *American Journal of Public Health, 100,* 272–275.

Lenhart, A., & Horrigan, J. B. (2003). Re-visualizing the Digital Divide as a Digital Spectrum. *IT & Society, 1,* 23–39.

Lieberman, D. Z., & Huang, S. W. (2008). A technological approach to reaching a hidden population of problem drinkers. *Psychiatric Services, 59*(3), 297–303.

Lipkus, I. M., Lyna, P. R., & Rimer, B. K. (1999). Using tailored interventions to enhance smoking cessation among African-Americans at a community health center. *Nicotine Tobacco Research, 1,* 77–85.

Lorence, D. P., Park, H., & Fox, S. (2006). Racial disparities in health information access: Resilience of the Digital Divide. *Journal of Medical Internet Systems, 30,* 241–249.

Marcus, B. H., Emmons, K. M., Simkin-Silverman, L. R., Linnan, L. A., Taylor, E. R., Bock, B. C., et al. (1998). Evaluation of motivationally tailored vs. standard self-help physical activity interventions at the workplace. *American Journal of Health Promotion, 12,* 246–253.

Marrero, D. G., Vandagriff, J. L., Kronz, K., Fineberg, N. S., Golden, M. P., Gray, D., et al. (1995). Using telecommunication technology to manage children with diabetes: The Computer-Linked Outpatient Clinic (CLOC) Study. *Diabetes Education, 21,* 313–319.

Massachusetts Medical Society. (2010). *New England Journal of Medicine, 346*(6). Available from http://content.nejm.org/content/vol346/issue6/index.dtl.

Padilla, R., Bull, S., Raghunath, S. G., Fernald, D., Havranek, E. P., & Steiner, J. F. (2010). Designing a cardiovascular disease prevention web site for Latinos: Qualitative community feedback. *Health Promotion Practice, 11*(1), 140–147.

Pew Internet & American Life Project. (2006). *Latest Trends: February 15–April 6, 2006.* Retrieved from http://www.pewinternet.org/Shared-Content/Data-Sets/2006/FebruaryApril-2006-Gadgets-and-Internet-Typology.aspx

Piot, P., Bartos, M., Larson, H., Zewdie, D., & Mane, P. (2008). *Coming to terms with complexity: A call to action for HIV prevention. The Lancet, 372*(9641), 845–859. Retrieved from http://www.thelancet.com/journals/lancet/article/PIIS0140-6736(08)60888-0/abstract

Prochaska, J. J., Zabinski, B. A., Calfas, K. J., Sallis, J. F., & Patrick, K. (2000). PACE+: Interactive communication technology for behavior change in clinical settings. *American Journal of Preventive Medicine, 19,* 127–131.

Prochaska, J. O., DiClemente, C. C., Velicer, W. F., & Rossi, J. S. (1993). Standardized, individualized, interactive and personalized self-help programs for smoking cessation. *Health Psychology, 12,* 399–405.

Rainie, L., Horrigan, J., Wellman, B., & Boase, J. (2006). *The strength of Internet ties.* Retrieved from http://www
    .pewinternet.org/Reports/2006/ The-Strength-of-Internet-Ties.aspx

Rakowski, W., Ehrich, B., Goldstein, M. G., Rimer, B. K., Pearlman, D. N., Clark, M. A., et al. (1998). Increasing
    mammography among women aged 40–74 by use of a stage-matched, tailored intervention. *American Journal of
    Preventive Medicine, 27,* 748–756.

Rice, E., Stein, J., & Milburn, N. (2008). Countervailing social network influences on problem behaviors among
    homeless youth. *Journal of Adolescence, 5,* 625–639.

Rimer, B. K., Conway, M., Lyna, P., Glassman, B., Yarnall, S. H., Lipkus, I., et al. (1999). The impact of tailored
    interventions on a community health center population. *Patient Education and Counseling, 37,* 125–140.

Rodgers, A., Corbett, T., Bramley, D., Riddell, T., Wills, M., Lin, R. B., et al. (2005). Do u smoke after txt? Results of a
    randomised trial of smoking cessation using mobile phone text messaging. *Tobacco Control, 14,* 255–261.

Rogers, E. M. (1995). *Diffusion of innovations theory.* New York, NY: Free Press.

Rosenstock, I. M. (1974). Historical origins of the health belief model. *Health Education Monographs, 2,* 328–335.

Rosenthal, A., Mork, P., Li, M. H., Stanford, J., Koester, D., & Reynolds, P. (2010). Cloud computing: A new business
    paradigm for biomedical information sharing. *Journal of Biomedical Informatics, 43*(2), 342–353.

Sanders, A. E., Lim, S., & Sohn, W. (2008). Resilience to urban poverty: Theoretical and empirical considerations for
    population health. *American Journal of Public Health, 98,* 1101–1106.

Siek, K., Khan, D., & Ross, S. (2009). A usability inspection of medication management in three personal health
    applications. *Proceedings of Human Computer Interaction International, 1,* 129–138.

Skinner, C. S., Siegfried, J. C., Kegler, M. C., & Strecher, V. J. (1993). The potential of computers in patient
    education. *Patient Education and Counseling, 22,* 27–34.

Skinner, C. S., Strecher, V. J., & Hospers, H. (1994). Physician recommendation for mammography: Do tailored
    messages make a difference? *American Journal of Public Health, 84,* 43–49.

Spek, V., Nyklicek, I., Smits, N., Cuijpers, P., Riper, H., Keyzer, J., et al. (2007). Internet-based cognitive behavioral
    therapy for subthreshold depression in people over 50 years old: A randomized controlled trial. *Psychological
    Medicine, 37,* 1791–806.

Strecher, V. J. (1999). Computer-tailored smoking cessation materials: A review and discussion. *Patient Education and
    Counseling, 36,* 107–117.

Strecher, V. J., Kreuter, M., Den Boer, D. J., Kobrin, S., Hospers, H. J., & Skinner, C. S. (1994). The effects of computer-
    tailored smoking cessation messages in family practice settings. *Journal of Family Practice, 39,* 262–268.

Sun, X., Wang, N., Li, D., Zheng, X., Qu, S., Wang, L., et al. (2007). The development of HIV/AIDS surveillance in
    China. *AIDS, 21,* S33–S38.

Swindle, S., Baker, S. S., & Auld, G. W. (2007). Operation Frontline: Assessment of longer-term curriculum effectiveness,
    evaluation strategies, and follow-up methods. *Journal of Nutrition Education and Behavior, 39,* 205–213.

Tate, D. F., Wing, R. R., & Winett, R. A. (2001). Using Internet technology to deliver a behavioral weight loss
    program. *JAMA, 285,* 1172–1177.

Taylor, C. B., Houston-Miller, N., Killen, J. D., & DeBusk, R. F. (1990). Smoking cessation after acute myocardial
    infarctions: Effects of a nurse-managed intervention. *Annals of Internal Medicine, 113,* 118–123.

Taylor, J. J. (2007). Assisting or compromising intervention? The concept of "culture" in biomedical and social
    research on HIV/AIDS. *Social Science and Medicine, 64*(4), 965–975.

Thyrian, J. R., & Ulrich, J. (2007). Population impact—Definition, calculation and its use in prevention science in the
    example of tobacco smoking reduction. *Health Policy, 82,* 348–356.

Turner, C. F., Ku, L., Rogers, S. M., Lindberg, L. D., Pleck, J. H., & Sonerstein, F. L. (1998). Adolescent sexual
    behavior, drug use, and violence: Increased reporting with computer survey technology. *Science, 280,* 867–873.

van den Berg, M., Schoones, J., & Vliet Vlieland, T. (2007). Internet-based physical activity interventions: A
    systematic review of the literature. *Journal of Medical Internet Research, 9,* e26.

Wallace, L. S., Buckworth, J., Kirby, T. E., & Sherman, W. M. (2000). Characteristics of exercise behavior among
    college students: Application of cognitive theory to predicting stage of change. *Preventive Medicine, 31,* 494–505.

Weinstein, P. K. (2006). A review of weight loss programs delivered via the Internet. *Journal of Cardiovascular
    Nursing, 21,* 251–258.

Zhang, D., Bi, P., Hiller, J. E., & Lv, F. (2008). Web-based HIV/AIDS behavioral surveillance among men who have
    sex with men: Potential and challenges. *International Journal of Infectious Diseases, 12,* 126–131.

2 ⬛

Ethical Issues
in Technology-Based
Health Promotion

CHAPTER OVERVIEW

This chapter offers an overview of the unique ethnical issues that confront health promoters and program evaluators when doing technology-based work. It covers anticipated ethical benefits that can be realized with technology-based work and considers specific ethical challenges to this field. We consider the best ethical practices that are currently employed in technology-based health promotion and examine emerging trends with regard to ethics and technology.

WHAT ARE UNIQUE AND BENEFICIAL
ETHICAL CONSIDERATIONS FOR
TECHNOLOGY-BASED HEALTH PROMOTION?

Beneficence

Beneficence is presented in the Belmont Report as "acts of kindness or charity that go beyond strict obligation" (U.S. Department of Health, Education, and Welfare, 1979, Part A, Section 2, para. 1). In this document, beneficence is understood, in a stronger sense, as an obligation. Two general rules have been formulated as complementary expressions of beneficent actions in this sense: (a) do not harm and (b) maximize possible benefits and minimize possible harms (U.S. Department of Health, Education, and Welfare, 1979). As mentioned in the previous chapter, one of the unique advantages that technology-based health promotion affords is reach. If we can effectively reach larger numbers of people with technology than we could with stand-alone programs, there is ethical support to do so. Of particular interest is offering reach where it has not previously been available. An example of this is the Wyoming Rural AIDS Prevention Project, an HIV prevention intervention with demonstrated efficacy that targets men who have sex with men living in rural areas (Bowen, Williams, Daniel, & Clayton, 2008). This is an example of extending the beneficence of programs to areas that might otherwise not have a program—rural areas are not only limited by fewer structural resources where programs can be delivered; in addition, the ongoing stigma related to HIV and homosexuality in rural areas may even preclude delivery of such programs when resources are available.

Similarly, the advent of mobile phones and ubiquitous access to the Internet via other portable devices may extend program services in rural and resource-poor settings that have never been reached by traditional programs. Such is the case in many of the programs detailed in current assessments of cell phone use (Fjeldsoe, Marshall, & Miller, 2009; Krishna, Borren, & Balas, 2009).

Transparency

Researchers using the Internet to collect data have developed a process for informed consent (S. Rosser, personal communication, September 25, 2009) that can serve as an example for increased transparency for informing participants in health promotion programs as well. An example of a page from a study of sexual risk behavior is shown in Figure 2.1. This figure shows that the researchers have divided up the informed consent. The page shows a segment typically covered in the informed consent: procedures for study participants. In this example, the researchers presented the information as a question ("What will I be asked to do as a study participant?") and only covered this topic on this page. They created two buttons: "I consent and wish to enter the study" and "I do not consent and wish to leave the study." Participants can read each segment easily—it is presented in a relatively large font and simple language, and the page has quite a bit of white space. The page also includes a picture, intended by the researchers to break up the monotony of text.

In addition to making this process more appealing to potential participants, we can employ these methods to understand more about precise motivations for disenrollment. By having a button stating "I do not consent and wish to leave the study," we can identify exact segments where participants declined to enroll and may be able to infer that the page where a person declined represents a particular aspect of the program that causes concern or discomfort among potential participants.

Equity

We have the opportunity given the reach of technology to consider the equitable distribution of our technology-based efforts. As will be discussed in Chapter 3, there is good evidence about technology usage available that suggests not all modes are equally popular and accessed by all groups. For

Figure 2.1 Example of an online consent form that is easy to read and uses technological tools to facilitate the process

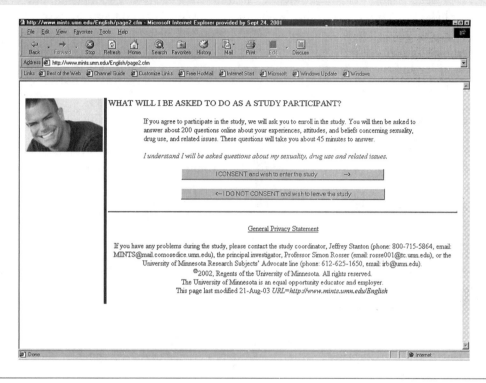

Source: S. Rosser (personal communication, September 25, 2009).

example, we have already mentioned the digital divide related to access of Internet-based technology programs and, additionally, the relative lower amount of bandwidth available for high-density graphics when the Internet is available in resource-poor settings. Given the data on popularity and use of mobile phones, however, it is now possible to distribute programs across various modalities to increase equity in access to technology-based health promotion. Additionally, we need to consider that the digital divide has separated populations from technology and may serve to reinforce perceptions that segments of the population "don't like," "won't use," or "reject" technology wholesale. Rather than assuming this is the case, it is worth exploring whether technology, when accessible and appealing, is indeed a viable option for populations heretofore cut off from it and if it is valuable to offer technology as a mechanism in and of itself to reduce digital divide and access issues.

Confidentiality

While much has been written about concerns regarding privacy online, and the issues of security for data are considerable, we now operate with technological advances that allow for greater and greater protections of data and user personal information. Combining greater complexity in creating passwords with other security measures such as data encryption and screen captures that are designed to detect the difference between a real person and a web robot, we have ample tools at our disposal to make sure information that participants give to us in the course of program implementation and evaluation stays private. In addition, also mentioned earlier, is the recognition that interacting with a computer offers some a greater sense of privacy and allows them to be more forthright than they might be in a traditional face-to-face health promotion program (Turner et al., 1998).

Working With Special Populations

This benefit of technology-based health promotion is the same as that mentioned above in the discussion of beneficence. It may be difficult for traditional health promotion programs to extend adequate reach to populations that are given special protections under research regulations (e.g., pregnant women, children, prisoners, the mentally incapacitated). To the extent that this is the case and technology can overcome the limitation of reach, we have an advantage. Consider, for example, delivery of health promotion programs to prison inmates. With the growing numbers of persons incarcerated in the United States, there is also growing attention to inmate health. However, it is likely that health promotion in prison settings faces substantial challenges due to cost and security. Technology-based programs could overcome both of these challenges and extend reach to this group.

WHAT ARE ETHICAL CHALLENGES WE FACE WITH TECHNOLOGY-BASED HEALTH PROMOTION?

Beneficence

One of the primary ethical challenges we face with technology-based health promotion is the consideration of *beneficence*. Just because you *can* reach more people and collect data more efficiently with a technology-based health promotion program is not an adequate reason to do so. As with any health promotion effort, technology use should be justified as having intrinsic value to participants. Technology-based health promotion may be attractive because of convenience—it may be easier to put up a webpage or send out text messages than to go into community settings with a multisession program.

In terms of observational work in preparation for program development, the experience of researchers conducting observational studies is instructive. They have acknowledged that there is an abundance of personal information that could be useful for health-related research offered by young adults when they create profiles on social networking sites that detail their sexual behavior, alcohol and drug use, or other behaviors (Moreno, Fost, & Christakis, 2008). While some have argued that this information is in the public domain and therefore available for use in research, the counterargument from an ethical standpoint suggests that persons who create profiles either may not fully be aware of the availability of their information for public view or did not intend for the information to be used for research purposes. This is also true for using these data for program planning purposes. For researchers, it is imperative that they—and the institutions that support their work—set a high standard for their work and take extra steps to ensure that their own protocols follow established ethical standards. We endorse the same for those using observational means to collect data for health promotion program planning.

Transparency

Health promotion experts using technologies in their work may never see their participants; they may enroll them through a website on the Internet or over the telephone. Alternatively, they may enroll them face-to-face and then follow up online or on the telephone. In the latter case, as well as with a more traditional face-to-face program protocol, we can rely on immediate verbal feedback from participants as well as body language and facial expression to ensure that participants clearly understand all the risks and benefits associated with the program and what their role is in the process. They can follow up immediately with questions to clarify any part of the process that they don't understand. We must ensure that there are adequate procedures and processes in place to ensure *transparency* in the research process for participants. Consent procedures and forms need to be simple and easy to understand, and need to include information about how to access resources for further information.

In addition to the need for transparency in the process of obtaining informed consent for research, technology-based health promotion implemented without face-to-face enrollment procedures opens up possibilities for fraud, both from the promoter and from the participant. Health promoters using technology need to offer detailed information on who they are and what they are doing, and this information needs to be readily accessible for people engaged in these programs. They should offer detailed information on where participants can call or e-mail if they have a concern and also offer third-party contact information for complaints or concerns to show impartiality. Health promoters may consider the utility of offering links for participants to further information—participants may appreciate being able to access detailed information on the condition the program focuses on or on ways they can link to support groups for the program. There are legal requirements as well that obligate providers to report participant disclosure of abuse or violence planned against oneself or another—any technology-based health promotion program needs to make it clear that this will occur if such disclosures are made.

Under certain circumstances, if researchers are collecting information from participants that could be potentially damaging or criminal—for example, information about drug use or prostitution—it is possible to apply for a certificate of confidentiality (COC) if they are federally funded to conduct their work. If a technology-based health promotion program is being delivered as part of a research study, this document will allow additional protection of particularly sensitive information that participants may otherwise choose not to disclose. COCs are only available through the federal government and must be approved by a project officer on a federally funded grant.

Participants need to be verifiable as being who they say they are; technology-based research opens up the possibility that people could lie about their age, gender, or other characteristics to enroll in an attractive study. Steps need to be taken by researchers to verify that participants are who they say they are and to limit opportunities for misrepresentation.

Equity

Researchers examining chronic illness, cancer, and infectious disease have been criticized for their failure to include diverse populations in their research samples (Djomand et al., 2005; Ford et al., 2008; Oddone et al., 2004; Peterson, Lytle, Biswas, & Coombs, 2004). By limiting enrollment to any one specific demographic group (e.g., White men or college students), researchers and health promoters alike not only run the risk of not being able to generalize their findings to other population groups, but they also unfairly limit both the rewards and the risks associated with research and program participation to specific groups. The National Institutes of Health (2001) have adopted standards set by the U.S. Office of Management and Budget to require investigators with federal research funding to document the demographic characteristics of those they intend to enroll and subsequently those they actually enrolled, and institutional review boards (IRBs) usually require researchers to justify why they plan to limit enrollment to any given demographic.

Given evidence that there is a digital divide, where groups with more financial and structural resources and cultural norms around rapid adoption of technology use these modalities more frequently and in greater numbers (Lenhart & Horrigan, 2003), we need to pay close attention to approaches for recruitment, enrollment, and retention of harder-to-reach populations that can both benefit from research and programs and share risks associated with each. For technology-based health promotion in particular, this means paying careful attention to who has access to the technological modality you wish to employ. For example, what ethical questions do you raise when conducting an HIV prevention program on the Internet, when it is well established that the fastest growing group of people infected with HIV includes minorities, the poor, and women, all of whom have limited access to computers, the Internet, and broadband and cable systems for high-speed downloading of graphics and data? If you proceed, what obligations do you have to ensure access to technology and address inequities in access?

Confidentiality

Researchers are ethically bound to guard the information they obtain from participants through their work as *confidential*. Using technology for research or health promotion programs doesn't automatically mean that confidentiality will be breached. However, having sensitive data of any kind collected electronically or shared electronically means that we must take care to avoid disclosure of such data. While technology has made it simpler to exchange information, there are also numerous opportunities for confidential information to be mishandled. For example, keeping detailed personal information on portable devices such as laptop computers or USB drives opens up the option for sensitive data to be lost or stolen. Transferring data from one institution to another can result in data being intercepted. Any technology-based health promotion program efforts involving data collection should take specific steps to set up technical firewalls, implement password protection for files and folders, and use encryption to transfer data remotely.

Working With Special Populations

When working with special populations in research studies, those engaged in research are required by IRBs to justify the need to recruit protected groups (e.g., prisoners, children, pregnant women). This is relevant for technology-based health promotion as well. However, with the concerns outlined above related to participant verification, it is possible that people who enroll are not who they say they are. For example, a child aged 13 may pretend to be age 16 to participate in a program online and receive an incentive. Until additional technologies such as thumbprint and retinal scanning are widely available—and these carry their own unique ethical issues—we cannot definitively determine an individual's true identity on the Internet or over the telephone. Note, however, that participant fraud does occur in face-to-face settings as well, lest there be increased anxiety related to technology-based programs. Participants can learn what the eligibility criteria are for a program and lie to enroll; if they meet the demographic requirements for eligibility, one may not know they are lying and may have no way to redress this circumstance.

When enrolling or obtaining program consent from young people, recall that persons younger than 18 are considered minors and that you may be required to obtain parental consent unless the project is one where you can obtain a waiver of parental consent.

The circumstances described previously that are relevant to obtaining consent for low-literate or nonnative English speakers extend to youth, particularly younger people. Program consent documents and processes should be as accessible as possible using the procedures described here.

Of particular concern for young people on the Internet is the increase in attention to online predation, where older adults try to entice young people or engage them in inappropriate interactions either online or offline. This represents another reason to offer as much transparency about your programs as possible so that young people or their parents or guardians can reassure themselves of your legitimacy. In addition, it may offer motivation to include along with the content of your program additional steps and tips for participants in your program on how they can protect themselves and their personal information online.

Other groups that you may work with using technology-based health promotion include jail or prison populations and the developmentally disabled. We consider that the same issues apply to these groups as to youth; consent processes need to be developed to ensure comprehension, and transparency in program protocols should be a priority. In addition, it is important to review state and local laws as well as institutional procedures to ensure that you do not violate any data collection norms or security procedures, also described here.

Other chapters in this book specifically address the methods to employ in technology-based health promotion development, implementation, and evaluation using modalities such as computers, the Internet, and mobile phones. Key ethical issues related to technology-based work are reiterated in Text Box 2.1, which represents the primary considerations to address before embarking on your technology-based health promotion endeavor.

TEXT BOX 2.1
Unique ethical issues related to technology-based health promotion

Ethical issue	Issues unique to evaluation in technology-based health promotion	Traditional health promotion program evaluation
Beneficence	• Special care needs to be taken to justify why the technology modality chosen is the best for the *participant,* not the health promoter.	• Researchers are required to demonstrate that their work will contribute to science.
Transparency in informed consent	• Lack of immediate and real-time engagement with participants at the time of program enrollment if enrolling online means researchers must take extra care to ensure that program information is understood because participants have no verbal or visual cues to assist them.*	• Health promoters have the opportunity to immediately answer questions to clarify any aspect of the program protocol. • Health promoters can rely on body language and facial expression to infer understanding or confusion.
Transparency related to participant veracity	• People may lie about who they are to enroll. • Extra procedures for participant verification should be employed.*	• Health promoters enrolling face-to-face can ascertain visually whether participants meet demographic enrollment criteria. • Where needed they can ask for identification.
Equity	• Ongoing digital divide issues mean that the benefits and risks associated with Internet-based health promotion are not equally shared across groups.*	• Benefit of rewards and burden of risk are theoretically shared.
Confidentiality	• There is little control over privacy in situations where evaluation data are collected online or over the phone. • Participant responses may be seen after data collection ends through review of cached material.	• Data collection activities are usually implemented in private settings. • Data with identifiers are stored separately from other data.
Data security and privacy	• Data collected in a therapeutic setting are HIPAA (Health Insurance Portability and Accountability Act) regulated. • When collecting data in community settings or online, health promoters	• Data are HIPAA regulated; when stored on paper, usually only one copy is placed in a locked file cabinet. When stored electronically, data need to be password protected and behind firewalls.

Ethical issue	Issues unique to evaluation in technology-based health promotion	Traditional health promotion program evaluation
	may need to follow HIPAA regulations and store and transfer electronic data using current standards for encryption, password protection, and storage behind firewalls.	
Special populations	• Ongoing concerns regarding participant verification may require additional standards to verify people are who they say they are when they enroll or participate in a program.	• Regulations exist to protect special populations wherein researchers must offer additional justification for recruitment of these groups (e.g., prisoners, children, pregnant women, the mentally incapacitated).

Note: The topics marked with an asterisk are covered in more detail later in this chapter and in other chapters in the book.

WHAT ARE THE CURRENT AND BEST ETHICAL PRACTICES IN TECHNOLOGY-BASED HEALTH PROMOTION?

Working With IRBs

When conducting health research, universities are usually required to obtain approval for their research protocols from an external review board known as an IRB. These boards are established to independently review research protocols to ensure that biomedical and behavioral research involving human subjects or participants is conducted ethically. If you are working with technology to deliver a health promotion program and have no intention to conduct research, you will never encounter or be asked to obtain approval from an institutional review board, or IRB. However, if there is a time when you wish to share your findings with colleagues and peers in a scientific journal, you will likely be required to document following ethical guidelines in program delivery and evaluation, and you may be limited in publishing if you do not obtain IRB approval for any data collection you do related to program development, implementation, or evaluation.

Although there has been a proliferation of technology-based research in the past decade, not every university with an IRB will be familiar with the ethical issues that are unique to technology-based research identified here.

Figure 2.2 offers a flowchart to illustrate procedures that can help in introducing your IRB to technology-based research.

Using Technology to Improve the Informed Consent Process

While researchers have specific procedures to follow within institutions that are required to obtain informed consent from potential research participants, data show that making informed consent documents easier to read for low-literacy populations and persons for whom English is a second language increases both their comprehension of the research they participate in and their satisfaction with the research process. Researchers have made calls to improve the

Figure 2.2   Steps involved in engaging the IRB in technology-based program evaluation

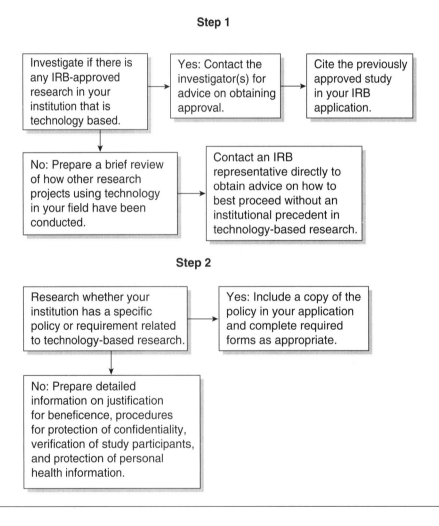

informed consent process to ensure comprehension and satisfaction, especially for vulnerable populations (Coyne et al., 2003; Elks, 1993; Flicker, Haans, & Skinner, 2004; Koo & Skinner, 2005; Marquez, Muhs, Tosomeen, Riggs, & Melton, 2003; Raich, Plomer, & Coyne, 2001; Santelli, 1997; Santelli et al., 2003). As mentioned above, one advantage health promoters have already demonstrated is how the informed consent process can be redesigned for the Internet environment, using multiple pages with brief sentences and pictures to convey information, and asking participants to agree to continue before moving on to the subsequent page (Pequegnat, Rosser, Bowen, Bull, & DiClemente, 2007). Although we haven't seen evidence of using audio to facilitate informed consent among low-literate populations, this technology is available— rather than requiring participants to read complicated text, a voice-over program could be utilized that reads text for participants—this is also a feature that can be embedded and used as needed, where participants can choose to enable or disable an audio voice-over.

As with other ethical issues, these data are relevant for technology-based health promotion as well. We have a unique opportunity to use technology to our advantage in facilitating the process of educating program participants about the program process. Readers are probably well aware of "terms of service" presented in small text boxes like the one shown in Figure 2.3 that they may be required to review and agree to before signing up for a service online. These terms of service are not generally presented in an easy-to-read or -understand format.

Figure 2.3   Example of "terms of service" frequently seen online

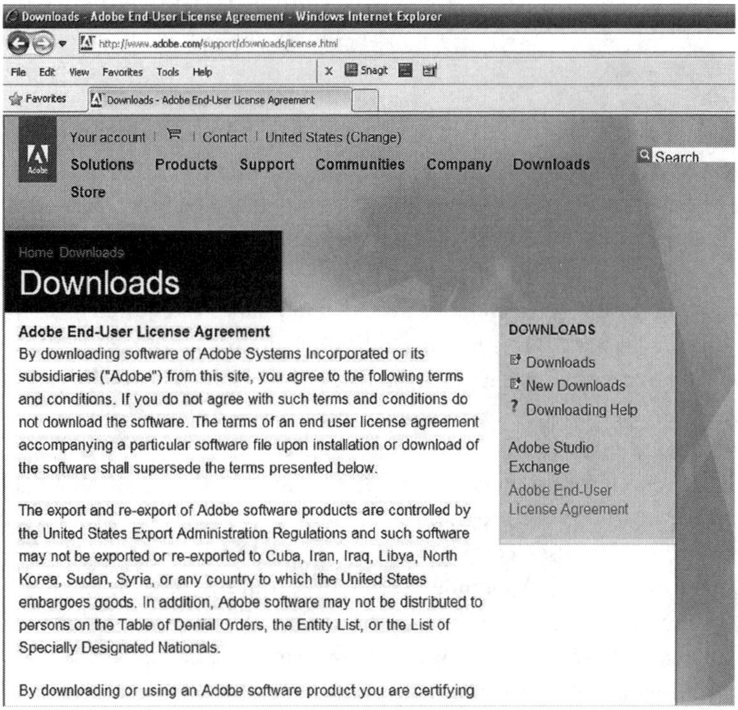

While it is tempting to put all the informed consent information in one area or on one page to minimize the navigation participants are required to perform to get into a computer- or Internet-based program, data from more traditional face-to-face settings show that having more—not fewer—pages on a consent form, having more white space, and having a bigger font all contribute to better comprehension and satisfaction with the informed consent process (Coyne et al., 2003; Raich et al., 2001).

As mentioned above, technology offers us new opportunities to overcome limitations in obtaining informed consent—and indeed in delivery of any program content—by using graphics, pictures, and audio to assist with participant comprehension.

To date, we know of no health promotion program that has used a mobile phone as the modality for enrollment and obtaining consent. We consider, however, that it will not be long before this does occur. Because of small screen size on mobile devices, paying particular attention to issues of page layout, font, and white space within such a small viewing area will be vital for researchers. We urge health promoters contemplating the use of mobile phones to deliver consent documents to consider the practices described here for obtaining computer- and Internet-based consent as a starting point, and then we also urge them to pretest and validate the process to document comprehension of program procedures before employing these methods. Of course, when using mobile phone technology for intervention delivery, it is always possible to obtain consent in a relatively "old school" manner—that is, through a telephone call! Obtaining a verbal consent over the telephone also has the potential advantage of reducing bias for those low-literate or limited English-speaking populations who otherwise may have difficulty with a written consent (Lloyd et al., 2008).

Security and Issues of Program Data Protection

As mentioned above, there are specific technical tools to employ to maximize data security. The elements described here are considered standards of practice in information technology (IT) departments within many institutions. In general, research studies and health promotion programs use data security standards that are equivalent to those required by the Health Insurance Portability and Accountability Act (HIPAA), inasmuch as HIPAA compliance is required for any entity offering a therapeutic program. In part, this is because HIPAA standards are recognizable to the public as strict standards for privacy and confidentiality. Using these standards will produce a sense that technology-based health promoters understand privacy and confidentiality and are adhering to regulations. Additionally, many institutions have upgraded their IT security training and devices to incorporate HIPAA requirements. Finally, even if you do not intend to gather personal health information (PHI) as a part of your program, such information may be transmitted by participants as part of their electronic responses, comments, or other communications.

The implementation of HIPAA included the publication by the U.S. Department of Health and Human Services of standards for privacy of health information, nicknamed the "Privacy Rule," as well as standards for security of health information, called the "Security Rule." The Security Rule is implemented via three broad categories of action: administrative, physical, and technical safeguards. In order to be in compliance with the Security Rule, institutions must have implemented the required elements of each of these categories, and further security measures are recommended in each. There also are requirements for organizational structures and documentation, policies, and procedures. Those will not be covered here but are explained in a number of sources on the Internet.

Administrative safeguards are generally the responsibility of the groups or units conducting the research, acting in accordance with the information security and privacy officers at their institutions (such as universities or hospitals). One requirement is that the organization must assign responsibility for security issues to a security officer, a person who is ultimately held responsible for the security of data. All staff must be routinely trained on security awareness issues, and security must be evaluated regularly. The security officer must routinely review the activity of the information system to assess security threats. The organization is required to conduct risk analysis, examining the potential threats to security that may arise, and to develop plans for risk management, incorporating a plan response and reporting as well as sanctions. All "business associates" of the organization must also be aware of security issues and must sign agreements regarding the proper maintenance of information security.

One administrative requirement is especially noteworthy: All HIPAA-compliant organizations must have a data backup plan as well as a contingency plan that can be implemented in the event of disaster, emergency-mode operations, and other system failures. System failures can occur at any time for a number of reasons, so it is critical to develop a contingency plan and train staff on the implementation of it. During some system failures or disasters, it may be impossible to get into offices or computer storage facilities, so plans should incorporate the possibility of remote implementation.

Physical security is another aspect of information security. If workstations and users are not protected from intrusion or physical hazards, then the data cannot be secure, so technology-based health promotion programs must use the most secure facility possible. Physical security can be especially difficult to address if technology-based programs are taking their data or data collection computers into the field. Laptops are notoriously easy to steal, so they must be protected accordingly; we anticipate the same concerns related to theft will emerge with mobile devices such as the iPad™. However, with these mobile devices, there are now features available that include global positioning system (GPS) software and remote access that will allow a user to (a) identify where the device is if lost and (b) turn it off remotely so others cannot use it. Those hoping to utilize these devices should have a detailed plan and protocol for how to turn off a device remotely so no one can access data stored on it; ideally they will also develop a plan for retrieving a device that has been lost or stolen. They may consider a reward or amnesty system that will allow someone to return a device without repercussion and potentially for a reward.

Physical security of data encompasses another area that is easily overlooked: the disposal of old machines and media (CDs, hard disks, removable storage, etc.). Organizations must have plans for the "wiping" of all data from computers or media that are being retired from service.

The final measure of data security safeguards outlined in the Security Rule involves technical security. This section describes the technical structures that must be put into place to keep data private and protected and to ensure that only authorized individuals have access to it. Technical safeguards are required to have audit controls associated with them so that constant corrections can be made. One technical safeguard is related to ensuring that users are authorized and are "authentic," or "who they say they are." Often, the technology that is used to allow individuals to log on to a system consists of one or more of three parts, which are informally called "something you know" (such as a password), "something you have" (such as a key or key fob with log-in numbers that change every 30 seconds), and "something you are" (such as a thumbprint). In addition to standard user identification and authentication, organizations need a procedure for emergency access by authorized persons.

Finally, it is important to employ technical safeguards to ensure that data are secure when they are being transmitted from one computer (or network, or entity) to another. Data may be stored on a *server,* and an individual *client* computer may need to upload or download information from it. In order to ensure that the transmission is secure, a Transport Layer Security (TLS) protocol must be initiated. While the technical specifications of a TLS protocol (or its very similar predecessor, the Secure Socket Layer, or SSL, protocol) are beyond the scope of this text, it is important to understand the overall procedure. The TLS protocol provides a method for the client to authenticate the server and ensure private communications using cryptography. When encrypting data, the contents are scrambled according to schemes that are very complex, and require "encryption keys" to be unscrambled. The two computers decide on encryption schemes and keys only after authenticating each other's identities.

In many Internet applications, only the server is authenticated; thus, your personal computer authenticates the bank's server to ensure that data are being sent to your bank account and not to a fraudulent server. Mutual authentication occurs when the server also authenticates the client, which requires an additional level of technological protocols. It is important for security officers and researchers to understand how stringent the security of the client–server connection is. The client and the server authenticate one another and determine how the data will be encrypted through a "handshake" negotiation. Essentially, the client and server provide each other with information about the types of encryption each can understand, their digital certificates, and public encryption keys. Once the server (and sometimes the client) is authenticated, the server and client work together using random numbers to generate a "Master Secret" from which all other encryption and key data for the subsequent interaction is derived. They then verify that their negotiated encryption and decryption schemes are accurate and that the rest of the interaction is encrypted accordingly.

These technical safeguards seem quite intricate and demanding, and for good reason. These are the processes that ensure that data are safe from tampering, fraud, and eavesdropping. Even with the security measures in place, security can be compromised by a number of events, so security officers, policies, and accountability are important considerations. Working with information-security officers can prevent an array of problems and prevent security breaches.

In addition to employment of the strictest technological standards for data security, it is also helpful to consider offering what may be more transparent to study participants regarding your confidentiality policy and procedures for an Internet-based study. Consider Figure 1.2 from Chapter 1. This shows an example of a webpage used in a diabetes prevention initiative. The figure allows participants to click on a link and get additional details related to privacy (e.g., "frequently asked questions," or FAQ; whom to contact for additional information or to raise a concern).

Specific procedures that we endorse for maintaining privacy for the Internet environment include the assignment of screen names and reminders for participants to maintain confidentiality during study sessions.

Screen Names and Personal Identity

It has been documented in the literature that some populations may not be aware of the ease with which their personal information is essentially made public when they post it online (Moreno et al., 2008). If you are enrolling participants in a program that will require them to (a) interact with multiple staff during the process and/or (b) interact with other research participants, you can improve confidentiality by assigning an unidentifiable screen name to each participant. You can choose to regulate the creation of the screen name (e.g., comprising the first letter of participants' first name, the last letter of their last name, and the first and last digit of their Social Security number), but this may be cumbersome for participants and difficult for them to remember. You can ask participants to create their own screen name, but then encourage them to ensure that they cannot be identified through the name they choose (e.g., *beachlover* is easier to remember and less identifiable than *youngmom80201*).

Screen names can be linked in one database to participant identifiers, and access to this database can be limited, with password protections, to a small number of program team members.

In addition to limiting access to linkages between screen names and participant identifiers, be careful to remind participants who engage with other participants during the course of a program (e.g., as they enroll in an online support group) that they should limit personal disclosures while online. You may choose to post reminders about screen names and privacy on program session pages and/or on the privacy page.

With regard to mobile phone interventions, we need to be aware that people may share cell phones or may be near others when they are talking on the phone or sending and receiving text messages. Indeed, researchers cannot assume that the person on the phone is the person with whom they intend to communicate, either by voice or by text message.

The same suggestions for creating a screen name apply to the mobile environment; participants should be encouraged to create an ID that is unique and does not identify them; it may be possible for participants to use their telephone number as their ID, since it is unique, but this does not ensure that the person using that ID is the participant. Therefore, participants using their phone number as an ID should also have a unique password that they can say in a verbal conversation or send using a text message.

WHAT ARE EMERGING AND EVOLVING ETHICAL TRENDS IN TECHNOLOGY-BASED HEALTH PROMOTION?

GIS and Tracking of Individuals

There are several important technological trends emerging that have implications for ethics in the conduct of health promotion. With the advent of geographic information systems (GIS), it is possible to track participants in programs if devices used have GIS-enabled features. Mobile phones, for example, have such features, and they may be used to track user location—if health promotion efforts are attempting to educate consumers about the negative health outcomes associated with consumption of fast food, they may send messages programmed for delivery when a person enters a fast-food establishment. If such programs are to be used, it is imperative to consider implications for participant privacy and the importance of full disclosure and informed consent before implementing such programs.

Also on the horizon are biomedical verification features that will be available to identify individuals. Readers may recall a scene from the movie *Minority Report* (Spielberg, 2002), where the lead character, played by Tom Cruise, enters a retail store. Upon entry, his irises are scanned, and an announcer welcomes him to the store and invites him to try on clothing that matches preferences identified from previous purchases made in retail stores. This may be in the distant future, but biotechnology does indicate that such biomarkers as thumbprints and iris scans may be more commonplace to establish individuals as unique and eligible for any number of things (security access, program access, etc.). While this may simplify participant verification, it is likely to raise many additional concerns about how individual privacy is protected and confidentiality is guaranteed.

Data Sharing Across Agencies

We briefly mentioned the concept of "cloud computing" in Chapter 1, where we may soon be able to access large servers via rental to quickly process data. Similarly, technology already exists for file sharing, where people can post documents online and access them from anywhere. Google maintains this service through "Google Docs," and there are other, similar services offered by Microsoft.

All of the current considerations we have for maintaining data security and participant privacy and confidentiality extend to circumstances when we share files or use cloud computing. It is our ethical obligation to ensure that when documents are not protected by firewalls and when data are transmitted, either they are devoid of participant identifiers or identifiers are encrypted, and access to files with data are password protected.

SUMMARY

The use of technology in health promotion poses some unique ethical challenges that need specific attention. We must take extra care to consider beneficence; while technology may make it easier for us to collect, manage, and analyze data, it doesn't mean this is the best way to reach and engage diverse populations. We must assess what is the most appropriate way to reach an audience. If we are working on a health issue where there is a racial/ethnic or class disparity, and/or with populations that are affected by the digital divide, we need to consider both ways to increase access to technology and approaches to reach them using the technologies they access now—for example, use mobile phones instead of the Internet if that is what your target audience has access to and prefers! We also need to take additional care with special populations such as children, prisoners, or the mentally impaired. Because relatively less technology-based health promotion has been done with these groups, extra care must be taken to ensure these potentially vulnerable groups receive extra protection related to consent and confidentiality of data.

Overall, the procedures to protect and maintain data confidentiality are highly sophisticated and effective. However, because they represent a very specialized field, bringing in experts in data security will allow you additional confidence that your data cannot be accessed by unauthorized persons. While it may be remotely possible that a very diligent individual can access data that are encrypted, password protected, and stored behind firewalls, it is much more likely that your data will fall into the wrong hands if you do not take care to implement all these steps up front to both protect your data and reassure your participants that you have done all you can to secure their sensitive information.

You should take extra care to ensure that participants in your programs are who they say they are and to pay attention to the common practices such as maintaining multiple e-mail accounts that could allow participants to fraudulently enroll in research. At the time of enrollment, take extra care to ensure you obtain *informed* consent. Simply using the typical text boxes with complex legal language does not offer confidence that any consent obtained is informed. Care should be taken to make consent documents easy to read, understand, and opt in and out of as desired.

Finally, be sure to set yourself up for success early by developing and maintaining a good relationship with your IRB if your project is considered research or you wish to publish your data. Meet with your IRB representatives and offer them as much detail as you can find about how others have utilized technology for research and program evaluation. Showing precedence can assist you in achieving approvals with fewer modifications or revisions. Table 2.1 offers a summary of the key terms associated with the ethics and technology-based programs covered in this chapter.

Table 2.1 Key terms related to ethics unique to technology-based programs

Term	Definition
Terms of service (TOS)	Legal terms users must agree to before participating in activities on a website; usually presented in small font that may be complicated and difficult to read and understand.
Frequently asked questions (FAQ)	On websites you will often find a FAQ link to take you to a separate page offering more detail on information about the site that isn't offered on the home page.
Webmaster	On an Internet site this is often the person whom you should contact with questions or concerns about the site.

(Continued)

(Continued)

Term	Definition
Privacy guidelines	On an Internet site or for other technology-based programs, you can offer a specific set of guidelines or policies that you will adhere to in the delivery of your program. This can lend credibility to your program.
Screen name	For any technology-based program, persons may have a name or number used to identify them as a participant. It is valuable to pay attention to the need to keep screen names separate from real names to protect individual privacy of participants.
HIPAA and PHI	The Health Insurance Portability and Accountability Act (HIPAA) established legal guidelines for the protection of personal health information (PHI) so that people would not have their confidentiality compromised when changing medical providers. Adherence to HIPAA and protection of PHI is required for technology-based programs that handle patient data.
Public domain	Information that is not secured through encryption or behind a password, a firewall, or another mechanism. This information is accessible to anyone with access to the technology you are using for a program. While readily available, not all users are aware how much and what of the information they provide is in the public domain. Steps should be taken to raise awareness about accessibility of sensitive information.

? CONCLUDING QUESTIONS

1. Is there precedence for technology-based health promotion within your institution? Do you have access to technology-based protocols that have been approved by your IRB that you can use as a template in applying for IRB approval?

2. What are the information technology security systems within your institution? Are there existing requirements to use encryption, TLS, firewalls, and password protection? If not, is there someone within your institution who can assist you in implementing such security measures?

3. What are special ethical considerations you need to address in your own technology-based program?

 ## CHAPTER EXERCISE

Your task is to consider a health promotion program you wish to deliver using technology. It can be the same program you thought of to complete the exercise for Chapter 1, or a different program.

Answer the following questions:

1. How can I demonstrate that the technology I choose is beneficent? How is delivering this program using technology an improvement over using a traditional health promotion format?

2. How will I maintain data security? Specify which elements you will employ from this list:

   a. Firewalls

   b. Transport Layer Security

   c. Data encryption

   d. Password protection on files

   e. Password protection on databases

3. Identify the specific ways you plan to obtain informed consent. How can you increase the likelihood that participants will read and comprehend your consent materials?

4. How will you verify that participants are who they say they are, both at the time of enrollment and when you deliver specific program content?

5. How will you establish and maintain your own credibility for program participants?

ADDITIONAL RESOURCES

Books, Articles, and Other Peer-Reviewed Literature

Resource	Description
Anderson, J., & Goodman, K. (2002). *Ethics and information technology: A case-based approach to a health care system in transition.* New York: Springer-Verlag.	This book uses a case study approach to introduce the reader to specific ethical considerations in delivery of computer-based health services.
Demiris, G., Afrin, L. B., Speedie, S., Courtney, K. L., Sondhi, M., Vimarlund, V., et al. (2008). Patient-centered applications: Use of information technology to promote disease management and wellness. A white paper by the AMIA knowledge in motion working group. *Journal of the American Medical Informatics Association, 15*(1), 8–13.	This white paper offers some "best practices" related to the use of computers in care settings for promotion of better self-management of chronic illness.
Lee, L. M., & Gostin, L. O. (2009). Ethical collection, storage, and use of public health data: A proposal for a national privacy protection. *JAMA, 302*(1), 82–84.	This brief paper raises considerations related to the collection and storage of sensitive health information.

(Continued)

(Continued)

Resource	Description
Meingast, M., Roosta, T., & Sastry, S. (2006). Security and privacy issues with health care information technology. *Conference Proceedings of the IEEE Engineering in Medicine and Biology Society, 1*, 5453–5458.	This paper raises some of the key security issues that one may consider in protection of data and privacy of health records and personal health information.
Robinson, T., Patrick, K., Eng, T., Gustafson, D., & the Science Panel on Interactive Communication and Health. (1998). An evidence-based approach to interactive health communication: A challenge to medicine in the information age. *JAMA, 280*, 1264–1269.	This report considers the opportunities and challenges we face with regard to the use of technology in care and health promotion. Although over a decade old, it still offers relevant cautions and appropriate considerations for work using technology today.
Sindall, C. (2002). Does health promotion need a code of ethics? *Health Promotion International, 17*(3), 201–203.	This article offers important questions for health promoters to consider in general related to the ethical delivery of health promotion interventions.
Spinello, R. (2002). *Case studies in information technology ethics* (2nd ed.). Upper Saddle River, NJ: Prentice Hall.	This book uses a case study approach to consider ethical issues related to information technology in the delivery of care and health promotion.
Tavani, H. (2007). *Ethics and technology: Ethical issues in an age of information and communication technology.* Hoboken, NJ: Wiley.	This book offers a broad look at emerging ethical considerations related to the use of technology to retrieve and send information and for communication between individuals and organizations.

REFERENCES

Bowen, A. M., Williams, M. L., Daniel, C. M., & Clayton, S. (2008). Internet based HIV prevention research targeting rural MSM: Feasibility, acceptability, and preliminary efficacy. *Journal of Behavioral Medicine, 31*(6), 463–477.

Coyne, C. A., Xu, R., Raich, P., Plomer, K., Dignan, M., Wenzel, L. B., et al. (2003). Randomized, controlled trial of an easy-to-read informed consent statement for clinical trial participation: A study of the Eastern Cooperative Oncology Group. *Journal of Clinical Oncology, 21*, 836–842.

Djomand, G., Katzman, J., Tommaso, D. D, Hudgens, M. G., Counts, G. W., Koblin, B. A., et al. (2005). Enrollment of racial/ethnic minorities in NIAID-funded networks of HIV vaccine trials in the United States, 1988 to 2002. *Public Health Reports, 120*, 543–548.

Elgesem, D. (2002). What is special about the ethical issues in online research? *Ethics and Information Technology, 4*, 195–203.

Elks, M. L. (1993). The right to participate in research studies [Review; 15 refs]. *Journal of Laboratory & Clinical Medicine, 122*, 130–136.

Fjeldsoe, B., Marshall, A. L., & Miller, Y. D. (2009). Behavior change interventions delivered by mobile telephone short-message service. *American Journal of Preventative Medicine, 36*, 165–173.

Flicker, S., Haans, D., & Skinner, H. (2004). Ethical dilemmas in research on Internet communities. *Qualitative Health Research, 14,* 124–134.

Ford, J. G., Howerton, M. W., Lai, G. Y., Gary, T. L., Bolen, S., Gibbons, M. C., et al. (2008). Barriers to recruiting underrepresented populations to cancer clinical trials: A systematic review. *Cancer, 112,* 228–242.

Haigh, C., & Jones, N. A. (2005). An overview of the ethics of cyber-space research and the implication for nurse educators. *Nurse Education Today, 25,* 3–8.

Keller, H. E., & Lee, S. (2003). Ethical issues surrounding human participants research using the Internet. *Ethics & Behavior, 13,* 211–219.

Koo, M., & Skinner, H. (2005). Challenges of Internet recruitment: A case study with disappointing results. *Journal of Medical Internet Research, 7,* e6.

Krishna, S., Borren, S. A., & Balas, E. A. (2009). Healthcare via cell phones: A systematic review. *Telemedicine and e-Health, 15,* 231–240.

Lenhart, A., & Horrigan, J. B. (2003). Re-visualizing the Digital Divide as a Digital Spectrum. *IT & Society, 1,* 23–39.

Lloyd, C. E., Johnson, M. R., Mughal, S., Sturt, J. A., Collins, G. S., Roy, T., et al. (2008). Securing recruitment and obtaining informed consent in minority ethnic groups in the UK. *BMC Health Services Research, 8,* 68.

Marquez, M. A., Muhs, J. M., Tosomeen, A., Riggs, B. L., & Melton, L. J. (2003). Costs and strategies in minority recruitment for osteoporosis research. *Journal of Bone & Mineral Research, 18,* 3–8.

Moreno, M. A., Fost, N. C., & Christakis, D. A. (2008). Research ethics in the MySpace era. *Pediatrics, 121,* 157–161.

National Institutes of Health. (2001). *Policy and guidelines on the inclusion of women and minorities as subjects in clinical research.* Retrieved from http://grants.nih.gov/grants/funding/women_min/guidelines_amended_ 10_2001.htm

Oddone, E. Z., Olsen, M. K., Lindquist, J. H., Orr, M., Horner, R., Reda, D., et al. (2004). Enrollment in clinical trials according to patients race: Experience from the VA Cooperative Studies Program (1975–2000). *Controlled Clinical Trials, 25,* 378–387.

Pequegnat, W., Rosser, E. R. S., Bowen, A. M., Bull, S., & DiClemente, R. J. (2007). Conducting internet-based HIV/STD prevention survey research: Considerations in design and evaluation. *AIDS and Behavior, 11,* 505–521.

Peterson, E. D., Lytle, B. L., Biswas, M. S., & Coombs, L. (2004). Willingness to participate in cardiac trials. *American Journal of Geriatric Cardiology, 13,* 11–15.

Pittenger, D. J. (2003). Internet research: An opportunity to revisit classic ethical problems in behavioral research. *Ethics & Behavior, 13,* 45–60.

Raich, P. C., Plomer, K. D., & Coyne, C. A. (2001). Literacy, comprehension, and informed consent in clinical research. *Cancer Investigation, 19,* 437–445.

Santelli, J. (1997). Human subjects protection and parental permission in adolescent health research. *Journal of Adolescent Health, 21,* 384–387.

Santelli, J. S., Smith, R. A., Rosenfeld, W. D., DuRant, R. H., Dubler, N., Morreale, M., et al. (2003). Guidelines for adolescent health research: A position paper of the Society for Adolescent Medicine. *Journal of Adolescent Health, 33,* 396–409.

Spielberg, S. (Director). (2002). *Minority report* [Motion picture]. United States: Twentieth Century Fox.

Turner, C. F., Ku, L., Rogers, S. M., Lindberg, L. D., Pleck, J. H., & Sonenstein, F. L. (1998). Adolescent sexual behavior, drug use, and violence: Increase reporting with computer survey technology. *Science, 280,* 867–873.

U.S. Department of Health, Education, and Welfare. (1979). *The Belmont Report: Ethical principles and guidelines for the protection of human subjects of research.* Retrieved from http://ohsr.od.nih.gov/ guidelines/belmont.html

PART II ▟

Unique Aspects of Technology-Based Program Development, Implementation, and Evaluation

3 ▪▪

Technology-Based Health Program Development

CHAPTER OVERVIEW

In this chapter, readers are oriented to the initial steps they need to pursue if contemplating a technology-based intervention. Note the emphasis here is on issues relevant for health promotion program development; by this we mean the steps needed to take before you actually implement a program—instruction in the creation of content for programs is beyond the scope of this work. However, we offer multiple suggestions and resources for those readers who do wish to create their own content.

First, we consider the benefits afforded by different modalities for health promotion—specifically, CD-ROM and computer kiosks, the Internet, and mobile phones and devices—and how to maximize sustainability of programs given rapid evolution in technology. We then consider limitations with using each approach. We offer examples of best practices in program development, and consider emerging innovations with regard to technology-based program options.

The information covered in this chapter is relevant for all types of technological modalities (i.e., computer, Internet, mobile phone, and handheld devices). We cover the issues unique to implementation and evaluation of using each of these types of modalities for health promotion in subsequent chapters.

WHAT ARE UNIQUE AND BENEFICIAL CONSIDERATIONS FOR EACH TYPE OF TECHNOLOGICAL MODALITY?

The CD-ROM/DVD

This modality is one that can be ideal for use when you have a program that you wish to distribute to a network of organizations with ample computer access, such as schools, clinics, hospitals, or jails/prisons. The primary advantage of this modality is that once it has been developed, it is a low-cost method to get your product wisely distributed.

The CD-ROM/DVD is also a highly structured modality. You can develop the program with a great degree of complexity, allowing for multiple branching and tailoring that will allow a program user to individualize content for greater relevance. The high degree of structure also allows for greater confidence in program fidelity; users cannot change the program structure, so it will be delivered in a consistent fashion each time.

The Computer Kiosk

This modality is ideal for delivering technology-based programs in settings where users have limited access to technology and less familiarity with technology-based health promotion. The primary advantage of this modality is that it is a good way to extend the reach of your program to populations that may have not been reached previously with technology-based health promotion.

As with the CD-ROM/DVD, a computer kiosk is also very structured. Your program can have a good deal of complexity, including branching and tailoring that will maximize a personalized message for the user. The high degree of structure also allows for greater confidence in program fidelity; users cannot change the program structure, so it will be delivered in a consistent fashion each time. The structure on a kiosk, however, can be more flexible; if written in hypertext markup language (HTML) or extensible hypertext markup language (XHTML), programming languages often used in Internet programming, you have the added benefit of being able to regularly update content and make it more current.

If your program would reach a population that has heretofore not had access to technology, and can effectively engage that population, it may be the ideal option for you. Consider those populations most affected by the digital divide when thinking about the computer kiosk, or perhaps populations in resource-poor settings domestically or internationally for whom the computer kiosk can double as a valuable resource above and beyond the technology-based health promotion program.

The Internet

As access to the Internet proliferates, so does the appeal of an Internet-based health promotion program. This modality offers the advantage of extensive reach, in that you could reach people in multiple cities, states, and nations with a health promotion endeavor. Of particular interest is the possibility to "scale up" using the Internet. As mentioned in Chapter 1, one of the primary appeals of technology-based health promotion is the possibility of increasing the impact of our programs—if we can reach more people, even with modest effects we can anticipate greater impact on morbidity and mortality. The Internet has strong potential for contributions here, inasmuch as access to the medium is continually growing, and taking a program that works on a small scale to a larger audience is possible with this medium.

The modality also offers a way to deliver and evaluate programs very rapidly, and to do so at any time of day or night depending on user preference. The Internet offers the same advantages as the CD-ROM/ DVD and computer kiosk with regard to program structure and fidelity. The Internet also offers a relatively low-cost programming option, inasmuch as the HTML programming often used is easy to update and keep current, although costs can and do increase when using heavy graphics and applications.

Mobile Phones and Other Portable Devices

The primary advantage of the mobile phone is coverage and reach. Even in resource-poor settings where there is no infrastructure to support landlines for telephones there are numerous mobile phone users. A mobile phone-based program has the advantage of portability—users can receive program content anywhere, and do not need to be in front of a computer. As mentioned earlier in this chapter, minorities are among the most frequent users of mobile phones and, given their overrepresentation among those with chronic and infectious conditions, may be ideal populations for mobile phone–based health promotion. The mobile phone has the same "scale up" potential as the Internet, and could even surpass the reach of the Internet, as the portability has made it widely used and adopted globally.

As of this writing, we are aware that other mobile devices such as the iPad™ are available that can allow users to access the Internet on a platform that is bigger than a phone but smaller than a laptop. We anticipate growth in interest and potential for using these devices to deliver health promotion content as well. However, they are still new to the Internet and computing environment, and we don't yet have information on their popularity or utility.

WHAT ARE CHALLENGES WE FACE WITH
EACH TYPE OF TECHNOLOGICAL MODALITY?

While each modality has advantages, there remain concerns for each that suggest careful consideration of both the pros and cons for each modality is needed before selecting one. Selection should further be influenced by two additional factors. First, anticipating and planning for obsolescence is perhaps more critical in this than other fields—technology evolves so quickly, and user appetite for new content and applications is large. Second, making content available beyond the life of an evaluation requires forethought and planning in addition to financial resources.

Challenges With Using Each Type of Modality

The CD-ROM/DVD

The primary disadvantages of this modality are cost and accessibility. It is generally more costly to produce a CD-ROM/DVD, and once it is finalized, it is more difficult to change or update it, making it more costly than other options. In addition, you must be confident that the end user will have the equipment that he or she needs to run the CD-ROM/DVD (i.e., a computer and monitor with a CD-ROM/DVD port). For those without equipment, the program is not usable. On balance, if you are working with a group of institutions and are confident they have the equipment needed and that your program will have relevance for some time, then this option is a good one for you.

The Computer Kiosk

The primary disadvantages of using a computer kiosk program are cost and equipment safety. It is costly to purchase, monitor, and maintain kiosks across multiple settings, or to move a kiosk from one setting to another. If delivering a program in a health care setting, for example, it may be cumbersome or awkward to move a kiosk from one room to another, or you may find that having a kiosk requires too much space. As we see availability of other portable devices such as the iPad™, these may be more appealing than a kiosk—you could easily move it from room to room and deliver the same content as you would on a kiosk. However, with the more portable device you are likely to face more chronic issues related to theft and security. Depending on where you deliver your program, it may be a safety risk to maintain your kiosk or portable device in the field.

Other concerns with the computer kiosk are related to data storage and transfer. If your kiosk is in a location with Internet access, either wired or wireless, then it may be possible to create a hybrid program that is run simultaneously on the Internet and delivered via computer kiosk. One real advantage here is the ability to store data on a remote server and avoid potential data loss or damage related to uploading it. However, many sites do not have regular and reliable Internet access, meaning that data will need to be stored on each individual machine and uploaded manually by a program staff person on a regular basis. This concern is actually minimized with a portable device such as the iPad™, which utilizes a wireless access to a 3G configuration (or "third generation" technology, which refers to the speed with which data are transferred online) and does not rely on Internet access through cable or other modem devices—as long as there is network service available.

The Internet

There are two primary disadvantages of the Internet. The first is accessibility. Even though access to the Internet appears to be increasing, a digital divide still persists, and some of those with the greatest need for health promotion related to a specific disease or condition may not have access to it if it is delivered online. Access is not simply access to a computer with an Internet connection—bandwidth speeds vary greatly and can be particularly slow in resource-poor settings, making program quality quite limited even when access is available. Another disadvantage is sampling. While it is certainly possible and advantageous to accrue large numbers of participants in an online program, we don't have—nor will we ever likely have—a complete list of all Internet users, which limits our ability to generalize results to a larger population if recruitment for programs is conducted online. One way to overcome this is to sample and recruit in face-to-face settings using traditional methods, and then deliver programs online to the population sampled for the program.

As with the computer kiosk, we can consider a hybrid approach with the Internet to overcome these difficulties. Consider resource-poor settings—particularly international settings, where there is substantial evidence of growing Internet use through Internet cafés, rather than through use at home, making delivery of a program in these settings attractive. It is important, however, to assess an individual café's equipment and broadband, cable, or wireless Internet access to ensure programs are not overly graphic-intensive resulting in prohibitively slow loading speeds for users.

Mobile Phones and Other Portable Devices

The main disadvantage for mobile phones is the lack of complexity available to the health promoter in program delivery. While tailoring and branching is certainly available through interactive voice response (IVR) programs, where the user will choose options and push different numbers on a keypad to go in multiple directions, the availability of and accessibility to the graphics and animation through other modalities is limited.

Another disadvantage in the United States is the cost associated with some mobile phone innovations. Users pay for a voice plan, and every time they send or receive a voice or text message, they are charged, making incoming program messages less appealing. In many international settings, users do not pay for incoming messages, be they voice or text, reducing this concern.

We have fewer examples of interventions that work for the mobile phone environment, probably due more to having had less time to develop these more novel approaches compared to the other modalities discussed here. We anticipate that there will be growing interest in using the phone, and that there are also many opportunities for hybrid programs that use the phone for specific program elements, such as text messages, to remind a participant to complete a program element online, or to call a clinic for test results, or to take a medication.

Text Box 3.1 outlines these specific pros and cons for each modality and allows the reader to consider them in the context of the unique advantages offered by technology.

Challenges in Technological Obsolescence

As we will discuss below, it is imperative to engage members of your target audience in the development of any technology-based program to learn what they will like and dislike, what will motivate them to use the program, and what will keep them coming back. However, it is

TEXT BOX 3.1
Unique considerations for each modality

Element	CD-ROM/DVD	Computer Kiosk	Internet	Mobile Phone	Handheld Device
Reach	Pro: With CD-ROM/DVDs, programs can be widely distributed although not as widely as with the Internet.	Con: While reach is expanded above what may be possible in the clinic, it is relatively less effective than other modalities.	Pro: With Internet you can reach hundreds or thousands of people quite quickly.	Pro: With a mobile phone you can reach hundreds or perhaps thousands, but you have less access to users compared to Internet.	Pro: With handhelds, programs can be widely distributed although not as widely as with the Internet.
Standardization	Pro: Programs can be highly standardized.	Pro: Programs can be highly standardized.	Pro: Programs can be highly standardized.	Pro: Programs can be highly standardized.	Pro: Programs can be highly standardized.
Individual Tailoring	Pro: Algorithms can be used to make information relevant to individual users.	Pro: Algorithms can be used to make information relevant to individual users.	Pro: Algorithms can be used to make information relevant to individual users.	Pro: Algorithms can be used to make information relevant to individual users.	Pro: Algorithms can be used to make information relevant to individual users.
Cost	Con: Compared to other modalities, CD-ROM/DVDs are generally more costly to produce.	Con: Compared to other programs, the equipment needed for computer kiosks is more expensive.	Pro: Programs on the Internet are relatively less costly to produce although high-end graphics and applications do drive up cost.	Pro: Using text messaging is perhaps the lowest-cost approach of all the modalities.	Con: Compared to other programs, the equipment needed for handhelds is more expensive, although less than kiosks.
Accessibility and Sampling	Pro and Con: If you have control over who has access to the CD-ROM/DVD, you can increase accessibility to those	Pro: By providing all the equipment needed, you increase access for those who do not have it. You can also control who	Con: While access to Internet is growing, there remains a digital divide, and sampling is problematic.	Pro and Con: With the ubiquitous nature of the mobile phone, you may offer a program to a more diverse	Pro and Con: If you have control over who has access to the device, you can increase accessibility to those who may

(Continued)

(Continued)

Element	CD-ROM/DVD	Computer Kiosk	Internet	Mobile Phone	Handheld Device
	who may not have Internet access, but they do need a computer to run the program.	has access to the program depending on where it is placed.		audience; however, sampling is problematic.	not have Internet access, but only a limited number can have the device.
Program Complexity	Pro: The program can have a high concentration of graphics, audio, and animation.	Pro: The program can have a high concentration of graphics, audio, and animation.	Pro and Con: The program can have a high concentration of graphics, audio, and animation; however, the more of this, the less access to content by those without high-speed Internet.	Con: Small screens and expensive phone contracts for users mean complexity in programming is not widely available.	Pro and Con: While you can have greater complexity than on a phone, you are still limited by screen size and power of the device to less complex programs.
Data Transfer and Portability	Con: It is more challenging to store and transfer data from a CD-ROM/DVD.	Pro and Con: Data storage is easier than with CD-ROM/DVD, but transferring data can be problematic with multiple kiosks.	Pro: Data transfer can be instantaneous; care needs to be taken to ensure confidentiality and security.	Pro: Data transfer can be instantaneous; care needs to be taken to ensure confidentiality and security.	Pro and Con: Data can be downloaded from a handheld or transferred over the Internet—may require additional equipment.
Ease of Updating	Con: It is difficult to update or change a program once developed for CD-ROM/DVD.	Pro: If written in HTML language, it can be as easy to update a computer kiosk program as it is to update an Internet program.	Pro: The Internet offers easier options for updating content.	Pro: With simpler programming, updating content for voice- or text-delivered messages is easy.	Pro: If written in HTML language, it can be as easy to update a program for a handheld as it is to update an Internet program.
Equipment Safety	Pro: An individual CD-ROM/DVD costs little to replace if lost or stolen.	Con: If a computer or kiosk is damaged or stolen it is costly to replace.	Pro: There is no equipment per se for an Internet program, assuming the user has the computer needed to run the program.	Pro and Con: While mobile phones are cheaper than a computer, if lost or stolen they do incur a charge to replace.	Pro and Con: While handhelds are cheaper than a computer, if lost or stolen they do incur a charge to replace.

also important to develop programs in such a way as to allow for the interchange of photos and text that may quickly become dated, and to update modules with fresh content on a regular basis in anticipation that users will become bored if they see the same content multiple times.

A concept called "modular programming" is in use in response to the potential problem of obsolescence. Programmers develop segments of code that perform a singular task—for example, calculate body mass index (BMI). This is done to break up a large program into manageable units and to create code that can be easily reused in other programs or replaced with different or newer code when possible. Readers will recognize the concept of versioning— where a new version of a software program is released as a "new and improved" version, or one that is augmented with newer content. These processes are motivated by desires to simplify testing and debugging among programmers and have been in use for decades. In addition to modular programming there is an evolving field called "object-oriented" programming. The Ruby programming language offers a good example of object-oriented programming with its "Ruby on Rails" concept, also called RoR. The idea here is similar—programmers only want to write code for new elements of a program. Whenever possible, by compartmentalizing programming language, it allows for programmers to reutilize code for all conventional aspects of a program and to develop new code for customization or for new program elements.

Consider a typical Internet site for web-based shopping. There are conventional elements on all these sites—for example, a shopping cart, checkout procedures, log-in procedures. Some elements are typically used but not always, such as product search capabilities or a "new in stock" feature. Each of these elements can be developed in modular format, so when developers create a new site they can copy and paste the code and avoid having to rewrite complex algorithms. Furthermore, they can add in new elements or modules much more easily. Note, as described above, the opportunities for updating content are fewer for CD-ROM/DVD programs, so take that into consideration when planning what modality to use.

Make sure to develop your programs with chapters or modules where possible—this can allow you to exchange a more outdated module with a new one while still retaining other content that remains current. Also, make sure that you keep graphics, flash, audio, and other design elements separate. For example, if you have photos of people in your program dressed in sweaters and coats when the content is shown in summer, you may want to keep all other elements but find new pictures that match the season—so you can change a photo while keeping audio and flash if need be.

Making Content Available Beyond the Life of an Evaluation

Technology-based programs for health promotion are arguably still in their infancy. We are still learning best practices for program development, implementation, and evaluation, and have yet to identify multiple programs with efficacy that can be "scaled up" and disseminated widely to realize the promise of technology to improve program impact. A common criticism of traditional health promotion efforts is the lack of dissemination of effective programs—we do a poor job of translating "what works" to wider audiences and sustaining effective programs over time.

We have a unique opportunity to address this limitation in technology-based health promotion. If we develop our programs initially with the intent of scaling up once we know what works, we can build in plans from the time of program initiation for sustainability. Key issues to consider to achieve this will be (a) how to disseminate content once you know it works, (b) how to quickly adapt effective programs for different audiences in different settings, and (c) how to ensure consistent access to program content.

WHAT ARE THE CURRENT AND BEST PRACTICES IN TECHNOLOGY-BASED PROGRAM DEVELOPMENT?

Be as Informed as Possible About Expectations of Your Audience

To facilitate obtaining the best information on what is current among members of your target audience, identify preferences from representatives whenever possible. We advocate having a complete formative research process, where you conduct focus groups, in-depth interviews, observations, or other qualitative efforts with your target audience to determine such things as (a) what, if any, technology they use and like to use and, if they don't use any, what barriers exist to their use; (b) how often and where they use technology; and (c) what attracts them to their technology of choice—convenience? Access? Entertaining and artistic content? New and current content?

Text Box 3.2 offers an example of a topic guide for technology-based program development. As with other formative work, you should plan on collecting data from multiple groups or individuals until you reach saturation—that is, consistently hear the same messages about design, content, and presentation of information (Strauss & Corbin, 1990).

The focus of your formative work may differ given what you already know about your target audience. If, for example, there is ample literature on expectations for design and content delivery (e.g., there is a growing literature on youth preferences for design and "look and feel" for technology-based programs; Bull, McFarlane, Phibbs, & Watson, 2007; Myint-U et al., 2008), then your focus during your formative phase may be more on how to best direct users to your program. If your program is intended as a web-based program, the focus may be more on where youth spend time online so you can ascertain the feasibility of embedding a program into a popular existing site. If you already have identified a mechanism to distribute your program to an audience (e.g., you have all the cell phone numbers of students in an inner-city job training program), then your focus can be more on how to design elements of your program to make it as compelling as possible.

Make Sure Your Program Works in the Manner You Intended

In addition to the formative work that we advise to ensure that your program has elements and content relevant and appealing to your audience, you should beta test any technological program with members of your target audience. The beta testing process is not intended as a process to refine design or content elements—these should be established through your

---

TEXT BOX 3.2
Sample topic guide for technology-based program development

1. Tell us what you like and do not like about these sites on the Internet:

   (Moderator should show URLs—e.g., www.co.quitnet.com; http://www .nhlbi.nih.gov/health/prof/heart/latino/lat_8pub.htm)

Probes:

   a. What do you like best and least about the sites?

      (Moderator should "surf" the web with participants to the sites named and identify specific characteristics of preferred sites—e.g., color, font, pictures, and animation.)

   b. Of these sites, can you tell the difference between things you like and things that might make you take action?

      (Moderator should, for example, show a smoking cessation website.)

   c. Do you "like" the content? Would the website make you think about not smoking, change your attitudes toward smoking, or get you to stop? Why? What exactly was it on the site that would make you change?

   d. What things on the site are so interesting you'd tell your friends about them?

2. Tell us about reading information about heart disease online:

Probes:

   a. What kind of information do Latinos most need about heart disease online?

   b. How can this information help them prevent heart disease?

   c. What aspects of the website are most helpful for prevention—for example, audio (music, testimonials), video, role models (stories of prevention), links to other sites, statistics, information about prevention programs, games, or risk assessments (quizzes or tests)?

3. We want to see how well programs like this can work to help Latinos prevent heart disease. To do this, we need to test the program in different places in the community. Please tell us:

   a. How comfortable would you be to participate in such a test of the program? (Probe: What if we had to contact you later to try the program again?)

   b. What might make you more comfortable with participating? What can we do to encourage people in the community to try the program?

   c. Where are the places you go in the community (probes: shopping, recreation, church, exercise, activities with children)? We'd like to know where would be the best place to approach people and encourage them to test this program.

---

formative work. Rather the beta test process is intended to (a) determine if the program elements operate as intended, and (b) see if users can easily navigate through the program with minimal errors or problems. Text Box 3.3 offers an example of a beta test log. This is one example of a tool that can be used to document user experiences with your program. The first element of the beta test log allows an interviewer to capture participant reactions to the experience of the program. The idea is to ask the people using your program to "talk aloud" and just say out loud what enters their mind about the program as they use it. You should encourage participants not to modify their reactions but to speak honestly and openly. Table 3.1 shows examples of reactions to site design from such a "talk aloud" process that was employed for a social networking site developed for persons living with HIV (R. Rothbard, personal communication, October 15, 2008).

In addition to having a "talk aloud" option, your beta test process should include documentation of site navigation. This allows you to understand if the pages are loading as intended, if a text message is received and easy to read, and so forth. It allows you to see if users are easily able to navigate through and be exposed to all elements of your program as intended. If, for example, participants don't see a button instructing them to link to a separate part of the site, they may miss a critical element of the program—having this information could lead to a decision to forego using a link and instead embed the linked content directly into a subsequent program page. Observing site navigation can also allow you to see if the program freezes or pages take a long time to load, or if there is any confusion on the part of users as to where they are supposed to go or how they need to get where they want to be.

Development of Program Databases and Tailoring Algorithms

While the use of electronic databases is certainly not unique to research on technology-based health programs, it is imperative to ensure that the program can link to your databases and that data are stored appropriately. Most programs such as SurveyMonkey, Zoomerang, and other electronic survey programs that collect data will allow you to develop your own database, or the creation of a database to store data is integrated into the survey program. If you are not using this—and even if you are—part of your beta testing should include an assessment of whether all the data elements you are collecting are getting stored as intended in your databases. Issues related to data security mentioned in Chapter 2 may require you to encrypt some data elements—be certain to determine before you begin any data collection that these elements are being encrypted as intended, but also that they can be decrypted.

In addition to the great potential that technology-based health programs have to reach large samples, they have an advantage of being able to tap into computer algorithms to make information reaching large numbers of people simultaneously personally relevant. There is a substantial body of literature showing that if health information is personally relevant participants will be more responsive and consider it more appropriate and applicable, which in turn translates into higher likelihood that an individual will adopt healthy behaviors (Campbell et al., 1994; Kreuter & Strecher, 1996; Strecher, 1999; Strecher, Shiffman, & West, 2005).

Tailoring can be used to operationalize theoretical precepts; take, for example, the theoretical idea promoted by Bandura (1986) and Rogers (1995) that role models and popular opinion leaders are important motivators for behavior change. The role model is considered someone whom a person looks up to—for example, a teacher, parent, coach, or minister.

TEXT BOX 3.3
Example of a beta test log

	Navigation Log-in	*Comprehension/ Content Log-in*	*Navigation Page 1*	*Comprehension/ Content Page 1*
Participant 1234	1	0	2	3
Comments:	Couldn't log on with password assigned		Literacy— instructions for navigation not easy to follow	Wanted to be able to skip right to diabetes information
Participant 1235	1, 3	3	0	0
Comments:	Page didn't load; refresh didn't work	Didn't like having to reboot and start again		
Participant 1236	0	0	3	3
Comments:			Couldn't find material she wanted on diabetes	Didn't like the pictures of men— wanted to see some women like her
Participant 1237	2	2	2	2
Comments:	Didn't know how to create password	Didn't know how to create password	Literacy— instructions for navigation not easy to follow	Didn't understand the quiz questions

Key: 0 = no problems noted or observed; 1 = technical problems (e.g., content didn't load, algorithm didn't work, page timed out); 2 = participant comprehension difficulties (e.g., instructions not clear, literacy issues); 3 = participant frustration (e.g., didn't like procedure or content, was impatient with process, preferred to skip to next page/item).

A popular opinion leader is likely to be similar to participants demographically and represents someone they can identify with. Tailoring algorithms can be used to create various role models. If the participant is a middle-aged woman, the computer algorithm could direct the program to display pictures of middle-aged women in subsequent program elements. The role model could easily be changed based on such characteristics as gender, age, and race/ethnicity.

In addition to tailoring for role models, it is now common practice to tailor feedback to individuals based on information offered by participants on their behaviors. For example, if

Table 3.1   Data from a "talk aloud" process to assist with site design and navigability for a site targeting persons living with HIV

Topic Discussed	Quotes/Data
Reactions to home page	It's a lot brighter. It seems to stand out a lot more. Like scrolling down there's a lot more different information that will help out, a lot more current information. It looks like it has dates of medical news if you ever want research ideas . . . a lot more pictures, pictures always grab people and all of that. And um, it looks like you can log in and be a specific member, so that must mean that there's specific things you get benefit from if you're a member for the website and all that.
Motivations to participate	Um, I would only register on a website if I was directly connected to the information on there . . . such as this or job-related and stuff like that. I wouldn't not necessarily register just, you know, to get newsletter information . . . or you know. If I'm directly related to the information or if there's information that I can get that directly benefits me then I think I would definitely register for it.
Reactions to graphics and design	My first general impression is the pictures are way better than the previous one, because they're natural. They're showing athletic people, healthy people. Not like the sexual feeling I got from the other [site I reviewed] that it was more [focused just for the] gay community. [This I like because] there's a woman, there's a man, there's White people, there's Black people, there's females, males. It just feels more open to the [whole HIV+] community.
Using testimonials	Testimonials are always good to have. I mean, obviously if you're promoting a product, you know, testimonials always help. It helps people to understand that there's somebody out there like me who has tried this product or logged on to this website or gone to this clinic and this is their experience. So it's not hurtful or harmful, like it's not harmful to your credibility, but you know, it's a fine line. You have to kind of, for me, I don't want to see too many of them. And I don't want to see them on every single page of the website, [if] you know what I mean.

Source: R. Rothbard, personal communication, October 15, 2008.

you are assessing levels of participant physical activity, you could offer graphical feedback on how well their activity matches guidelines for the same. This feedback is dependent on—and will change based on—variations in responses to questions for individuals on weekly and daily moderate and vigorous physical activity.

Figures 3.1 and 3.2 show examples of tailoring using algorithms. In the first case, we are building on the theoretical concept developed by both Bandura (1986) and Rogers (2003) that health promotion material can be more relevant to participants when delivered by someone they admire and respect and/or by someone they can personally identify with (i.e., a role model). In Figure 3.1 we show you the simple algorithm that you can write in SAS to generate a role model that would match the gender and age of the participant. Role models can match other demographics as well (e.g., sexual orientation, ethnicity). Also in Figure 3.1 we show you an example of how an algorithm for a role model was used in a kiosk program for Latinos.

In Figure 3.2 we offer an example of the programming language you would need to tailor information associated with feedback on participant physical activity. In the case shown here, we compared actual participant physical activity to U.S. Surgeon General recommendations for the same. Each question on a survey is assigned a variable name, shown in brackets in the figure—for example, [PAVIGDAYS] is the variable assigned to the response to Question 1, the amount of vigorous physical activity the participant did over the past 7 days. The algorithm adds up the total vigorous and moderate physical activity along with the amount of time walking to produce feedback for participants on whether they exceed, meet, or do not meet the Surgeon General recommendations.

These examples in Figures 3.1 and 3.2 use programming language for SAS (SAS Institute, n.d.), but any software package such as IBM® SPSS® Statistics (formerly called PASW® Statistics) or Stata will have similar syntax.

Teamwork—The Information Technologist, Creative Developer, Health Promoter, and Evaluator— and Their Diverse and Varied Skill Sets

One of the most important considerations when designing your technology-based health promotion program is to consider the skill set of your team, regardless of the modality you employ. It is highly likely that the special skills required to develop programs will not be concentrated in one or two persons; rather, teams will often require the talent and skills of multiple people.

As with traditional health promotion programs, the content for the program will most likely be developed by individuals trained in health promotion and theories of health behavior change. They may have specialized experience and training in communication and development of health messaging. Since technology-based health promotion is a relatively new field, having specific experience in developing programs for use on computers, the Internet, or mobile phones may be rare. However, the field is growing, and it is likely health promotion experts will develop this capacity quickly.

In addition to health promotion experts, teams will require persons with expertise in program evaluation who can pay adequate and appropriate attention to designing your health promotion effort so that it can be evaluated appropriately. As with traditional programs, bringing in expertise in evaluation before a program starts is critical, so plans for appropriate data collection and analysis can be implemented that are synergistic with program delivery.

The new skills required for well-implemented technology-based health promotion programs are that of an information technology (IT) expert and a creative designer with expertise in technology-based content design and layout. The information technology expert will have appropriate skills in computer programming so that design ideas can be translated to the technology environment you choose—called the "front end" of a program, it is what end users

Figure 3.1   Sample tailoring algorithms for role models

ROLE MODELS

Q1. What is your gender? Please check one.
- ☐ Male
- ☐ Female

Q2. Please fill in your age in years _____

Q3. What is the primary language you speak at home?
- ☐ $_1$ English only or English more than Spanish
- ☐ $_2$ English and Spanish equally
- ☐ $_3$ Spanish only or Spanish more than English

ROLE MODEL ALGORITHM—Choose one of EIGHT

If Q1=1 and Q2 >(44) and Q3=1 or 2 then VAR1 [where the variable name will represent the older male English speaking role model];

Else if If Q1=1 and Q2 <=44 and Q3=1 or 2 then VAR2 [younger male English speaking role model];

Else If Q1=0 and Q2>44 and Q3=1 or 2 then VAR3 [older female English speaking role model];

Else If Q1=0 and Q2<=44 and Q3=1 or 2 then VAR4 [younger female English speaking role model];

Else If Q1=1 and Q2 >(44) and Q3=3 then VAR5 [older male Spanish speaking role model];

Else If Q1=1 and Q2 <=44 and Q3=3 VAR6 [younger male Spanish speaking role model];

Else If Q1=0 and Q2>44 and Q3=3 then VAR7 [older female Spanish speaking role model];

Else If Q1=0 and Q2<=44 and Q3=1 or 2 then VAR8 [younger female Spanish speaking role model].

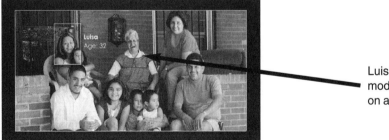

Luisa is one role model selected based on age, gender.

Figure 3.2 Sample tailoring algorithms for feedback on physical activity

1. During the last 7 days, on how many days did you do vigorous physical activities like heavy lifting, digging, aerobics, or fast bicycling? [PAVIGDAYS]
2. How much time did you usually spend doing vigorous physical activities on one of those days?

[PAVIGHOURS] [PAVIGMINS] ----- →COMBINE FOR NEW VARIABLE, [PATOTVIG], SO PATOTVIG=(PAVIGHOURS*60) + PAVIGMINS

3. During the last 7 days, on how many days did you do moderate physical activities like carrying light loads, bicycling at a regular pace, or doubles tennis? Do not include walking.[PAMODDAYS]
4. How much time did you usually spend doing moderate physical activities on one of those days?[PAMODHOURS][PAMODMINS], NEW VARIABLE IS [PATOTMOD]
5. During the last 7 days, on how many days did you walk for at least 10 minutes at a time? [PAWALKDAYS]
6. How much time did you usually spend walking on one of those days?

[PAWALKHOURS][PAWALKMINS] NEW VARIABLE IS [PATOTWALK]

PHYSICAL ACTIVITY ALGORITHM:

Exceeds recommendations=PAVIGDAYS*PATOTVIG>60 OR PAMODDAYS*PATOTMOD+PAWALKDAYS*PATOTWALK>150;

Meets Recommendations= PAVIGDAYS*PATOTVIG=60 OR PAMODDAYS*PATOTMOD+PAWALKDAYS*PATOTWALK=150;

Approaches Recommendations= PAVIGDAYS*PATOTVIG >45 and <60 OR PAMODDAYS*PATOTMOD+PAWALKDAYS*PATOTWALK >112 and <150;

Does not meet Recommendations= PAVIGDAYS*PATOTVIG <=45 OR PAMODDAYS*PATOTMOD+PAWALKDAYS*PATOTWALK <=112;

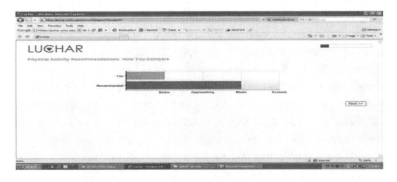

will see when they interact with the modality used to deliver content. A team member will also need skills in the "back end" elements of the program—the back end is where all data are stored. It is critical that the IT expert work with the evaluator to ensure that desired data are being captured and stored for later analysis. Typically, data will include pre- and post-assessments to ascertain program effects, but in addition, many other data can be captured, such as log-ins to a site and the "click trail," which pages a user views in what order, number of visitors to specific pages, and so forth.

Of course a creative element exists in any traditional program for health promotion and is not unique to technology. What is unique, however, is the delivery of content using creative strategies that are specific to the varied modalities available for technology-based health promotion. Graphic design skills are imperative to the team, along with skills in copywriting that are specific to a technological environment.

There are additional resources listed at the end of this chapter to access for greater understanding of IT and graphic design issues. This chapter and textbook are not intended to teach IT and graphic design but rather to introduce health promoters and health promotion program team leaders to the general issues relevant to the design of technology-based programs.

Partnerships for Technology-Based Health Promotion

In an era when we have multiple competing demands for our attention, our technology-based programs need to be designed to reach and hold the attention of users. You may be working with persons who have less familiarity with technology (e.g., the elderly, non-English speakers). You may be working with members of a technologically savvy group who will need something particularly compelling to attract them to your program (e.g., youth). Consider identifying organizations that work with your target audience—offering social, health, or community services—and meeting with them to help you in program development. Organizations could serve as a resource for recruitment, be it for recruiting target audience members to assist in program development (described in more detail in the section below on program implementation). They can also offer important insight on your target audience, giving feedback on your plans for recruitment, program content, and design elements based on their expertise working with the population of interest.

In some cases, they could also be a resource for program implementation. The LUCHAR (Latinos Using Cardio Health Action to Reduce Risk) project (NHLBI 1U01 HL79208) was a pilot program designed to increase physical activity, improve nutrition, and reduce smoking among Latinos in Denver, Colorado. Because our formative work revealed that both elderly and non-English-speaking Latinos would feel more comfortable having assistance in completing the program, we decided to place the program on computer kiosks and to place the kiosks in community-based organizations serving Latinos. This served to increase trust in the program, and self-efficacy for users. Latinos accessing services in trusted community organizations (including churches, a school, social service agencies, and a coffee shop) received encouragement from a recruiter to use the kiosk and complete the program. While this recruiter was available to offer technical assistance with the program, once participants began interacting with the technology, little further assistance with program completion was needed (Leeman-Castillo, Beaty, Raghunath, Steiner, & Bull, 2010).

As mentioned in the introduction to this book, one of the primary reasons why technology is so attractive for health promotion is that it offers enormous potential to increase reach to much larger numbers than those traditionally involved in health promotion programs. However, just because more people are connected to technology doesn't mean you can actually reach them—both because they may be distracted by all the media options they have and because you have limited options to actually reach people given costs associated with online advertising and sampling mechanisms that are currently suboptimal.

It may be possible to turn to work sites and other large organizations to tap into larger populations of people online. Employees of large organizations such as school districts, large private corporations, hospitals, government agencies, and so forth often have access to intranet services through their organization. It may be possible to partner with such organizations to deliver a technology-based program—this could offer a reasonable solution to some of the existing challenges we face with sampling, recruitment, and retention that will be discussed in more detail in Chapter 4. As mentioned above, using the CD-ROM/DVD modality may be ideal when working within institutions where there is already ample equipment available for program delivery.

The analogous organization to a community-based organization online is an advocacy site on the Internet for specific groups. Examples include Gay.com, an advocacy site for persons who identify as gay or lesbian—the site offers information on gay-friendly businesses, political advocacy, and news events relevant to the gay community. Gay.com has been used several times for Internet-related research on HIV prevention for men who have sex with men (Bull, Lloyd, Rietmeijer, & McFarlane, 2004; Rhodes, Diclemente, Cecil, Hergenrather, & Yee, 2002; Ross, Rosser, & Stanton, 2004)—the site is recognized as offering a good opportunity to connect with gay, lesbian, bisexual, and transgendered populations. Other examples of relevant sites on the Internet are Cancer.org (the American Cancer Society), AmericanHeart.org (the American Heart Association), AARP.org (the American Association for Retired Persons), BlackPlanet.com, MiGente.com, AsianAvenue.com, and GLEE.com (targeting gay, lesbian, bisexual, and transgendered individuals).

Know Your Population and What Modality It Uses

The *Healthy People 2010* goals include an overarching aim to decrease health disparities, and attention to this goal has often resulted in identification of disparities in health for racial and ethnic minorities in the United States (U.S. Department of Health and Human Services, 2000).

Literature on the extent and scope of disparities is ample; in brief, there is evidence that African Americans, Latinos, and Native Americans of all ages suffer disproportionately from negative health outcomes, limited access to care, and lower quality of health care. By disparity, we refer to overrepresentation of a group with a disease given the proportion group members represent in the general population.

For example, African Americans have significantly higher rates of colorectal, prostate, and cervical cancer compared to Whites, yet there are fewer African Americans than Whites in the general population. Latinos have higher rates of stomach, liver, and cervical cancer compared to Whites. African Americans have higher rates of hypertension and heart disease compared to Whites, and they have higher rates of HIV/AIDS compared to Whites.

Latinos, African Americans, and Native Americans all face limitations in accessing care and in insurance coverage compared to their White counterparts, and there is evidence that they suffer from relatively lower quality of care in comparison (Centers for Disease Control and Prevention, 2006; Committee on Understanding and Eliminating Racial and Ethnic Disparities in Health Care, 2003; Cooper et al., 2000; Cubbin et al., 2002; James, 2003; McGruder, Malarcher, Antoine, Greenlund, & Croft, 2004).

As mentioned in the introductory chapter, technology-based health promotion has proliferated in the past decade. Yet there has been little specific attention to making an appropriate match delivering technology to specific risk groups to maximize the potential of technology to address health disparities. If we are to do so, we need to take a careful look at how people use technology in order to capitalize on the reach of these modalities to better effect changes in health outcomes for populations at high risk for negative health outcomes.

Technologies Used by Persons Facing Health Disparities and Chronic and Infectious Diseases

While the growth in technology-based applications for health promotion is exciting and dynamic, we must take extra care not to leave those with greatest need for attention behind in our health promotion efforts. In past decades we have observed that there is differential access to technologies such as computers, the Internet, and mobile phones given differences in education and income—termed the "digital divide," there were concerns that the revolution in technology would forever leave the poor and less educated marginalized (Bernhardt, 2000; Chang et al., 2004; U.S. Department of Commerce & National Telecommunications and Information Administration, 1999). There is debate, however, on whether the digital divide is indeed shrinking or whether it persists and is simply shifting to different groups—for example, non-English speakers (Latino Issues Forum, 2004; Lenhart & Horrigan, 2003; Lorence, Park, & Fox, 2006)—while other groups—for example, youth aged 12 to 17—enjoy almost universal access to technology (Lenhart, Madden, Rankin Macgill, & Smith, 2007).

We therefore should not assume universal access to all technology is forthcoming, nor should we assume that universal access automatically translates into universal use. In several instances we have noted that increased access to the Internet doesn't necessarily increase use of the medium for some groups, for example. Increased access by virtue of access to machines and technology at work or libraries doesn't necessarily translate into increased use, and there are obvious differences in use patterns for technology that are likely for those with computer and broadband technology in the home compared to those without (Jackson et al., 2008; Lorence et al., 2006).

A critical consideration, therefore, for those wishing to develop and evaluate health promotion programs using technology is to appropriately match the technology to their target audience—does the audience currently have access to and use the modality they hope to employ? If not, is there evidence or a trend that use of this modality is increasing?

Take the field of Internet-based HIV prevention, for example. This is an area where we have seen substantial growth in technology-based surveillance to document risk and interventions to promote safer sexual behavior—however, there is little evidence across multiple studies that these efforts have succeeded in enrolling substantial numbers of African Americans in their samples. Given that African Americans comprise over 60% of those infected with HIV, we are not doing an adequate job of harnessing the potential of technology to reach this underserved group (Benotsch, Kalichman, & Weinhardt, 2004; Bowen, Horvath, & Williams, 2007; Bull, 2003; Bull et al., 2004; Bull, Pratte, Whitesell, Reitmeijer, & McFarlane, 2009; Halkitis & Parsons, 2003; Rhodes, 2004; Ross et al., 2004; Ross, Tikkanen, & Mansson, 2000).

Another example is diabetes—we have seen no technology-based programs directly targeting Latinos for diabetes—yet Latinos have some of the most extreme disparities for this chronic condition (Barrera, Glasgow, McKay, Boles, & Feil, 2002; Glasgow, Boles, McKay, Feil, & Barrera, 2003; Gottlieb, 2000; Kim & Kim, 2008).

Table 3.2 highlights trends in usage of various technological modalities across different demographic groups. Note, for example, that African Americans comprise the fastest-growing group of cell phone users—now is the time to consider development and testing of health interventions using this modality for African Americans. Note, as well, that although a relatively small proportion of the elderly have access to and use the Internet, this proportion is growing—we cannot assume that the elderly will reject technology-based interventions. As a matter of fact, they have embraced interventions for diabetes and heart disease self-management (Glasgow et al., 2003; Leeman-Castillo et al., 2010). For example, elderly Latinos were among a sample of 300 users of a computer kiosk–based heart disease behavioral management intervention—they initially were reluctant to enroll in the program, but once offered an "infomediary" (Baur & Deering, 2000)—that is, a person standing at the kiosk to assist them as needed—they became more comfortable and completed the program with few problems.

Table 3.2   Technology user trends by demographic characteristics

User Demographic	Trends
Youth	Almost universal gamers; heavy users of social networking sites; extremely high Internet access and use. Heavy cell phone users and frequently use text messaging. Much less likely to use e-mail for communication.
Elderly	Growing access to and use of the Internet—close to a quarter of those aged 65+ have Internet access. While they have mobile phones, little data available on use of text messaging.
Whites	Close to two thirds have access to Internet and most use e-mail. Medium to high cell phone use compared to other groups.
African Americans	Have among the highest rates of cell phone usage of any group. Growing access to the Internet, but usage still significantly lower than that of Whites.
Latinos	Have high cell phone usage and over half have Internet access, but significantly fewer use Internet compared to Whites.

Source: Fox, 2004; Fox & Livingston, 2007; Lenhart et al., 2008; Lenhart, Madden, Rankin Macgill, & Smith, 2007.

Developing Your Program Content: Some Examples

While a detailed description of how to write and create content for your program is beyond the scope of this book, we can offer some basic "how-tos" and references here. As mentioned above, the information technology and graphic design team members are indispensable—the high level of professionalism that has emerged with technology-based programs means users often expect to see state-of-the-art content. Rather than concentrate on offering tutorials here on how to create content, we simply identify some of the language and content elements, offer some brief examples, and then identify good resources for readers to consider when designing their programs.

Some excellent and easy-to-use resources for programming are included at the end of the chapter under "Additional Resources." HTML and XHTML are special text files that include "tags" or information on how information is to be sequenced and presented. The tags are indicators (using the < and > symbols) that inform placement of content and type of content. Figure 3.3 shows an example of the XHTML used to create the graphic shown in Figure 3.2.

XHTML is considered a newer version of HTML, and many are moving to adopt this language. Cascading Style Sheets (CSS) is a way to add style to your HTML in the form of different font, color, and graphics. It allows you to distinguish your content and make it appealing to your audience. Finally, Java programming is a computer programming language often used by web designers to program content.

Programming on the mobile phone requires familiarity with SMS, or short message service, a method to send short messages (up to 160 characters) using text from one mobile phone to another. Many telephones are SMS enabled, meaning users can simply write and send text to each other without any need to know or understand an SMS programming language. Text messages are sent from the sender to an SMS center, which routes the message to the receiver. They can also be sent from the Internet, using an Internet-based application within a web browser or using applications such as Skype, an Internet-based communication service allowing for no- or low-cost phone communication. Programmers will use applications to program delivery of SMS so that they do not have to send and resend messages individually but can "blast" messages to hundreds or thousands of people simultaneously. An application programming interface (API) is one tool that can be used to automate message delivery. This option also allows for users to customize messages with such features as a web link embedded into the text message, a specialized ringtone to alert the recipient that the message is coming from a specific source, black-and-white pictures, or a logo.

WHAT ARE EMERGING TRENDS IN TECHNOLOGY-BASED PROGRAM DEVELOPMENT?

Four important trends are emerging with respect to technology-based program development, and they sit at opposite ends of a spectrum. The first is the development of very brief and focused interventions that can take multiple forms and be included as one element in a larger program or serve as a stand-alone single dose. The second is the development of technology-based components that are designed to be integrated into a more intensive, comprehensive educational curriculum. The third is the development of blended technology programs that utilize multiple modalities within a single intervention (e.g., Internet and mobile phone within

Figure 3.3   Sample XHTML language for tailoring and personalizing feedback

```
1   <!DOCTYPE html PUBLIC "-//W3C//DTD XHTML 1.0 Transitional//EN"
2           "http://www.w3.org/TR/xhtml1/DTD/xhtml1-transitional.dtd">
3
4   <html>
5       <head>
6           <title>Luchar</title>
7           <meta http-equiv=Content-Type content="text/html; charset=utf-8">
8           <link href="/stylesheets/luchar.css?1165443186" media="screen" rel="Stylesheet" type='
9           <link href="/stylesheets/print.css?1163648091" media="print" rel="Stylesheet" type="te
10          <script src="/javascripts/prototype.js?1163113305" type="text/javascript"></script>
11          <script src="/javascripts/effects.js?1163113305" type="text/javascript"></script>
12          <script src="/javascripts/dragdrop.js?1163113305" type="text/javascript"></script>
13          <script src="/javascripts/controls.js?1163113305" type="text/javascript"></script>
14          <script src="/javascripts/protoplus.js?1163648286" type="text/javascript"></script>
15          <script src="/javascripts/application.js?1163648336" type="text/javascript"></script>
16      </head>
17      <body>
18          <div id="header">
19              <div id='indicator' style="float: right; margin-right: 20px; margin-top: 20px; displc
    #3058a0;">
20                  Loading...    <img alt="Indicator" src="/images/indicator.gif?1163]
21              </div>
22
23              <div id="progress" style="float: right; margin-right: 20px; margin-top: 20px; text-c
24                  <div id="graph"><div class="graphBar Blue"style="width: 30px"></div></div>
25              </div>
26
27          </div>
28          <div id="content" style="margin-left: 15px; margin-right: 15px;">
29              <h2 id="title">Physical Activity Recommendations: How You Compare</h2>
30
31
32
33              <div align="center" style="margin: 0px auto;">
34                  <object classid="clsid:D27CDB6E-AE6D-11cf-96B8-444553540000"
35                          codebase="https://download.macromedia.com/pub/shockwave/cabs/flash/swflash.
36                      WIDTH="710"
37                      HEIGHT="150"
38                      id="charts"
39                      ALIGN="">
40                      <PARAM NAME=movie VALUE="https://luchar.uchsc.edu/flash/charts.swf?library_path=|
    luchar.uchsc.edu/flash/charts_library&xml_source=https://luchar.uchsc.edu/flash/en/pc
41                      <PARAM NAME=quality VALUE=high>
42                      <PARAM NAME=bgcolor VALUE=#666666>
43                      <PARAM NAME=wmode VALUE=transparent>
44                      <param name="allowScriptAccess" value="always" />
45                      <EMBED src="https://luchar.uchsc.edu/flash/charts.swf?library_path=https://luchc
    charts_library&xml_source=https://luchar.uchsc.edu/flash/charts/en/pa/below.xml"
46                          quality=high
47                          bgcolor=#666666
48                          WIDTH="710"
49                          HEIGHT="150"
50                          NAME="charts"
51                          ALIGN=""
52                          wmode="transparent"
53                          TYPE="application/x-shockwave-flash"
54                              PLUGINSPAGE="http://www.macromedia.com/go/getflashplayer">
55                      </EMBED>
56                  </OBJECT>
57              </div>
58              <br/>
59              <br/>
60              <div class="operations">
61                  <form action="/page/next_page" method="post">
62                  <input name="commit" onclick="Element.show('indicator'); Element.hide('progress');" +
    value="Next  &gt;&gt;" />
63                  </form>
64              </div>
65
66          </div>
67      </body>
68  </html>
```

one program). The fourth is the use of technology to extend or expand existing clinical services, referred to as "hybrid" programming (e.g., using cell phones to remind people to take medications or having an "ask the expert" online forum available to all people engaged in a clinic-delivered behavioral intervention).

Very Brief, Focused, and Targeted Interventions

In considering some of the challenges we face with technology-based health promotion, we have discussed those of technological obsolescence, where we can develop a detailed intervention only to find that it is obsolete by the time we demonstrate its efficacy.

In response, some practitioners are developing interventions that are designed to be very brief, single-session interventions. A specific example is a 3-minute intervention designed for men who have sex with men at risk for hepatitis B (HBV). The intervention was designed to increase intentions to get an HBV vaccine. Researchers were able to show that a message delivered using a brief personal narrative online was more effective in increasing intentions to get vaccinated than messages delivered using statistics or messages using assertions that vaccination was important (deWit, 2009).

With increasing competition for our attention online, the notion of having a brief, focused intervention can have appeal.

"Blended" Programs That Utilize Multiple Technological Modalities Within One Program

While we have yet to see technology-based health interventions that test the use of multiple technologies incorporated into one intervention, it is possible to consider the development of programs that do just that. As mobile phones evolve technologically to incorporate access to the Internet, for example, one could easily imagine a program that could be delivered using text messages that incorporate links to the Internet, making it possible to go online as part of a health promotion program.

"Hybrid" Programs That Utilize Technology to Enhance or Extend Face-to-Face Programs

As mentioned in Chapter 1, the historical evolution of technology-based health promotion has been to develop and implement stand-alone programs, designed to be delivered in their entirety using technology. However, if one considers the ways that we have integrated technology into other facets of our life, this stand-alone approach could be considered shortsighted. Ultimately, we should consider ways to link technology to the myriad of efficacious and effective health promotion efforts that take place through traditional means. Technology could be used to offer reinforcement and to follow-up on in-person counseling sessions, for example. In this example, individuals attending a group counseling session could go online after the session to pursue questions they may have been reluctant to voice in a more private and confidential way with a counselor.

We have several good examples about how technology can be used to extend clinic services. Persons can receive reminders to take medications via mobile phone and text messaging; they could log on to a website and upload home blood pressure readings for a nurse to review; they could opt in to receive test results online or via text messaging. All these are examples of some simple interventions that can enhance and support clinical practice (Brennan, 1998; Brennan, Moore, & Smyth, 1991; C. Rietmeijer, personal communication, November 2007).

We envision hybrid programs that are much more integrated, using technology for skills-building exercises introduced in classroom settings, or using technology for social support among persons enrolled in a program. While stand-alone programs have some evidence they can be beneficial, hybrid programs also have substantial potential, and can contribute immensely to expanding reach of health promotion.

Use of Geographic Information Systems (GIS) in Program Planning

GIS has been used by epidemiologists to identify "hot spots" or geographic locations where there is greater concentration of disease or infection—for example, in relation to sexually transmitted infections (Potterat et al., 1999; Rothenberg et al., 2000).

With regard to program development, GIS has been used to identify locations within communities where there are structures, organizations, or businesses of interest. For example, as shown in Figure 3.4, the Medical Foundation and the Massachusetts Tobacco Control Program (MTCP) endeavored to ascertain the level of tobacco retailer compliance with regulations regarding advertising to minors. They used GIS to identify schools and nearby tobacco retailers, and then went to these areas to collect data using handheld devices and camera phones. They used GIS programs that could help with visual display of data. Figure 3.4 shows the result of the proximity of tobacco retailers to schools.

Figure 3.4   GIS base map with schools, buffers, and tobacco retailers

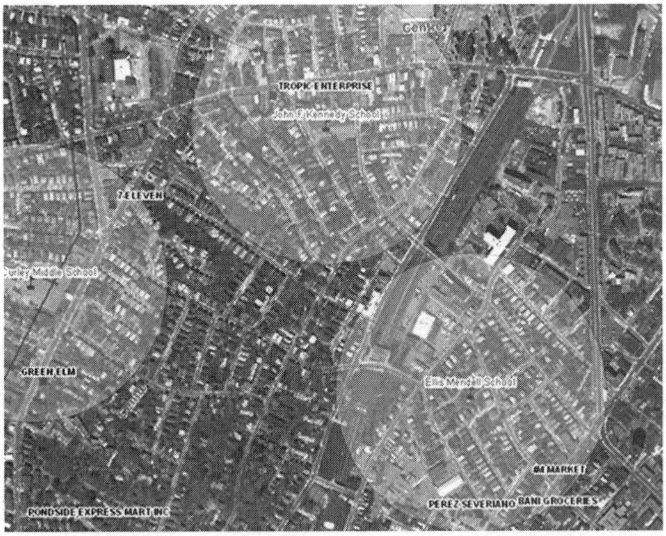

Source: http://gis.harvard.edu/icb/icb.do?keyword=k235&pageid=icb.page138032

SUMMARY

Program development for technology-based health interventions involves careful understanding of multiple elements. First, researchers need to be particularly careful in understanding the best technological modality to use in their program. We urge researchers to use what makes the most sense for the population they work with. It certainly isn't appropriate to use technology because it is convenient and attractive for the health promoter—it needs to be convenient and attractive for the audience. With substantial attention to health disparities, we face an opportunity to consider how to use these technologies to address health disparities. There is evidence that diverse audiences are using technologies such as the Internet, computers, and mobile phones—but consider what they use the most, whether they are already integrating technology into their lives, or if they need assistance in technology use before launching into a technology-based health promotion effort.

Remember how quickly technology changes and evolves, and be prepared to make your program flexible enough to adapt as these evolutions emerge. By using such approaches as modular programming you can make this process easier—swap out one program element when a newer, more attractive version emerges without having to rewrite the entire program.

Remember also that you are probably more familiar with and aware of your program than the naïve user. Just because you can navigate your program doesn't mean a participant can with the same ease and understanding. Use the beta testing and "talk aloud" processes here to ensure that the intended audience can use your program easily and finds it compelling.

When planning your program, do all you can to tap into existing resources to reach your target audience. Regardless of whether your program is on a computer kiosk, the Internet, or a mobile phone, you can identify members of organizations and workplaces who are potential program users to facilitate access to and use of your program. Working with professional or community- or computer-based organizations can give you access to large communities of people within your target audience to engage with as you plan and prepare your program.

Table 3.3 offers a summary of terms and definitions covered in this chapter.

Table 3.3   Key terms relevant for technology-based program development

Term	Definition
Alpha version	Usually the most preliminary version of a program. Serves to offer potential participants some concrete examples of program design and content, but doesn't have fully functioning components.
Beta version	An almost complete version of the program. Beta testing will generally occur to assist program planners in understanding how well the program works. Does it capture data from participants as intended? Can participants navigate the program easily? Do they understand the program content?

Term	Definition
Broadband capabilities	Broadband capabilities refer to the amount of data a participant can receive over time. The greater the broadband speed, the easier it will be for participants to load complex graphics, video, and audio. In resource-poor settings, it is critical to pay attention to the broadband capabilities of your audience, since a program with complex graphics that take a long time to load may mean users may not be able to access program content.
Hypertext and extensible hypertext markup language (HTML and XHTML)	Programming languages used to develop content on the Internet that use special text files with "tags" or information on how information is to be sequenced and presented.
Infomediary	The name given to an individual who can help users connect with a program. In the event that someone is not familiar with how to use a technology, this person can coach and assist program users. Infomediaries can offer encouragement, support, and troubleshooting to increase access and confidence among users.
Java	A computer programming language often used to develop Internet content.
Modular programming	The process of creating program content in chapters or modules. This allows for easy updating of outdated content when only a section of the program needs changing and other elements can remain the same.
Ruby on Rails (RoR)	RoR allows for compartmentalizing programming language so programmers can reutilize code for all conventional aspects of a program and to develop new code for customization or for new program elements.
SMS	Short message service, the technical name for text messages on a mobile phone.
User trends	The current practices of different demographic groups with regard to technology use. For example, user trends have shown the greatest use of cell phone minutes is among youth, social networking applications are gaining in popularity on the Internet, and so forth.

? CONCLUDING QUESTIONS

The following questions can assist you in thinking about how to utilize best practices in program development.

1. Who is the audience you wish to serve through your work? Is this the most appropriate audience given what you know about health disparities?

2. What technology or technologies is your audience using? Computers? The Internet? Mobile phones? What do you know about the digital divide and access to these modalities? Is your chosen technology the most appropriate given use patterns and health disparities? Is a technology-based intervention even appropriate given what you know about use patterns?

3. How will you involve your target audience in program design and testing? What instruments will you use?

4. What technology experts are you engaging to develop your program content?

5. How will you monitor changes in and trends for technology and use of technology within your target audience? How will you adapt your program when these changes occur?

 CHAPTER EXERCISE

Imagine you are the head of a community-based agency in a resource-poor community. The most recent data from the health department show rising incidence of tuberculosis (TB). Problems that members of your community face include TB and diabetes. Many of the population do not speak English, or it isn't their primary language. Many are elderly and have little to no experience with technology.

Your organization is concerned because the health department doesn't have adequate resources to conduct directly observed therapy for adherence to TB medications among persons diagnosed with the disease. You think technology might offer some potential to bridge this gap.

1. From what you read in this chapter, what do you think might be appropriate modalities to use with this population? Why?

2. What types of interventions would you consider using to increase compliance with medication regimes?

3. What challenges do you anticipate?

4. How will you partner with the health department?

5. Design a brief focus group topic guide to gather preliminary program ideas from your target audience about what you might do.

 ADDITIONAL RESOURCES

The following are Internet-based resources for technology-based programming and for obtaining up-to-date details on technology users:

Resource	Description
Barksdale, K., & Turner, E. S. (1999). *HTML & JavaScript programming concepts.* Florence, KY: Course Technology.	This book will give the reader an orientation to webpage design using the Java language.
Castro, E. (2006). *HTML, XHTML, and CSS: Visual quickstart guide.* Berkeley, CA: Peachpit Press.	This book will give the reader an orientation to webpage design using HTML, XHTML, and CSS languages.
Duckett, J. (2008). Beginning *web* programming with HTML, XHTML, and CSS. Indianapolis, IN: Wrox, an imprint of Wiley.	This book will give the reader an orientation to webpage design using XHTML and CSS languages.

Websites

Resource	Description
http://www.cs.cf.ac.uk/Dave/PERL/node250.html	Internet page; basic HTML programming
http://www.w3.org/2002/03/tutorials	Internet page; contains over 20 tutorials, on HTML and CSS; also contains slides and links to other tutorials
http://www.corewebprogramming.com/	Internet page and links to a PDF version of a book on web programming
http://www.smscountry.com/productdetails.asp	Internet page; contains information on SMS and API
http://www.pewinternet.org/	The Pew Internet & American Life Project explores the impact of the Internet on children, families, communities, the workplace, schools, health care, and civic/political life.
http://www.info4cellphones.com/cell-phone-trend.html	Offers product endorsements and descriptions for phones and some data on users
http://www.infoworld.com	InfoWorld analysts and editors provide both hands-on analysis and evaluation, as well as expert commentary on issues surrounding emerging technologies
http://www.marketresearch.com/	Market Research has a "technology and media" page offering up-to-date information on trends in technologies, new applications, and user trends

Note: All websites noted here are hot-linked at www.sagepub.com/bull; at this site you will also find newer resources relevant to the material in this and other chapters.

REFERENCES

Bandura, A. (1986). *Social foundations of thought and action*. Englewood Cliffs, NJ: Prentice Hall.

Barrera, M., Jr., Glasgow, R. E., McKay, H. G., Boles, S. M., & Feil, E. G. (2002). Do Internet-based support interventions change perceptions of social support? An experimental trial of approaches for supporting diabetes self management. *American Journal of Community Psychology, 30*(5), 637–654.

Baur, C., & Deering, M. J. (2000). *Proposed frameworks to improve the quality of health web sites: Review.* Retrieved from http://www.medscape.com/ viewarticle/418842

Benotsch, E. G., Kalichman, S., & Weinhardt, L. S. (2004). HIV-AIDS patients' evaluation of health information on the Internet: The digital divide and vulnerability to fraudulent claims. *Journal of Consulting and Clinical Psychology, 72*, 1004–1011.

Bernhardt, J. M. (2000). Health education and the digital divide: Building bridges and filling chasms. *Health Education Research, 15*, 527–531.

Bowen, A., Horvath, K., & Williams, M. (2007). A randomized controlled trial of Internet-delivered HIV prevention targeting rural MSM. *Health Education Research, 22*, 120–127.

Brennan, P. F. (1998). Computer network home care demonstration: A randomized trial in persons living with AIDS. *Computers in Biology and Medicine, 28*, 489–508.

Brennan, P. F., Moore, S. M., & Smyth, K. A. (1991). ComputerLink: Electronic support for the home caregiver. *Advances in Nursing Science, 13*, 14–27.

Bull, S. (2003). *The process of sex partner seeking online among men who have sex with men and related sexually transmitted disease risk.* Presentation to the 2003 STD/HIV Prevention and The Internet Conference: National Coalition of STD Directors and Centers for Disease Control and Prevention.

Bull, S. S., Lloyd, L., Rietmeijer, C., & McFarlane, M. (2004). Recruitment and retention of an online sample for an HIV prevention intervention targeting men who have sex with men: The Smart Sex Quest Project. *AIDS Care, 16*, 931–943.

Bull, S., McFarlane, M., Phibbs, S., & Watson, S. (2007). What do young adults expect when they go online? Lessons for development of an STD/HIV and pregnancy prevention website. *Journal of Medical Internet Systems, 31*(2), 149–158.

Bull, S., Pratte, K., Whitesell, N., Reitmeijer, C., & McFarlane, M. (2009). Effects of an Internet-based intervention for HIV prevention: The Youthnet trials. *AIDS and Behavior, 13*(3), 474–487.

Campbell, M. K., DeVellis, B. M., Strecher, V. J., Ammerman, A. S., DeVellis, R. F., & Sandler, R. S. (1994). Improving dietary behavior: The effectiveness of tailored messages in primary care settings. *American Journal of Public Health, 84*, 783–787.

Centers for Disease Control and Prevention. (2006). *Racial/ethnic disparities in diagnoses of HIV/AIDS—33 states, 2001–2004* [Rep. No. 55(05)]. Atlanta, GA: Author.

Centers for Disease Control and Prevention. (2010, April 5). *Reducing health disparities in cancer.* Division of Cancer Prevention and Control, National Center for Chronic Disease Prevention and Health Promotion. Retrieved from http://www.cdc.gov/cancer/ healthdisparities/ basic_info/disparities.htm

Chang, B. L., Bakken, S., Brown, S. S., Houston, T. K., Kreps, G. L., Kukafka, R., et al. (2004). Bridging the digital divide: Reaching vulnerable populations. *Journal of the American Medical Informatics Association, 11*, 448–457.

Committee on Understanding and Eliminating Racial and Ethnic Disparities in Health Care, B. o. H. S. P. I. o. M. (2003). *Unequal treatment: Confronting racial and ethnic disparities in health care*. Washington, DC: National Academy Press.

Cooper, R., Cutler, J., Desvigne-Nickens, P., Fortmann, S. P., Friedman, L., Havlik, R., et al. (2000). Trends and disparities in coronary heart disease, stroke, and other cardiovascular diseases in the United States: Findings of the national conference on cardiovascular disease prevention. *Circulation, 102*(25), 3137–3147.

Cubbin, C., Braveman, P. A., Marchi, K. S., Chavez, G. F., Santelli, J. S., & Gilbert, B. J. (2002). Socioeconomic and racial/ethnic disparities in unintended pregnancy among postpartum women in California. *Maternal and Child Health Journal, 6*, 237–246.

deWit, J. (2009). *Intentions to increase HBV vaccination through computer mediated intervention*. Presented to the AIDS Impact Conference, Gaborone, Botswana.

Fox, S. (2004). *Older Americans and the Internet*. Pew Internet & American Life Project. Retrieved from http://www.pewinternet.org/PPF/r/117/ report_display.asp

Fox, S., & Livingston, G. (2007). *Latinos online: Hispanics with lower levels of education and English proficiency remain largely disconnected from the Internet*. Pew Internet & American Life Project. Retrieved from http://eric.ed.gov/ERICDocs/data/content_ storage_01/0000019b/80/28/ 06/54.pdf

Glasgow, R. E., Boles, S. M., McKay, H. G., Feil, E. G., & Barrera, M. (2003). The D-Net diabetes self-management program: Long-term implementation, outcomes, and generalization results. *Preventive Medicine, 36*, 410–419.

Gottlieb, S. (2000). Study explores Internet as a tool for care of diabetic patients. *Western Journal of Medicine, 173*, 8–9.

Halkitis, P. N., & Parsons, J. T. (2003). Intentional unsafe sex (barebacking) among HIV-positive gay men who seek sexual partners on the Internet. *AIDS Care, 15*, 367–378.

Jackson, L. A., Zhao, Y., Kolenic, A. , Fitzgerald, H. E., Harold, R., & Von Eye, A. (2008). Race, gender, and information technology use: The new digital divide. *Cyberpsychology & Behavior, 11*, 437–442.

James, S. A. (2003). Confronting the moral economy of US racial/ethnic health disparities. *American Journal of Public Health, 93*, 189.

Kim, S. I., & Kim, H. S. (2008). Effectiveness of mobile and Internet intervention in patients with obese type 2 diabetes. *International Journal of Medical Informatics, 77*, 399–404.

Kreuter, M. W., & Strecher, V. J. (1996). Do tailored behavior change messages enhance the effectiveness of health risk appraisal? Results from a randomized trial. *Health Education Research, 11*, 97–105.

Latino Issues Forum. (2004). *Latinos, computers and the Internet: How Congress and the current administration's framing of the digital divide has negatively impacted policy initiative established to close the significant technology gap that remains*. Retrieved from http://www.lif.org/download/ digitaldivbrief.pdf

Leeman-Castillo, B., Beaty, B., Raghunath, S., Steiner, J., & Bull, S. (2010). LUCHAR: Using computer technology to battle heart disease among Latinos. *American Journal of Public Health, 100*(2), 272–275.

Lenhart, A., & Horrigan, J. B. (2003). Re-visualizing the Digital Divide as a Digital Spectrum. *IT & Society, 1*, 23–39.

Lenhart, A., Kahne, J., Middaugh, E., Rankin Macgill, A., Evans, C., & Vitak, J. (2008). *Teens video gaming and civics: Teens' gaming experiences are diverse and include significant social interaction and civic engagement*. Washington, DC: Pew Internet & American Life Project.

Lenhart, A., Madden, M., Rankin Macgill, A., & Smith, A. (2007). *Teens and social media: The use of social media gains a greater foothold in teen life as they embrace the conversational nature of interactive online media*. Washington, DC: Pew Internet & American Life Project. Retrieved from http://www.pewinternet.org/pdfs/PIP_Teens_Social_Media_Final.pdf

Lorence, D. P., Park, H., & Fox, S. (2006). Racial disparities in health information access: Resilience of the Digital Divide. *Journal of Medical Internet Systems, 30*, 241–249.

McGruder, H. F., Malarcher, A. M., Antoine, T. L., Greenlund, K. J., & Croft, J. B. (2004). Racial and ethnic disparities in cardiovascular risk factors among stroke survivors: United States 1999 to 2001. *Stroke, 35*, 1557–1561.

Myint-U, A., Bull, S., Greenwood, G., Patterson, J., Rietmeijer, C., Vrungos, S., et al. (2008). Safe in the City—Developing an effective, video-based intervention for STD clinic waiting rooms. *Health Promotion Practice, 11*, 408.

National Center for Health Statistics. (2009, April 2). *Fast stats*. Centers for Disease Control and Prevention. Retrieved from http://www.cdc.gov/nchs/ fastats/default.htm#H

Potterat, J. J., Zimmerman-Rogers, H., Muth, S. Q., Rothenberg, R. B., Green, D. L., Taylor, J. E., et al. (1999). Chlamydia transmission: Concurrency, reproduction number, and the epidemic trajectory. *American Journal of Epidemiology, 150*, 1331–1339.

Rhodes, S. D. (2004). Hookups or health promotion? An exploratory study of a chat room-based HIV prevention intervention for men who have sex with men. *AIDS Education and Prevention, 16*, 315–327.

Rhodes, S. D., Diclemente, R. J., Cecil, H., Hergenrather, K. C., & Yee, L. J. (2002). Risk among men who have sex with men in the United States: A comparison of an Internet sample and a conventional outreach sample. *AIDS Education and Prevention, 14*, 41–50.

Rogers, E. M. (1995). *Diffusion of innovations theory.* New York: Free Press.

Rogers, E. M. (2003). *Diffusion of innovations.* New York: Free Press.

Ross, M. W., Rosser, B. R., & Stanton, J. (2004). Beliefs about cybersex and Internet-mediated sex of Latino men who have Internet sex with men: Relationships with sexual practices in cybersex and in real life. *AIDS Care, 16*, 1002–1011.

Ross, M. W., Tikkanen, R., & Mansson, S. (2000). Difference between Internet samples and conventional samples of men who have sex with men: Implications for research and HIV interventions. *Social Science and Medicine, 51*, 749–758.

Rothenberg, R. B., Long, D. M., Sterk, C. E., Pach, A., Potterat, J. J., Muth, S. Q., et al. (2000). The Atlanta Urban Networks Study: A blueprint for endemic transmission. *AIDS, 14*, 2191–2200.

SAS Institute. (n.d.). *About SAS.* Retrieved from http://www.sas.com/

Strauss, A., & Corbin, J. (1990). *Basics of qualitative research: Grounded theory procedures and techniques.* Newbury Park, CA: Sage.

Strecher, V. J. (1999). Computer-tailored smoking cessation materials: A review and discussion. *Patient Education and Counseling, 36*, 107–117.

Strecher, V. J., Shiffman, S., & West, R. (2005). Randomized controlled trial of a web-based computer-tailored smoking cessation program as a supplement to nicotine patch therapy. *Addiction, 100*, 682–688.

U.S. Department of Commerce & National Telecommunications and Information Administration. (1999). *Falling through the Net: Defining the Digital Divide* [Rep. No. July]. U.S. Department of Health and Human Services. (2000). *Healthy people 2010* (Vol. 2, 2nd ed.). Washington, DC: Office of Disease Prevention and Health Promotion.

4 ∷

Technology-Based Program Implementation

CHAPTER OVERVIEW

In this chapter, we discuss specific techniques used for *implementation* of technology-based health interventions. After reading Chapter 3, you will have chosen a technological modality, considered the audience you wish to reach, and made plans to engage with members of that audience to obtain feedback on your program design ideas. You will have considered how to tailor your program using algorithms and how to use specific programming language.

We now turn our attention to the issues that you will face in the day-to-day delivery of a technology-based program. We first consider the unique aspects of technology-based program implementation that are beneficial—that is, the ability to recruit very large numbers of people to programs, the ability to standardize content, and the ability to readily adapt program content for use in different settings. We consider the challenges we face with program implementation, which are often the same as the benefits; we still face challenges in recruiting, enrolling, engaging, and retaining the right people in programs. We also have inevitable challenges when our technologies fail. We look at best practices in program implementation, including the use of (a) an "infomediary," a person who can motivate enrollment in a kiosk, computer-based, or mobile phone program; (b) strategies to enhance banner advertising online; (c) chat room-based recruitment to diversify and appropriately sample; and (d) respondent-driven sampling online. As with other chapters, we close with a list of additional resources for program implementation, along with questions and exercises to assist your own efforts in this area.

WHAT ARE UNIQUE AND BENEFICIAL CONSIDERATIONS FOR TECHNOLOGY-BASED PROGRAM IMPLEMENTATION?

Recruitment of Large Numbers of Program Participants

One of the largest benefits of technology-based health promotion is that your program can be delivered to large numbers of people who may otherwise not be exposed to it. In a traditional program, you are limited to the physical locations where you have staff and brick-and-mortar buildings or physical community settings (e.g., if you deliver your program as an outdoor theater, you will likely not use a building). By making your program available through technologies such as the Internet and/or mobile phones and portable devices, you can greatly extend the reach. We discuss best current practices in reaching large numbers of people and challenges to doing so below.

Delivery of Standardized Content

A second important benefit to be realized through technology-based health promotion is the standardization of content. Often our traditional programs are as good as the staff delivering them. Many are fortunate to have gifted staff members with the ability to connect emotionally with their clients and the ability to motivate behavior change. However, once a program expands to reach more people and new staff members are hired, those qualities may not always be present in each one; or, if a staff member retires or resigns and needs to be replaced, it isn't always possible to find someone with enough similar qualities to make the program delivery consistent. This consideration is particularly important when we think about "scaling up" of programs for maximum effect and greater impact. As we have discussed in earlier chapters, if a program has efficacy, in order to create greater impact it should be delivered and disseminated on a larger scale. Technology offers the opportunity to scale up without fear of losing fidelity to the original approaches for program implementation.

With technology-based content, you have the assurance that the content can be implemented the same way whether it is delivered 10, 100, or 1,000 times.

Ease of Adoption for Implementation in Diverse Settings

Related to the issue of standardization of program content for fidelity of delivery is the notion that content can be adopted easily when appropriate to reach diverse audiences. Health promoters are well aware of the need to make adaptations to materials to make them more culturally relevant and appealing across groups. Changes in language, spokespersons, exercises, and other program elements may be required in order to achieve this. By using the modular programming concept and the Ruby on Rails programming discussed in Chapter 3, making these changes is potentially simpler than redesigning an entire program. Program planners can review modules and revise a single module or multiple modules as appropriate, perhaps without having to redesign the entire program.

WHAT ARE CHALLENGES WE FACE WITH TECHNOLOGY-BASED PROGRAM IMPLEMENTATION?

Sampling and Generalizability of Samples Recruited in Virtual Settings

While recruitment of large numbers of people to participate in programs is a key advantage of using technology for health promotion, on balance it is most critical to consider whom you are reaching with your programs, and whether these participants are those most in need of the program. This challenge is not unique to technology-based health promotion—indeed, traditional programs constantly face the challenge of getting persons at highest risk for a given condition enrolled in prevention or self-management programs.

It is important to note, however, that there may be a type of seduction in seeing large numbers of people enrolled in a program and a tendency to assume that because there are many people they are the most appropriate persons engaged with your program.

Fundamentally, if we reach large numbers of people with our technology-based programs but these people are not at substantial risk or will not benefit from the program, then we will have no hope of realizing the potential of technology to affect the impact of health promotion programs.

Currently, work in the field of technology-based health promotion is at a crucial juncture. We have examples of excellence and best practices for program development to address diabetes, heart disease, smoking, substance use, and HIV prevention. These programs all have demonstrated capacity in reaching more people than they otherwise may have in a traditional health promotion program. However, recruitment, enrollment, and retention of persons at highest risk for morbidity and mortality using a technology-based program have not been achieved consistently. In some instances, we have seen participants enrolled in technology-based programs who have relatively low risk.

Management of Large Numbers of Participants Enrolling Simultaneously

The potential downside with being able to reach and enroll large numbers of participants in health promotion programs is the challenge in managing them once they engage with the program. If you have a program that requires multiple communications with and interactions with participants by staff, then you will have to either plan for additional staff or establish automated systems to track interactions or both. For example, consider if you have a program that offers rewards or incentives for completing each module or program segment. If you have thousands of people enrolled, it may be important to automate a process that can track when each person has completed a module or segment. This way, each time individuals complete a segment, their name or program ID would be automatically entered into a database that could be checked daily. Then staff would check the database and send out incentives to everyone in it on a predetermined periodic basis.

Retention of Program Participants

The management of large numbers of program participants is critical to achieving adequate retention in programs. If people drop out before the program ends, it is likely to reduce program efficacy. Some recent publications outline some best practices in retention of health promotion program participants engaged in programs delivered through the Internet (Abdolrasulnia et al., 2004; Chiasson et al., 2006; Hatfield et al., 2009; Pequegnat et al., 2007). These are outlined in the section titled "Care and Support of Participants During Program Implementation."

WHAT ARE THE CURRENT AND BEST PRACTICES IN TECHNOLOGY-BASED PROGRAM IMPLEMENTATION?

Use of an Infomediary to Orient Potential Program Participants

The "infomediary" is a person designated to assist participants in technology-based programs to get oriented with the equipment, technical program aspects, and program elements, and can be designated to do so in face-to-face or virtual settings. In the face-to-face environment, intermediaries offer a useful connection to the kiosk, desktop, or laptop computer program, especially for the technology novice. In face-to-face encounters, infomediaries can invite people to consider enrolling in a computer kiosk or computerized health promotion program and can guide them through the enrollment process. They can troubleshoot enrollment by helping resolve technical issues such as difficulty in logging on, Internet connection issues, or issues with a monitor, printer, or mouse. They can answer questions posed by potential participants, and give them detailed information about what the program is about, how long it will take, and what benefits can be gained through enrollment.

Program planners may consider using a face-to-face infomediary for programs where they plan to enroll novice users or users with limited experience in technology. Planners for the LUCHAR (Latinos Using Cardio Health Action to Reduce Risk) program, a kiosk-based healthy lifestyle promotion program targeting Latinos in community settings, learned in the process of their program development that although the computerized elements of the program were attractive and culturally relevant for Latinos, there needed to be a live person at the kiosk to encourage them to use the program. Feedback planners suggested that members of the target audience would not approach a kiosk or computer on their own, even in a trusted community setting such as a church or social service agency, because they felt the need for invitation, permission, and encouragement to engage with the program (Padilla et al., 2010). Data showing that Latinos lagged behind other technology adopters suggested they may need more hands-on training to feel comfortable navigating the program (Fox & Livingston, 2007).

As a health promotion program planner, you may hear the argument that members of your intended audience are so technically naïve that they will not approach a computer kiosk on their own and that using technology is therefore not appropriate. Consider, however, that your technology-based program could be one element in a larger program, or could be an effort in and of itself to increase technology capacity within your target audience. Just because users are naïve to technology doesn't mean we should perpetuate a digital divide by limiting exposure to it—one could argue that it is only by making technology available and familiar that we can reduce disparities in access.

Certainly a disadvantage of using an infomediary is that it can increase program cost and potentially reduce program reach. If you need to train and pay an individual to assist participants in accessing your program, there will certainly be an added cost, and you are limited to being able to reach people only when the infomediary is on hand. On balance, however, you should consider the potential for added benefit if having this person will make the difference in whether individuals choose to enroll or not. Figure 4.1 offers a decision aid in making the choice to use an infomediary, and Text Box 4.1 outlines the key skills and competencies this person will need.

If you are confident your program can be attractive and appealing without an individual to promote it and recruit participation, it is certainly possible to forego the use of an infomediary for your program. Readers are probably all aware of examples of passively delivered technology-based content or examples of content delivered through programs that can be self-initiated. One example, although not necessarily related to health, is messages received at the gas pump through LCD screens. A program connected to injury prevention in Minnesota used LCD screens at gas pumps to promote a "Click It or Ticket" seat belt campaign (Governors Safety Highway Association, 2010).

TEXT BOX 4.1
Skills and competencies needed for an infomediary

Ability to engage and motivate participation. Depending on the target audience you wish to engage, consider recruiting staff members who

- are bilingual or multilingual to communicate effectively with diverse participants;
- have experience working with this audience;
- have training specific to the cultural considerations related to working with this audience; and
- have an engaging and outgoing personality.

Strong technical skills. Your infomediary may need to troubleshoot technical difficulties on-site. Look for or offer training to staff members so they

- are competent with all the program equipment;
- can easily reboot, clear paper jams, and navigate to different parts of the program;
- can address Internet connection issues and reestablish connections easily; and
- can configure equipment as needed to deliver the program.

Figure 4.1   Decision-making aid to use infomediary

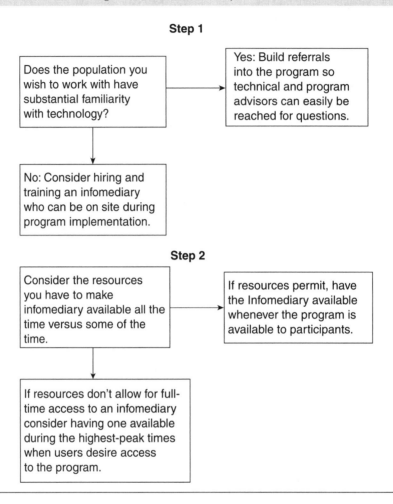

This is perhaps the simplest, easiest way to engage people in a technology-based health promotion endeavor; reach them passively with a relevant message at a time when they are captive such as at the gas pump or waiting for cash at the ATM.

When the program is not passively delivered but requires the individual to engage with a computer kiosk or desktop, it may be more challenging to motivate members of your audience, because they may not have the time or inclination to approach the device, they may not have confidence in ease of use, or they may simply not be aware that the device is available and open for use. A group of primary care doctors and cardiologists in Denver, Colorado, developed a computer-based kiosk program for users to quickly assess their risk for heart disease using an algorithm based on the Framingham risk assessment (Koenig, Löwel, Baumert, & Meisinger, 2004). Users complete a short assessment and get instant feedback on their risk for heart disease over time (Colorado Prevention Center, n.d.). Program implementers have learned that the kiosk is utilized more readily at health fairs, where it can be part of a booth where people are accessing information and other health-related services; placing the kiosk in community settings without an infomediary reduced use, primarily because people didn't know what the kiosk was for and/or didn't think they had time to use it.

Recruiting the Most Appropriate Audience to Maximize Program Reach

Banner Advertising

Health promoters have successfully used banner advertisements to recruit large numbers of participants for technology-based health promotion in a short time frame. The primary advantages of using banner advertising are reach—you can expose thousands to an ad—and time—you can enroll very large numbers of people in your program in a very short period of time. Blas et al. (2007) recruited over 700 men into their online HIV prevention program in a short time; Bull, Vallejos, and Ortiz (2008) recruited and enrolled over 3,000 people in 2 months for an online HIV prevention program; Ross, Rosser, and Stanton (2004) recruited over 1,000 men for an Internet HIV prevention initiative.

We have learned from these researchers and other literature that there are key strategies to developing and delivering good banner advertisements to recruit participants in your technology-based health promotion program. First, as mentioned in Chapter 3, be sure to engage your target audience in the development of these and other types of recruitment materials. Banner advertisements need to be large enough to attract people, and should be colorful but not too busy or wordy. Research on the factors that influence people to click on a banner advertisement shows that when users perceive synergy between the website and the ad they are more likely to click on it; they are also more likely to click on ads they find personally relevant, so it is critical to understand what might motivate your target audience (Cho & LaRose, 1999). Consider choosing an Internet service provider (ISP) or website that has a large number of subscribers from your target audience or one that specifically targets your audience—for example, MTV targets young people; BET.com (Black Entertainment Television) targets African Americans; Gay.com targets the gay, lesbian, bisexual, and transgendered community. Banner advertisers have the option to geotarget their ads—meaning deliver them to audiences in specific geographic areas—and optimize the "run of service" for days of the week and times of the day when the most people will be exposed to them.

Figure 4.2 shows banner ads developed for the Youthnet program, an Internet-based HIV prevention program for youth. These ads resulted in enrollment of more than 3,000 people in the Youthnet program in one month (Bull, Vallejos, & Ortiz, 2008). Note that the ads contain pictures and colors, information about the University of Colorado where the program was housed, and a logo, which offered credibility by linking the ad to a respected institution. Table 4.1 offers some key considerations for persons developing a banner advertising campaign when enrolling participants in their program online.

While banner advertising is indeed effective in reaching many more people in a short time than could be reached using face-to-face recruitment methods, a significant caution regarding the use of banner ads is warranted. Evidence shows that only a very small proportion—ranging

Figure 4.2   Examples of banner advertisements

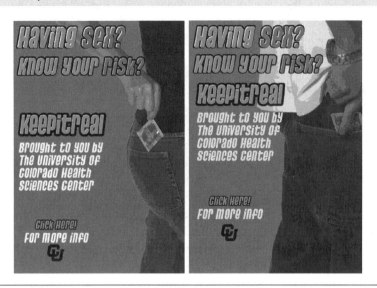

Table 4.1   Considerations for developing banner advertisements

Consideration	*How-tos*
Banner design elements	• Engage members of your target audience in developing ad content. • Use a logo if available for enhanced credibility. • Include a link to your site if possible. • Use large font and minimal text. • Use pictures and flash if possible.
Banner size and shape	• Talk with your ISP regarding the size and shape of ads that generate the highest click-through rate—that is, the number of people seeing the ad who click on it.
Choosing your ISP (Internet service provider)	• Consider who the ISP serves. • Is an adequate proportion of the ISP's subscribers people from your target audience? • Are there other ISPs or sites that serve more of the population you wish to reach?
Cost of ads	• Some ISPs are willing to run ads that are relevant to health for free or reduced cost. • Be sure to negotiate with the company to see if this is possible.
Geotargeting	• Check with your ISP to see if it has the capability to geotarget (i.e., run ads only in certain geographic areas) and consider if this will offer you any advantage in reaching your audience.
Run of service	• Check with your ISP to learn whether you can run ads during the highest use times among subscribers.

from 0.01% to 0.06%—of people exposed to banner advertisements actually click on the advertisement, and only a proportion of those clicking on the ad will be eligible for a program, enroll, and complete it. The Youthnet study, whose banner advertisement is shown in Figure 4.2, offers a case in point. For a month in late 2005 banner advertisements were purchased on BlackPlanet.com and MiGente.com, two different sites on the Internet. Banners were posted a total of 1,780,000 times (each posting is called an "impression"), and 1,158 persons from BlackPlanet.com and MiGente.com clicked on the banner ad (this is called "clicking through"). Thus, the "click through" rate was .06%. An additional 1,778,503 banner advertisement impressions were made on Yahoo!, and a total of 8,196 persons from Yahoo! clicked on the ad (.46%). While this did yield a very high number of enrollees in the program (more than 3,000), Youthnet cannot be said to have enrolled a group representative of 18- to 24-year-olds in the program.

With the millions of people on the Internet, engagement of fewer than 1% of persons exposed to an advertisement may still result in high numbers of program participants—indeed, recruitment for any program using more traditional media recruitment methods may face the same challenges in ensuring that a high proportion of those exposed will enroll in a program.

Ways to facilitate better click-through rates include the following:

- Placement of the banner ad on a website where your target audience can be found
- Placement of ads at times of day and during days of the week when your target audience is more likely to be online
- Placement of an ad on a specific part of the site where a user may be expecting more advertisements or may be more willing to engage (Cho & LaRose, 1999)

Program planners need to be aware, however, as mentioned above, that enrollees recruited through banner advertisements are not representative of those in their target audience. If program planners seek to enroll large numbers in their program without regard to representation, then banner advertisements do hold promise and potential. However, when it is important to pay attention to representation and generalizability, banner advertisements may not be an adequate approach. As mentioned in Chapter 2, the issues of beneficence and equity should be considered when planning for recruitment. If your program seeks to engage persons at high risk for the health condition of interest or persons overrepresented among those with a health disparity, then a "take all comers" approach offered through banner advertising may not be appropriate. Health researchers have raised the concern that we shouldn't be recruiting individuals for technology-based health promotion in large numbers just because we can (Pequegnat et al., 2007). If we can only enroll people who have Internet access and high-speed connections, we may be addressing our programs to users who do not have the risk for a condition that would warrant a substantial outlay of resources for Internet-based program delivery.

Chat Room Recruitment

There are several examples of using chat rooms on the Internet as a way to connect with people to facilitate enrollment in technology-based health promotion. Connecting with individuals in chat rooms could be considered analogous to meeting them face-to-face when doing so isn't possible. Many ISPs and websites have chat rooms, where multiple users can hold a public or semipublic conversation. To chat, ISPs or websites often require users to create a profile, where they offer information about themselves that others can access. Chatters may also be subject to the terms of service (TOS) on a site, which can limit the types of language or activities occurring in chat rooms. For example, chatters may be expected to avoid solicitation of others for commercial purposes (e.g., to buy a car or go to a website selling a product); they may be expected to avoid using inflammatory or derogatory language. Chat rooms are often moderated by individuals employed by the ISP or website to ensure adherence to these TOS, or chatters themselves can self-monitor and send a complaint to a webmaster for persons they perceive as violators of the TOS.

There are several examples from the HIV prevention literature where outreach workers have developed profiles on a chat room housed on a gay-friendly or gay-oriented site, and then participate in chat in their outreach capacity either to offer instant educational messages to other chatters or to refer chatters to services. Howard Brown Health Center in Chicago, Illinois, conducts outreach in venues such as Manhunt.net, Gay.com, and AOL chat rooms. In Houston, Texas, Montrose Clinic staff conducts online outreach as part of Project CORE (Cyber OutReach Education). A handbook and protocols have been developed for online recruitment and interventions (McFarlane, Kachur, Klausner, Roland, & Cohen, 2005). The handbook contains material contributed by other sites and is a valuable resource for the project staff.

Another form of online outreach is "auditorium"-style chat, where there is a moderator who can set up a date and time for people to come into a chat room and pose questions. This is a program-driven rather than user-driven mechanism, but can be an effective way to recruit people for online health education. It was used by the San Francisco (California) Department of Public Health (SFDPH) and Internet Sexuality Information Services (ISIS), who collaborated to establish seven auditorium-style chats with online visitors to Gay.com. They recruited for the auditorium chats in the Gay.com chat rooms by letting chatters know there would be an "expert" on the site and named the date and time when users could log on to participate. The sessions were real-time, 1-hour interactions facilitated by a physician from SFDPH. Online chatters entered questions that were then selected by a moderator for expert response. The moderator posted the question, and the expert then posted an answer as quickly as possible.

In Florida, United Foundation for AIDS (UFA) actively conducts Internet-based outreach to men who have sex with men using a specific topical chat room. Thus, rather than being a user-created chat room or an auditorium-style "meet the expert" organized chat, the topical chat room is designed to focus on a specific topic all the time. UFA has used this approach to communicate with users of crystal methamphetamine ("crystal meth"). The Crystal Alert program is a chat room–based educational program with 25 to 30 attendees on the site daily.

When using chat rooms for recruitment, program planners may consider using this mechanism to recruit for a program that is to be delivered offline (e.g., recruitment in chat rooms to encourage people to get tested for syphilis at their local health department) or for programs that are intended for online delivery (e.g., the Crystal Alert program). Figure 4.3 offers an example of a chat room profile from the Chicago-based Howard Brown Health

Figure 4.3 Screenshot of a chat room profile

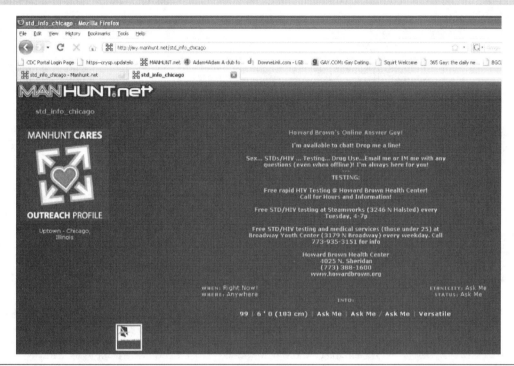

Center, which uses chat room outreach to increase access to its clinical services. Regardless of the type of program delivery you plan, there are some important considerations for recruiting participants using chat rooms. They include profile development and presence online, training of recruiters, timing of recruitment, and management of complaints or TOS violations. Table 4.2 offers more detail about each of these.

Chat room-based program recruitment has the advantages of being able to connect directly with your target audience for a program—similar to an infomediary, you can help potential users become aware of and access your program content, be it online or offline. This type of recruitment for programs has the disadvantage, however, of limiting reach to populations. As with computer kiosk, desktop, handheld, and mobile phone programs, the chat room program is limited only to those you can reach in rooms. An exception would be if you were to use banner advertising in chat rooms—which may yield a larger number of participants, but has the disadvantage of not being able to recruit a representative group from your population to participate in your program. One approach to facilitate better sampling of populations—particularly those who might be at higher risk or harder to reach online—is to use venue-based sampling. This approach will yield a probability sample; while not necessarily representative of the population you wish to serve, the improvement with a venue-based sampling approach is that it will allow you to enroll people who have had an equal probability of being included, therefore allowing you to generalize your program findings to those within your sampling

Table 4.2   Considerations for chat room–based recruitment

Consideration	How-tos
Creating your profile	• Be completely honest about your organization and what you want. Deception can result in violations of the TOS on the site and loss of credibility with your audience. • Include logos from your organization and, when allowed, links to your site. • Keep language simple and easy to read. This is not a place to be wordy!
Management of complaints and TOS violations	• Train recruiters to respond professionally and politely no matter what kind of communication they have with chatters. • Make sure recruiters know the TOS for a room; chatters may report a recruiter for perceived violations of TOS. In some instances recruiters may have unintentionally done so—either because they were not aware of all details of the TOS or because the TOS changed. In such instances you may have your profile blocked, meaning you cannot access the site until you have resolved the violation with the ISP.
Presence online for a topic-specific chat room	• Welcome chatters as they join, either directly in the room or through an instant message (IM) that only they can see. • The IM can be standardized to offer a brief intro to the room, or more detailed to describe your purpose. • Include information in your profile regarding your program.
Presence online for a user-created chat room	• Once in the chat room, introduce yourself and invite chatters to read your profile. Do that again only when a large number of the chatters originally in the room have left and there are new chatters. • Respond to questions, but do not initiate conversations about your program; this can be perceived as self-serving. • Do work to establish rapport with chatters—thank people for interest, and offer to answer questions.
Timing of recruitment	• You may need to recruit outside a traditional Monday–Friday, 9 a.m.–5 p.m. window. Review the chat room traffic to ascertain what days of the week and times of day are the busiest, and plan your recruitment for those times. • You may need to offer flex or release time to staff to recruit. In some cases, busy times occur very late at night (e.g., 12 a.m.–3 a.m.) or on weekends.
Training of recruiters	• Recruiters should always be professional—if they have been selected because they have specific connections to the target audience, they may need reminding that when recruiting they are representing your program, not engaging with people as an individual. • Often, program delivery will be tied to the agency rather than an individual recruiter, so recruiters will not include a picture or personal information about themselves, and will often use a standardized program profile, screen name, and user ID.

frame. Note that venue-based sampling is an approach that can also be used to identify and recruit a probability sample of participants in face-to-face settings—much has been written on this method and is available for review elsewhere (Muhib et al., 2001a, 2001b).

Another form of recruitment for technology-based programs that holds promise is called respondent-driven sampling (RDS). This involves selecting a "seed" or a participant who can then recruit his or her friends/acquaintances into your program for you. RDS is gaining a great deal of credibility for targeting and enrolling "hard to reach" individuals who may be at risk for a condition (Malekinejad et al., 2008; Platt et al., 2009), but it has yet to be tested and validated as a technology-based approach. We discuss both venue-based sampling and RDS with the emerging trends for program implementation below.

Care and Support of Participants During Program Implementation

Participant Verification

Once you have enrolled your program participants, there are important technical considerations to address in program implementation that are common to technology-based programs. First is the issue of participant verification. With no face-to-face recruitment and enrollment process, you should establish protocols to verify participants are who they say they are. You can employ both electronic and human verification processes to accomplish this. First, using a database program such as Microsoft Office Access™ you can "flag" participants with the same IP (Internet protocol) address and/or similar name, address, e-mail address, and telephone number. Because many people could share the same IP address, you can also ask for detailed contact information. A visual check of all this contact information for individuals flagged can reveal participants, for example, who have similar names (e.g., Sue Wilson, Susan Wilson, and S. Wilson), e-mail addresses (e.g., suewilson@yahoo.com, swilson@yahoo.com, and suewilson@hotmail.com), and telephone numbers.

If you need to ensure that all participants are unique individuals, then you will need to identify instances when it appears that participants have attempted to enroll multiple times. They may do so if you offer an incentive for program participation, for example. Participants who have attempted to enroll multiple times using variations on names and contact information can be contacted and asked to document their identity (e.g., by providing a faxed copy of their driver's license) so that they can be established as a unique individual. When telephoning participants to obtain correct addresses or remind them to return to your site to complete the next portion of the program, in some instances you may be able to ascertain if participants do not seem to fit within the eligibility criteria. For example, if your program is for persons aged 18 to 24 but the person on the phone sounds much older, you may flag him or her for verification. If the program is for men but the person sounds female, you can do the same.

In addition to the need for participant verification for persons enrolling online, you will need to take precautions when participants are already engaged in your program by establishing user identification and passwords, informing participants that these are the mechanisms you have

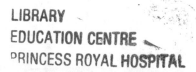

developed to ensure privacy and confidentiality. People may elect to share user IDs and passwords, however, so utilizing regular checks to make sure individuals are who they say they are is also important. You may be familiar already with this strategy, often employed to protect credit card users, for example. At enrollment, you can ask participants to give you their mother's maiden name or the name of the city where they were born, or some other datum that is likely known only to them. At the time of log-in, if you are concerned about participant identity being used by someone else, then you can also employ this level of verification to continue in the program.

Mobile phone–based programs may have additional problems, in that mobile phones may be shared, lent, or borrowed. If, for example, you implement a program using mobile phones to text individuals when their test results are available, you will need to make sure that the person receiving the text is the person enrolled in the program. Thus, it may be important to consider having a person text back a user ID or password prior to receiving a message. Alternatively, if you are sharing information that could be sensitive, you can send a more generic text saying "text 12345 if you wish to see the program results for today" so that people know there is information waiting for them. This could circumvent difficulties or violations in the Health Insurance Portability and Accountability Act (HIPAA) should an individual pick up a friend's telephone for him or her and get a message intended for the friend or should someone be looking over the shoulder of your participant and see a message he or she shouldn't.

Monitoring and Facilitating Program Elements

Technology-based health promotion programs may have the advantage of being able to recruit and enroll large numbers of people, but this can also serve as a challenge for program delivery. If your program requires that participants complete multiple activities at various times, then you should establish a tracking system to ensure that all are completing the steps required. This will also assist you in sending reminders to participants who have not completed specific steps to encourage them to do so. As with the participant verification process described above, the use of a database software program such as Microsoft Office Access™ is helpful in this process.

An example of program management for a large number of participants is the program described above for HIV prevention delivered on Facebook (RO1NR010492; Levine et al., in press). As part of the program evaluation, participants are asked to complete a baseline assessment of HIV-related attitudes and risk behaviors. They are then asked to visit the Facebook site a minimum of once each week for 8 weeks, and complete a follow-up evaluation at the end of 8 weeks to assess change in HIV-related attitudes and behaviors. Researchers wanted to ensure that each of these activities was accomplished and sent out reminders to participants *not* accomplishing any one of these steps. By using Microsoft Office Access™ to establish a participant tracking database, researchers could run queries on who had enrolled, completed their initial assessment, visited the site, and completed their 8-week assessment. Those who had not completed any one of these steps could be identified and sent a reminder. Figure 4.4 shows examples of some of the tables and queries created in Access™ that allowed researchers to easily

Figure 4.4 Microsoft Office Access™ tracking database examples

Query for finding participants who completed initial assessment:

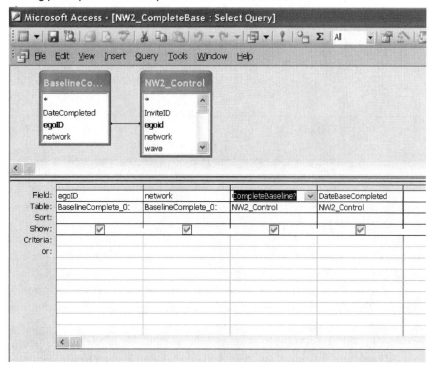

Result of query:

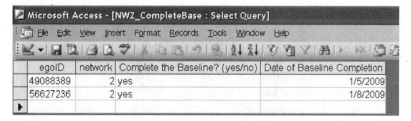

identify and track participants. This allowed them to ensure that people who were completing all program requirements were not bothered or hassled with reminder messages, while sending out only up to three reminders to those not completing any one program element to limit the annoyance factor of repeated reminders.

Managing Technical Difficulties in Technology-Based Program Implementation

With any technology-based health program, you should anticipate and be prepared for technical difficulties, such as computer crashes, Internet outages, electrical outages, and other

Table 4.3 Troubleshooting tips for technology-based health promotion

Modality	Issues	Resolution
Computer kiosk, desktop, handheld device Internet-based program	User-operated errors, power outages, equipment failures	If using infomediary, have him or her be very familiar with how to get device operating after failure due to user error, power outage, or other difficulty. If not, be sure to post easy-to-follow instructions in the event of difficulties on how to reboot or restart the program.
Mobile phone	Out of range or service area	Content will typically be restored when back in service area.
	Out of power	Have backup contact information for users to remind them to charge their phone.

types of equipment problems or failures. While it may be impossible to anticipate and plan for every technical difficulty, there are some obvious ones for each of the modalities we consider here (i.e., computer kiosk or desktop programs, Internet-based programs, mobile phone programs, and handheld programs). We will discuss considerations for each modality here. Note that Table 4.3 has specific troubleshooting tips for each modality.

For computer kiosks and desktop programs as well as those delivered using portable devices or mobile phones, technical difficulties can arise with regard to user operation of the device in turning it on or rebooting when needed. If using an infomediary with delivery of programs using these modalities, be sure to train this person to develop expertise in equipment management. Infomediaries should be adept at rebooting, getting the program started, and returning to where the participant was in the program when the problem occurred. If not using an infomediary, make sure that detailed instructions for troubleshooting are made available to users in the form of easy-to-read and -follow handouts. These could be laminated sheets or pages in a binder or folder. They could also be kept as electronic instructions that participants can click on the computer screen. One example of this is a program called "Health-e-Solutions," a kiosk program with a telephone that users could pick up to talk with a program staff person if they experienced difficulties. If not using an infomediary on-site this could be a way to help people connect with a program staff person for help (Colorado Prevention Center, n.d.).

For Internet-based programs, technical difficulties can arise (a) when there are graphic-intense program elements that are slow to load, (b) when connection to the Internet is lost, or (c) when the program freezes. Because there may often not be an infomediary on-site, it is critical that you inform users of what to do when any of these instances occur. Make sure that you have an obvious place on your site where users can click to obtain information on what to do if they have problems. Include detailed, easy-to-follow instructions. Try to ensure that participants will not be penalized in any way should they fail to complete a program element because of a technical difficulty. Always include the contact information for a webmaster or other program staff so that a participant can either e-mail or call an individual for help. When possible, include a toll-free number for participants to use, and staff that number as often as possible.

For mobile phone users, technical difficulties will arise when trying to use the device out of range, when the user cannot get a signal. Typically, users will be able to access any program communications when they get back in range—for example, if you send a text message to users who are out of range, when they get back into their service area they will find the message visible. Be sure to alert participants to this possibility. Additional challenges may arise when users do not charge their phone, making them inaccessible until the phone is charged. To ensure you have the capacity to communicate with your participants under these circumstances, make sure you have alternative contact information for them (e.g., landline telephone numbers, e-mail addresses, or social networking site addresses).

WHAT ARE EMERGING TRENDS IN TECHNOLOGY-BASED PROGRAM IMPLEMENTATION?

Venue-Based Sampling

Venue-based sampling offers an approach to identifying the volume of chatters and how well they represent your target audience. The first step in this process is identifying the chat rooms where you will recruit. Are you working with an ISP that has a specific number of rooms? Often users will add and create new rooms continually, so it may be necessary to identify a random cross section of all the rooms on a given day and use this as your initial sampling frame. Another approach would be to identify the universe of chat rooms on a given day—this will be possible only if the total number of chat rooms is small. On larger ISP sites, such as AOL or Yahoo!, there may be many hundreds if not thousands of chat rooms; not all these will be places of interest for your target audience, and cross-sectional sampling or random sampling among those rooms is possible.

Once you have defined the rooms where you wish to recruit, you will conduct a first-level enumeration. Enumeration allows for an objective count of people who frequent chat rooms that can be analyzed to identify those rooms with high traffic. In first-level enumeration, you will log in to a chat room and count the number of people within a specified time (e.g., 30 minutes) who are presumed to fit given eligibility criteria (e.g., African American women aged 25 to 45, ascertained based on a review of their profile) who enter the room. In this stage, you should be very liberal in your estimations, including any person who might fit the criteria. During first-level enumeration, you want to visit the chat rooms at various times of the day and days of the week to ascertain the highest-volume days and hours.

In second-level enumeration, you will return to the venues with highest yield of potential participants on days and times when participation in chat appeared highest during the first level of enumeration. You will review the profile of every nth person who enters the chat room to determine if he or she would fit your program eligibility criteria. If the potential yield of participants is adequate, that chat room as well as the day and time you are observing—known as a venue-day-time increment or VDT—is entered into the sampling frame. During recruitment, you can then randomly select VDT increments and go to each venue to recruit. Once you have identified high-volume and high-traffic chat rooms (level-1 enumeration) and recruited participants from randomly selected chat VDT increments, your enrollees will constitute a probability sample enrolled in your program.

In Figure 4.5 we illustrate an example of a data collection form for VDT enumeration. It allows for the researcher to document the venue, day and time; enumeration type (level 1 or level 2); and outcomes: the number of people clicked and, for level-2 enumeration, the number of those approached and the assumed or actual demographic characteristics of potential participants. This data collection sheet was developed for a social marketing campaign to increase female condom use targeting African American and Latina women (Bull, Posner, et al., 2008), and was used for face-to-face venue-based sampling. We have adapted it for use in the virtual world.

Recruitment Using Respondent-Driven Sampling

Another approach to recruitment is to use respondent-driven sampling, or RDS. As with venue-based sampling, this type of recruitment is not unique to the virtual world or technology-based programs, and is widely recognized as an acceptable method for program enrollment, particularly for hard-to-reach populations (Centers for Disease Control and Prevention [CDC], 2005). RDS was first employed in HIV prevention research to help with enrollment of particularly difficult-to-reach groups (e.g., injection drug users and commercial sex workers; Jordan, Tolbert, & Smith, 1998) in face-to-face settings. RDS is similar to the approach used by the CDC in identifying new cases of HIV infection. Called social networks testing, this approach similarly begins with an index case, or an individual testing positive for HIV. This individual is asked to identify others within his or her social network and participate in getting these individuals in for testing. The approach has been highly successful, yielding a 6% positivity rate on HIV testers using this method, a rate 6 times higher than through a typical clinic-based testing approach (CDC, 2005).

Applied to technology-based program delivery, RDS has the potential to overcome some of the challenges inherent when recruiting online or recruiting hard-to-reach populations for technology-based programs. Although we know of no instances where RDS has been applied for technology-based programs to date, we do know of several proposals for projects to use this approach. Hongjie Liu is planning a project using text messaging among money boys (MB), or male commercial sex workers in China. He plans to identify several MBs and then recruit others into his mobile phone text messaging project based on referrals to the program by the initial MBs (H. Liu , personal communication, December 20, 2008). Eric Rice is planning a project for homeless youth, whom he will contact at youth shelters and social service agencies in Los Angeles. Subsequent to enrollment in the program, he will ask youth to communicate

Figure 4.5 Example of a chat room–based VDT summary form

VDT number: ___[UNIQUE NUMBER]___ Chat room name/location: _____

Person Completing This Form: _____

Today's Date: _____ Day of Week: _____

Time in: _____ am / pm Time out: _____ am / pm

Type of Visit: ☐ Type I Enumeration ☐ Type II Enumeration

Total Number of people documented _____

Any notes about this chat room or suggestions for other chat rooms?

_____

_____

Estimation of demographics- % <15 ____ **% 15-17** ____ **% 18-20** ____ %

21-25 ____ **% 25+** ____ **% Gender-F** ____ **% M** ____ %

Ethnic/Racial Profile of those documented via profile review AA ____ % Lat ____ %

Other ____ % Venue Type[1]: _____

Other VDT Times					
Day	_Time_	VDT #	_Time_	_Time_	VDT #
M	___	___	___	___	___
T	___	___	___	___	___
W	___	___	___	___	___
Th	___	___	___	___	___
F	___	___	___	___	___
Sat	___	___	___	___	___
Sun	___	___	___	___	___

Recruiter Name

# chatters approached for screener (Column A)	# chatters completed screener (Column B)	# Eligible from screener (Column H)	# Enrolled in program

Note: 1. Venue Types include: schools, bars, community organizations, outdoor events, malls, transportation stops, restaurants, grocery stores, laundromat, festivals, etc

through MySpace to their friends and online acquaintances about strategies for risk reduction around drug and alcohol use, for example. His work on prosocial networks and high-risk youth shows both that these youth are well connected to others at high risk and that they do have low- or no-risk peers in their networks, who appear to positively influence behaviors of high-risk youth (Rice, Milburn, & Rotheram-Borus, 2007; Rice, Stein, & Milburn, 2008).

Strategies, then, for utilizing RDS include identifying the population you wish to enroll in your program and opportunities for engaging with its members. Are there agencies or clinics that serve your audience? Can you connect with individuals from your target population in these settings? If so, you may be able to identify initial "seeds" or index individuals who can assist in identifying others in their network whom you can recruit for your program. You may need to consider offering an incentive or small stipend or thank-you gift to your initial seed individuals to motivate them.

Some cautions regarding RDS are related to both sampling and confidentiality. While the approach may indeed yield participation by a greater proportion of people who are indeed at high risk or otherwise meet your criteria to be members of the program's target audience, RDS is not an approach that yields a representative sample. Because there are seldom, if ever, records or documentation for some hidden or hard-to-reach groups that can be used to identify a sampling frame (e.g., a roster or directory), we cannot know if those participating are representative of all in your target audience. With regard to confidentiality, program planners need to take precautions as needed when initial program recruits are aware that those they recruited are participating in a program. If eligibility for the program includes criteria such as illicit or stigmatized behaviors, then the initial recruit will know that those he or she enrolled are engaging in these behaviors if they are accepted into the program. For example, if the program is only open to recent injection drug users (IDUs), then an RDS seed will know that the person he or she recruited is a recent IDU. Presumably, the seed knows this already—but program planners should be extra cautious about protecting the confidentiality of all those recruited and enrolled in the program using this approach.

Recruitment of and Communication With Participants Using "FriendBlaster" on Social Networking Sites

A new but as of yet unproven tool for reaching individuals for program participation online is through social networking sites such as MySpace or Facebook. These are sites on the Internet where people can post information and share it on a large scale with others in their social network without having to repeat messages multiple times. Information individuals wish to share with everyone in their network is posted to their home page—so anyone in their network can see that they have just graduated from high school or just gotten a job. This way individuals can stay connected with others in their network without having to reiterate this information over and over to all in their social group. In addition, all members of an individual's network are exposed to everyone else in that network, so you can see not only what one person posts but also what everyone else within that network posts and shares online.

There are thousands of individuals on these network sites, and each is connected to thousands more. People connect to one another by sending out requests to be a "friend."

Friending is the term used when an individual invites others to be part of his or her network. Typically, individuals will "friend" those with whom they want to maintain regular contact, and links to these "friends" will appear on an individual's page on the social networking site. A network could thus incorporate hundreds of individuals—for example, say an individual has 20 friends linked to her page. If each of these individuals in turn has 20 friends, and these 20 friends have 20 friends each, then in four steps you can identify 160,000 people linked to this initial seed. It is possible to connect to each of these individuals or a subset of those who may fit the eligibility criteria for your program, and invite them to participate.

Following is a description of how this approach can work on MySpace, one of the biggest social networking sites in the United States. Note that MySpace has restrictions on the number of "friend" invites you can send without it being considered spam—users of MySpace can be inundated with friend requests from organizations or commercial interests, and the site wants to limit the annoyance factor that these introduce to its users. Therefore, you cannot simply identify thousands of individuals and ask them to "friend" you and enroll in your online program. You can, however, purchase a software application called "FriendBlaster," sanctioned by MySpace, that allows you to send invitations through personal messages to up to 250 persons daily to enroll in your program. Note, if you are sending 250 messages, it is to ask individuals to *add you* as a friend (i.e., they have to go to your page and send you a request to be your friend); if you want them to simply accept your invitation to be their friend (i.e., they don't have to leave their page and go to yours), then you are limited to 100 friend invitations daily. Figure 4.6 shows a screenshot from FriendBlaster with a sample invitation.

Note that on MySpace individuals can set up their accounts to automatically reject a mass mailing by installing a program to pop up a "captcha" code. This is a code that must be retyped manually by senders to ensure they are a real person (see example in Figure 4.6). Once individuals have received an invitation to either add you as a friend or accept your friend invitation, they can go directly to your MySpace page and participate in your program. As we have described in detail elsewhere, there are a number of lessons we are learning about recruiting and connecting with individuals through social networking sites (Wright, Breslin, Black, & Bull, forthcoming), summarized in Table 4.4. Also note that we do not know if utilizing a "blasting" program does indeed result in higher recruitment rates; it may not yield substantial gains in recruitment if persons receiving messages perceive your blast as spam. On social networking sites, it may be important to first establish a relationship with users and then utilize this tool for follow-up—we essentially know little about how to most effectively engage with and retain the attention of populations on social networking sites.

Use of Geographic Information Systems (GIS) to Facilitate Program Delivery

One of the most useful features of GIS for technology-based program delivery is the ability to geotarget your interventions if they are delivered on the Internet. It may be quite expensive to deliver program content indiscriminately to all users of the site where your program is housed. It may also be practical to limit access to your program material if you have intentions to evaluate program effectiveness and wish to compare people who haven't seen your program to others who have. ISPs will often facilitate delivery of program content by zip code or

Figure 4.6   "FriendBlasting" Using FriendBlaster Pro on MySpace

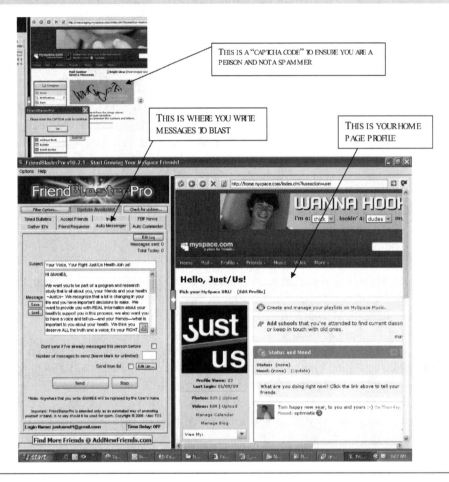

metropolitan statistical area (MSA) or some other geographic designation (e.g., state, city, region). This allows you to make your program accessible only to persons with an account for this ISP in a given region. This practice is emerging as a common approach to targeting health promotion services and programs online. A recent report in *Health Promotion Practice* reviewing hundreds of public health applications using GIS indicates that the majority of applications include surveillance activities, risk analysis, assessment of or planning for health care access, or community health profiling (Nykiforuk & Flaman, 2009). There is documentation that public health professionals perceive GIS as another tool to use to facilitate decision making for health promotion (Joyce, 2009). In the "Additional Resources" section at the end of this chapter are citations for several reviews of public health applications using GIS.

Table 4.4 Lessons learned related to social network recruitment and participation in health promotion programs on MySpace

Lesson	Details
Establishing a "friend" on the site requires trust.	• People use social networking sites to connect with others they know. If you are trying to connect with individuals without knowing them, you need to work to establish trust and credibility. • As mentioned in Chapters 2 and 3 you can do this through very visible personal identification and through soliciting opinions and ideas for trust building from your target audience.
Everything needs to be shorter and current.	• The MySpace page or the space on other social networking sites isn't very large, and certainly wouldn't allow for detailed surveys and text-based content. On the other hand, it does allow for graphics, video, and art. • Users expect pithy and easy-to-read content, and they expect regular updates to content.
Users may not want to leave a social networking site to go elsewhere.	• When users leave MySpace they receive a "warning" message telling them they are no longer going to be on the site. • This can be off-putting and serve as a deterrent for program planners to deliver program content elsewhere online.
While you can use FriendBlaster, do so judiciously.	• Even though you could send messages to up to 250 people daily, including reminders and program updates, beware that individuals annoyed by such tactics can report you and have your actions halted or shut down. • Be sure to determine how much contact is acceptable before people consider you spam.

SUMMARY

In this chapter, we have covered specific issues for technology-based health program recruitment and implementation. Key terms introduced in this chapter are available in Table 4.5.

When recruiting for any technology-based program delivered using a computer kiosk, desktop, or mobile device, be it a mobile phone or a portable device, consider whether or not to use an infomediary, or a person who can help you recruit participants and troubleshoot any technical difficulties that arise. Such a person can be invaluable for connecting with and recruiting participation by groups that haven't yet been reached with these programs and that may need assistance or encouragement. Recognize, however, that you may sacrifice reaching the large numbers of people accessing the Internet if you use an infomediary; this person can only communicate with a limited number of individuals. Having an automated program online may allow you to reach many more individuals and tap into the potential of technology to expand programs more rapidly.

Table 4.5   Key terms relevant for technology-based program recruitment and implementation

Term	Definition
Auditorium-style chat	Using a chat room at a predetermined time and inviting people to attend and chat about a specific topic
Banner advertising	Using graphic ads on a website to engage members of your audience and recruit them to your program
Blasting	Sending out friend invitations to multiple people simultaneously
Chat room recruitment	Using chat rooms online to engage your audience in an online program or offline services
Click-through rate	The proportion of people exposed to your banner who click on it
Flaming	When a person online uses rude or abrupt language directed at someone else online
Friending	Inviting an individual on a social network site to become a part of your network
Infomediary	A person trained to assist users in accessing a technology-based program either in person or through the Internet or phone. Usually very skilled and competent in recruitment as well as in technical troubleshooting for your equipment
Instant messages	Messages sent to people who are online that are not visible to others online—can be used to send private information to an individual in a chat room
ISP	Internet service provider—people pay ISPs to gain access to the Internet
Participant verification	The process used to ensure that persons enrolling in your program online are who they say they are
Profile	The mechanism used to present oneself or one's organization or program online; usually widely accessible, and offers information about an individual or a program to all viewers
Respondent-driven sampling	A method of connecting with and recruiting hard-to-reach or hidden populations for your program. Uses initial recruits to communicate with others like them in their social network to tell them about your program
Terms of service (TOS)	The agreements you agree to as a user of a given website. Violations of TOS can result in having your program shut down temporarily or permanently
Venue-based sampling	A method of obtaining a probability sample by identifying places where your target audience is likely to be found in large numbers. Can be used in chat rooms for recruitment

When recruiting online for technology-based programs, you can use banner advertising, chat room recruitment, or "blasts" to large numbers of individuals on social networking sites. While banner advertisements can assist you in enrolling large numbers of participants, remember participants often represent fewer than .01% of those exposed to the ad, so you cannot be confident your participants adequately represent the population you are trying to reach. Chat room recruitment may help target enrollment to the audience you want for your program, but also faces limitations in reaching the large numbers of Internet users because it requires human staff time.

Currently untested but newly emerging approaches for recruitment in technology-based programs are venue-based and respondent-driven sampling methods online. To increase the likelihood you are reaching participants who match your eligibility criteria, especially for hidden or hard-to-reach groups, you can consider respondent-driven sampling. Finally, new methods employed on social networking sites to reach individuals within networks include "blasting," or recruiting large numbers of people within a social networking site simultaneously.

When implementing your programs, be sure to anticipate and plan for technical difficulties such as computer crashes, Internet and electrical outages, and program freezes. If you have an infomediary, this person should have specific training to address these concerns. If you do not, make sure you offer users explicit and easy-to-read and easy-to-access information on how to troubleshoot. In addition, offer contact information for program staff in the event participants need or want to talk to a person to help them troubleshoot.

? CONCLUDING QUESTIONS

Consider the following questions that summarize material covered here:

1. Will the addition of an infomediary help your program? If so, how? If not, how will you facilitate enrollment and address any technical difficulties users will face?

2. If using banner advertisements, what ISPs reach your audience? When should the banners run? For how long? What design elements on your banner will appeal to your target audience?

3. If using chat room recruitment, what steps will you take to make your profile engaging and credible? What days of the week and times of day will you recruit? What chat rooms will you recruit in, and how were these chosen?

4. If using RDS, how will you identify your initial seed? How will you identify and recruit referrals?

5. If using a blasting program, how often will you send messages? How will you avoid appearing as spam? What will you do if people do not send you a friend request or accept your friend request?

6. How will you verify participants are who they say they are if not recruiting face-to-face for your program?

7. How will you manage and track large numbers of participants and ensure they are completing all program elements?

CHAPTER EXERCISE

The following exercises are designed to facilitate technology-based program implementation.

Choose one or more of these exercises to practice what you have learned in technology-based program implementation:

1. Venue-based sampling. Select a website that has multiple chat rooms. Using the VDT enumeration form (Figure 4.5 from this chapter) purposively select several chat rooms where you have already observed participation by persons that are of your target audience. Then, select several days of the week and times of the day, and observe how many people from your target audience participate in the chat room. Complete your TYPE I enumeration and forms based on your observations.

2. Respondent-driven sampling (RDS). Write a protocol (i.e., a detailed, step-by-step list of procedures) for the selection of "seeds" from an online site such as a forum or threaded discussion. How will you select your seed? Once selected, how will you attempt to engage with this person? (Please include examples of the types of messages you will post—either in direct e-mail communication or via public posts to the site.) What are the specific instructions you will give your seed about recruiting other people? How will you motivate their participation? How will you communicate with the people the seed refers? How long will your referral chain be?

3. Create messages to send via FriendBlaster about your program. Create "draft" (i.e., hand-drawn) banner ads that can be posted to sites where your target audience congregates.

4. Develop a detailed protocol (i.e., a step-by-step list of procedures) that you will employ to verify participant identity and uniqueness. Develop an access database to track participant activities in your program (e.g., number of times visiting site, number of pages viewed, number of postings made).

ADDITIONAL RESOUCES

Books, Articles, and Other Peer-Reviewed Literature

Resource	Description
Graves, B. A. (2008). Integrative literature review: A review of literature related to geographical information systems, healthcare access, and health outcomes. *Perspectives in Health Information Management, 5*, 11.	A review of GIS tools and applications in public health including assessment of impact on health outcomes
McLafferty, S. L. (2003). GIS and health care. *Annual Review of Public Health, 24*, 25–42.	A review of GIS tools and applications in public health

Resource	Description
Tuten, T. L. (2008). *Advertising 2.0: Social media marketing in a Web 2.0 world*. Westport, CT: Praeger.	A book offering details on how to get the most benefit from advertising on social networking sites, and also describing new approaches in addition to traditional ads for reaching customers online
Weber, L. (2007). *Marketing to the social web: How digital customer communities build your business.* Hoboken, NJ: Wiley.	A resource for selling products and materials using social networking sites online

Websites

Resource	Description
http://www.clickz.com/841811	A website with tips on how to create more effective banner advertisements
http://www.witiger.com/ecommerce/bannerads.htm	Offers data from multiple sources on why banner advertising is still relevant and can be useful
http://www.ncsddc.org/upload/wysiwyg/documents/IGO.pdf	Guidelines published by the CDC to facilitate Internet recruitment and program implementation in chat rooms

Note: All websites noted here are hot-linked at www.sagepub.com/bull; at this site you will also find newer resources relevant to the material in this and other chapters.

REFERENCES

Abdolrasulnia, M., Collins, B. C., Casebeer, L., Wall, T., Spettell, C., Ray, M. N., et al. (2004). Using email reminders to engage physicians in an Internet-based CME intervention. *BMC Medical Education, 4,* 17.

Blas, M., Alva, I., Cabello, R., Garcia, P., Carcamo, C., Redmon, M., et al. (2007). *Internet as a tool to access high-risk men who have sex with men from a resource-constrained setting: A study from Peru. Sexually Transmitted Infections, 83,* 567–570.

Bull, S., Posner, S., Ortiz, C., Lin, L., Pals, S., & Evans, T. (2008). Increasing POWER for reproductive health: A social marketing campaign promoting female and male condoms. *Journal of Adolescent Health, 43*(1), 71–78.

Bull, S., Pratte, K., Whitesell, N., Reitemeijer, C., & McFarlane, M. (2009). Effects of an Internet-based intervention for HIV prevention: The Youthnet trials. *AIDS and Behavior, 13*(3), 474–487.

Bull, S., Vallejos, D., & Ortiz, C. (2008). Recruitment and retention of youth online for an HIV prevention intervention: Lessons from the Youthnet trial. *AIDS Care, 20,* 887–889.

Centers for Disease Control and Prevention. (2005). *Use of social networks to identify persons with undiagnosed HIV infection—Seven U.S. cities* (Rep. No. 54).

Chiasson, M. A., Parsons, J. T., Tesoriero, J. M., Carballo-Dieguez, A., Hirshfield, S., & Remien, R. H. (2006). HIV behavioral research online. *Journal of Urban Health, 83,* 73–85.

Cho, H., & LaRose, R. (1999). Privacy issues in Internet surveys. *Social Science Computer Review, 17,* 421–434.

Fox, S., & Livingston, G. (2007). *Latinos online: Hispanics with lower levels of education and English proficiency remain largely disconnected from the Internet.* Washington, DC: Pew Hispanic Center. Retrieved from http://www.eric.ed.gov:80/RICWebPortal/search/detailmini.jsp?_nfpb=true&_&ERICExtSearch_SearchValue_0=ED495954&ERICExtSearch_SearchType_0=no&accno=ED495954

Governors Highway Safety Association. (2010). *Click it or ticket.* Retrieved from Retrieved from http://www.ghsa.org/html/projects/CIOT/08.html

Graves, B. A. (2008). Integrative literature review: A review of literature related to geographical information systems, healthcare access, and health outcomes. *Perspectives in Health Information Management, 5,* 11.

Hatfield, L. A., Ghiselli, M. E., Jacoby, S. M., Cain-Nielsen, A., Kilian, G., McKay, T., et al. (2009). Methods for recruiting men of color who have sex with men in prevention-for-positives interventions. *Preventive Science, 11*(1), 56–66.

Jordan, W., Tolbert, L., & Smith, R. (1998). Partner notification and focused intervention and a means of identifying HIV positive patients. *Journal of the National Medical Association, 90,* 524–546.

Joyce, K. (2009). "To me it's just another tool to help understand the evidence": Public health decision-makers' perceptions of the value of geographical information systems (GIS). *Health & Place, 15,* 801–810.

Koenig, W., Löwel, H., Baumert, J., & Meisinger, C. (2004). C-reactive protein modulates risk prediction based on the Framingham Score: Implications for future risk assessment: Results from a large cohort study in southern Germany. *Circulation, 109*(11), 1349–1353.

Levine, D., Madsen, A., Wright, E., Barar, R., Santelli, J, & Bull, S. (in press). Formative research on MySpace: Online methods to engage hard-to-reach populations. *Journal of Health Communication.*

Lim, M., Hawking, S., Aitkin, C., Fairly, C., Jordon, L., Lewis, J., et al. (in press). A randomised controlled trial of text and email messaging for sexual health promotion to young people. *International Journal of Epidemiology.*

Malekinejad, M., Johnston, L. G., Kendall, C., Kerr, L. R., Rifkin, M. R., & Rutherford, G. W. (2008). Using respondent-driven sampling methodology for HIV biological and behavioral surveillance in international settings: A systematic review. *AIDS and Behavior, 12,* 105–130.

Marcus, B. H., Owen, N., Forsyth, L. H., Cavill, N. A., & Fridinger, F. (1998). Physical activity interventions using mass media, print media, and information technology. *American Journal of Preventive Medicine, 15,* 362–378.

McFarlane, M., Kachur, R., Klausner, J. D., Roland, E., & Cohen, M. (2005). Internet-based health promotion and disease control in the 8 cities: Successes, barriers, and future plans. *Sexually Transmitted Diseases, 32,* S60–S64.

McLafferty, S. L. (2003). GIS and health care. *Annual Review of Public Health, 24,* 25–42.

Microsoft Office Access™ (Version 14) [Computer software]. Redmond, WA: Microsoft.

Muhib, F., Lin, L., Steuve, A., Miller, R., Ford, W., Johnson, W., et al. (2001a). Community Intervention trial for youth study team: A venue-based method for sampling hard-to-reach populations. *Public Health Reports, Supp. 16,* 216–222.

Muhib, F. B., Lin, L. S., Stueve, A., Miller, R. L., Ford, W. L., Johnson, W. D., et al. (2001b). A venue-based method for sampling hard-to-reach populations. *Public Health Reports, 116*(Supp. 1), 216–222.

Nykiforuk, C. I., & Flaman, L. M. (2009). Geographic information systems (GIS) for health promotion and public health: A review. *Health Promotion Practice.* Advance online publication. doi:10.1177/1524839909334624

Padilla, R., Bull, S., Raghunath, S. G., Fernald, D., Havranek, E. P., & Steiner, J. F. (2010). Designing a cardiovascular disease prevention web site for Latinos: Qualitative community feedback. *Health Promotion Practice, 11*(1), 140–147.

Pequegnat, W., Rosser, B. R., Bowen, A. M., Bull, S. S., Diclemente, R. J., Bockting, W. O., et al. (2007). Conducting Internet-based HIV/STD prevention survey research: Considerations in design and evaluation. *AIDS and Behavior, 11,* 505–521.

Platt, L., Wall, M., Rhodes, T., Judd, A., Hickman, M., Johnston, L. G., et al. (2009). Methods to recruit hard-to-reach groups: Comparing two chain referral sampling methods of recruiting injecting drug users across nine studies in Russia and Estonia. *Journal of Urban Health, 83*(Supp. 6), i39–53.

Rice, E., Milburn, G., & Rotheram-Borus, M. J. (2007). Pro-social and problematic social network influences on HIV/AIDS risk behaviors among newly homeless youth in Los Angeles. *AIDS Care, 19,* 697–704.

Rice, E., Stein, J., & Milburn, N. (2008). Countervailing social network influences on problem behaviors among homeless youth. *Journal of Adolescence, 5,* 625–639.

Ross, M. W., Rosser, B. R., & Stanton, J. (2004). Beliefs about cybersex and Internet-mediated sex of Latino men who have Internet sex with men: Relationships with sexual practices in cybersex and in real life. *AIDS Care, 16,* 1002–1011.

Wright, E., Breslin, L., Black, S., & Bull, S. (forthcoming). Recruiting for health related research and programs on social networking sites: Lessons learned.

5 ▪▪
▪▪

Program Evaluation for Technology-Based Health Promotion

CHAPTER OVERVIEW

This chapter covers issues relevant for evaluation of interventions using technology. In previous chapters we have discussed how to design and prepare your technology-based program (Chapter 3) and how to deliver your program on a daily basis (Chapter 4).

Note that specific instruction on methods for the very broad field of program evaluation is beyond the scope of this book, and this chapter in particular, and that there are numerous references that cover techniques for health promotion program evaluation quite ably (DiIorio, 2005; Steckler & Linnan, 2002). Thus, *we do not offer detail on specific health promotion program evaluation methods;* as with other chapters, our focus is on what aspects of program evaluation are unique or of particular importance for technology-based programs.

Material covered in this chapter includes a presentation of considerations regarding the design of your program evaluation, collecting evaluation data from participants, retention of program participants, and how to limit attrition from your technology-based programs. The chapter also covers management and delivery of incentives for program evaluation if you are using them.

We offer some specific suggestions for management of large and rapidly accruing data and discuss some of the opportunities for analysis that present themselves given the ability to collect data from larger samples using technology.

Because the promise of technology-based intervention includes the ability to standardize and easily replicate programs, part of the chapter is devoted to considerations of program reach, adoption, and sustainability, along with approaches for dissemination of program findings using technology.

WHAT ARE UNIQUE AND BENEFICIAL CONSIDERATIONS FOR TECHNOLOGY-BASED PROGRAM EVALUATION?

Design of Your Evaluation

Research related to the evaluation of program (or intervention) efficacy will typically require a rigorous experimental design that includes randomization of participants to either intervention or control status and more controlled conditions for participation in an intervention; for example, participants must take part in at least N sessions to be considered active and complete at minimum a baseline and follow-up assessment for inclusion in the analysis of program efficacy. While much of what we present here is relevant for those conducting research, our focus is on evaluation of a program, and thus we will limit our examples and considerations to program evaluation, not considering randomization and equivalent control groups. For more information on evaluation for research, there are detailed references that can guide you in research design, data collection, management, and analysis (DiIorio, 2005; Steckler & Linnan, 2002).

The basic premise for evaluating program outcome is to ascertain whether or not your program has produced the outcome you desire. In the case of program evaluation for health promotion, the types of outcomes can include changes in behavior (e.g., nutrition, physical activity, smoking, sexual behavior, drug or alcohol use, seat belt use, helmet use, sunscreen use, accessing screening, primary care) and changes in biomedical outcomes (e.g., cholesterol, weight, body mass index [BMI], blood pressure, fitness level, cotinine levels, presence of infection).

Additional types of program evaluation include formative evaluation and the steps needed to design and plan a program; we discussed specific issues relevant to evaluation for technology-based health program design in Chapter 3. Process evaluation, or the evaluation of how the program is being implemented, is also something we discussed in Chapter 3.

Typically, program evaluators are able to assess program outcomes by selecting either a nonexperimental or a quasi-experimental design. Nonexperimental and quasi-experimental designs are ones that do not include a control group or include a nonequivalent control group (i.e., one that hasn't had random assignment).

When making a decision about what type of design to use for a technology-based health program evaluation, important considerations include accessibility to your target audience for administration of evaluation tools, length of time for your program, accessibility to data regarding your participants from administrative or other sources, and the modality planned for data collection. These are general considerations relevant to multiple modalities for technology-based program delivery, but there are also modality-specific considerations, so we will consider each modality and the options available for evaluation when using that modality.

Designs for Computer Kiosk, Desktop, and Handheld Device in Clinic or Community Settings

First, consider the kind of accessibility you have to your target audience. Is your program delivered in a setting where you can approach and recruit evaluation participants face-to-face? Alternatively, can you recruit participants over the telephone? We offer specific ideas for employing technology to assist in data collection and for ensuring participant retention in your program and evaluation below.

Designs for Internet-Based Programs

As with programs delivered using computer kiosk, desktop, or mobile device, first consider access to your population. How likely is it that you will be able to connect with program participants, potentially for multiple assessments? As mentioned in Chapters 3 and 4, programs delivered exclusively online are at a disadvantage because they do not allow for the face-to-face time that can be valuable for establishing rapport. Literature on evaluations of Internet-based interventions for health promotion shows that participation in both program activities and evaluation activities seems to drop precipitously at about 3 months (McKay, Feil, Glasgow, & Brown, 1998) and programs experience higher attrition for Internet-based program evaluation compared to more traditional program evaluation (Bull, 2003; Bull, Levine, Vallejos, & Ortiz, 2008).

Evaluation designs that allow for passive data collection or collection of data from secondary sources may be possible for health promotion programs delivered on the Internet, but there are not many examples of programs that have accomplished this. One exception is a recent study where researchers viewed profile pages that are publicly available on MySpace for references to risky sexual behavior and drug use prior to intervening with youth by sending them an e-mail to ask them to consider dangers in doing so. Three months later they again reviewed profiles, including those of persons who hadn't received the e-mail, and collected the same data on references to risky sexual behavior and drug use, showing those who had received the e-mail were more likely to have made positive changes to their profile (Moreno et al., 2009). In this example, participants were not required to complete any assessments, but data on evaluation outcomes were publicly available and accessible to the researchers.

Design Options for Mobile Phones

As with the computer kiosk, desktop, or handheld device, pre- and postassessment, posttest only, and time-series designs are all possible using mobile phones. Certainly if you have participants' telephone numbers they can complete data collection evaluation activities over the telephone with a program staff member. Alternatively, they can respond to questions sent via short message service (SMS), also called text messaging. The challenge with the latter option is that you will likely not be able to ask participants many questions—first, as mentioned in Chapter 3, U.S.-based programs using text will be hampered by the charges users must pay for text, regardless of whether they receive or send it. Unless you plan to cover these costs with your program, you will have to consider how to motivate individuals to pay to participate in your evaluation. Second, the screen size and character limitations per text message (usually 160 characters) mean that you are limited on the amount of information you can provide or receive using SMS.

Automated Data Collection, Transfer, and Storage

Once you have determined the program design, if your evaluation will call for any data collection directly from participants in your program or from a comparison group, you may be able to take advantage of one of the nicest advantages of technology-based programs—automating your data collection. Automated surveys offer several advantages over pen-and-paper surveys. First, they require less paper and other equipment such as clipboards and pens. Second, they allow you to skip data entry and the possible errors that accompany that process. Third, they allow you to cut down on missing data and associated data cleaning. If you program your survey instrument to force users to answer questions before moving on, you can ensure you have no missing data—note that in this instance you will likely have to include a "don't know, don't want to answer" option for your questions. You can also program your survey instrument to automatically skip to questions based on user response rather than relying on users to find their next question.

Automated Data Collection for Internet- and Computer-Based Surveys

There are several excellent online survey design software programs that allow for construction of surveys, including SurveyMonkey (http:// www.surveymonkey.com/), Vovici (http://www.vovici.com/), and Zoomerang (http://www.zoomerang.com/). These allow you to develop sophisticated and complex surveys, include a back-end database for storage, and offer tracking of data for quality as they are being collected. See the section on data collection below for best practices and suggestions in how to utilize these resources.

Another software program available to facilitate design of surveys for use on desktop computers and kiosks is the audio computer-assisted self-interview, or ACASI, which uses a user-friendly application to assist you in designing a survey that can be administered over a computer with an audio component. An audio component can be particularly helpful for persons with lower levels of literacy or for those whose first language is not that employed in your survey.

Software programs such as these can also allow for data collection via a touch screen device. You will need to consider two things if choosing to use a touch screen device for your assessment. First, make sure you have a flat screen monitor. The rounded monitors can sometimes make it difficult to capture and record data depending on where the buttons are placed. Second, make sure the touch screen buttons are large enough and easy to read. If you have a graphics-heavy assessment tool, the user may be confused about what to touch in response to any question.

Note, for devices with smaller screens such as mobile phones, you will need to take extra care in ensuring that questions fit on the screen and are not cumbersome to answer. Make sure to pilot-test your evaluation instrument to make sure pages load as intended and participants see and can answer every question. See the section on current best practices in data collection below for further details on utilizing ACASI.

Automated Data Collection on a Mobile Phone

While you can collect data via text message using a mobile phone, this approach may be cumbersome and limiting given the small screen size available on the device. An alternative for collection of telephone-based data, which will be familiar to many, is known as interactive voice response, or IVR. This is an automated voice data collection system—using push buttons or voice, the user can answer questions posed by the computer. If you are delivering your technology-based health program via mobile phones, you could consider this option. Indeed, this is a viable evaluation option regardless of the program delivery mechanism.

The advantages of using IVR are the ability to complete more calls at various hours—you are not dependent on staff availability to complete calls. People are familiar with the technology and so may be accepting of it. It is similar to many voice mail systems that are more and more common in businesses and individual homes.

There are disadvantages to this method of data collection, however. Participants may feel less social desirability to respond to questions from an IVR system, and may be more likely to hang up or refuse to complete the assessment. They may not be able to understand or communicate effectively with the program. While software exists that allows for a human rather than digitized computer voice, there still may be difficulties in communication with the system.

Data Management, Security, and Participant Confidentiality

As already mentioned numerous times in this textbook, a primary advantage of using technology to deliver health promotion is the ability to enroll and deliver your program to large numbers of people, often larger numbers than are typically seen in traditional programs. The same holds true for program evaluation—you have the advantage of being able to collect evaluation data from large numbers of people in a short period.

Participant Tracking and Reminders

The rapid accrual of participants in a program and in a program evaluation can also be a drawback, unless you already have systems in place to ensure that data are well managed and participant activities and program protocols are easily tracked. The section on best practices in managing rapidly accruing samples offers more detail on participant tracking and reminders.

Automated Systems for Data Checks and Data Consistency

With rapidly accruing samples, having automated processes for cleaning data and checking for data consistency can facilitate excellence in data quality. You can build in data checks to make sure data are being captured as intended; you can also build in consistency checks to ensure that participants are reporting items as you would expect (e.g., asking birth date in one section, age in another, and year of birth in a third).

Pretesting Systems

Another benefit available technologically is the ability to pretest or beta test your site to ensure that data are being captured as intended and that all the systems work as planned. This process was first introduced in Chapter 3, Text Box 3.3, which shows an example of a beta test log that should also allow for identification of any items that are not being captured or elements on the site that are not appearing as intended with the program.

Protecting Participant Confidentiality

We detailed issues related to security of data generated through technology-based health programs in Chapter 2. Please refer to that chapter for specific suggestions for utilizing such tools as data backup plans, physical security of data, secure data transfers, and safeguards related to personal identification numbers (PINs), passwords, and security questions.

Table 5.1 offers a review of these security considerations by technologic modality.

Table 5.1	Security by modality for protection of data collected in technology-based health program evaluation
Modality	*Security measures to take*
Computer kiosk, desktop	1. Make sure the device is bolted or secured so that the equipment isn't stolen.
	2. Make sure the device has password protection so a person logging on outside your program cannot access program information.
	3. Make sure you store any data collected on a secure server. Ideally you will not store any data on the hard drive of the device unless you plan to download or upload it daily to a central location.
	4. Make sure you use encryption and decryption to protect sensitive information for any data transferred.
Internet	1. Make sure users are who they say they are; consider verification procedures identified in Chapter 4 (e.g., mother's maiden name, place of birth).
	2. Make sure the program has password protection so a person cannot log on unless he is enrolled.
	3. Make sure you store any data collected on a secure server, behind a firewall.
	4. Make sure you use encryption and decryption to protect sensitive information for any data transferred.
Mobile phone	1. Make sure you have a way to verify users are who they say they are—see notes in Chapter 4. Ask users to have a password or user ID and a security question (e.g., mother's maiden name, place of birth).
	2. Make sure the program has password protection so a person cannot log on unless he is enrolled.
	3. Make sure you store any data collected on a secure server, behind a firewall.
	4. Make sure you use encryption and decryption to protect sensitive information for any data transferred.

Advances in Statistical Analyses

While a discussion of how to conduct statistical analyses is beyond the scope of this textbook, it is worth considering the types of analyses that may now be open to program evaluators given large and rapidly accruing samples that are possible in evaluating technology-based health promotion. While these methods are certainly useable for other types of health promotion, they often require larger data sets and thus are not always feasible. We introduce each method and give a brief description of the circumstances under which you would use it. At the end of this chapter we also include additional statistical resources for those who wish to explore these options further. We cover factor analysis, structural equation modeling, and path analysis; social network analysis; and hierarchical linear modeling.

Factor Analysis, Structural Equation Modeling, and Path Analysis

Social science researchers often use factor analysis (FA) as a method to reduce large numbers of items used to measure a social construct or concept (e.g., gender norms) to a more manageable number of items, both for the participant and for later inclusion in statistical models. The procedure typically takes a large sample—while there is no agreed-upon minimum number of participants needed to respond to items hypothesized to relate to a construct, the literature has suggested anywhere from 5 to 10 participants responding to each item you wish to include in your FA should allow for an adequate sample. Thus, if you wish to factor analyze a 40-item scale, you should have between 200 and 400 persons (5×40 or 10×40). FA will determine how well each item is related to others on the scale you create, what "subscales" are related, and what items do not seem to fit. The process can help you reduce a potentially cumbersome 40-item scale, for example, to one with many fewer items, since you only keep those items that "hang together" as factors and eliminate others.

FA is used as a first step in structural equation modeling, or SEM, which uses FA as the first step in a two-step ordinary least squares regression (i.e., the measurement model). The factors identified in your FA can then be modeled in the SEM, and unlike a regular regression model, the SEM allows you to determine how well an a priori theoretical model with exogenous variables, endogenous variables (including mediators and moderators), and your primary outcome compares to the actual data from your evaluation. As with FA, SEM usually requires much larger sample sizes than other forms of regression, because of the added degrees of freedom with each item included in your model.

Path analysis is also a type of ordinary least squares regression that allows for temporal sequencing of variables, with exogenous and endogenous variables and mediators and moderators; however, path analyses only include single-item measures or indices, and not factors, so there is no measurement model.

Persons who wish to achieve good levels of reliability and validity with their measures used to document changes in constructs or concepts they hope to affect through their program may want to use factor analysis. SEM and path analyses are often considered excellent tools for developing and testing theories about how individual-level behaviors will be affected by the types of concepts we hope to promote and support in our health behavior programs.

With the advancement of technology-based health promotion we can make strides during the course of program evaluation in determining whether the theoretical frameworks frequently promoted for health behavior change hold true with the population we wish to serve. There are several theoretical constructs that have been shown to consistently impact behavior change in public health research; these include theoretical constructs such as perceived norms (the belief that others like you will perform a given behavior), attitudes (positive or negative feelings associated with performing a behavior), self-efficacy (the confidence to perform a behavior, even given difficult circumstances), and intentions (planning to perform a behavior in the near future; Albarracin, Fishbein, Johnson, & Muellerleile, 2001; Albarracin et al., 2005; Albarracin, Kumkale, & Johnson, 2004; Albarracin et al., 2003). Often these constructs are tested in multivariable models that do not take into account mediation or moderation, may not include all constructs in the same model, or may have been tested with limited samples. By using the larger and potentially diverse samples that you can accrue with technology-based health promotion, your program evaluations can help improve our theories of individual-level behaviors.

Social Network Analysis

Social network analysis (SNA) is a type of analysis that allows us to understand the relationships between multiple people in a sample, and to ascertain relationship density and the level of connectedness for individuals. SNA usually requires much larger samples and, when it is possible to employ, can assist in offering a much better understanding of the actual influence of peer relationships on behaviors, rather than simply the perceived influence heretofore examined through conceptual proxies such as perceived norms (a concept central to the theory of reasoned action and planned behavior; Azjen, 1991). If you have information on how people in your program are connected to one another (e.g., familial relationships, friends, new acquaintances), you can conduct an SNA. Steps in SNA include identification of each ego, or individual, in your data set. You can identify how many people each ego is connected to in the data set—this is called a 2-plex—and how many people are connected to each other. Persons with larger numbers of connections are rank ordered, and emerge as being in a denser part of the network. You can also identify how each 2-plex is connected to other 2-plexes or egos to ascertain closeness, centrality, and density of a network. Rank, centrality, closeness, and density are all variables that can be assessed in statistical models. For example, recent literature shows that relationships between family members and friends documented in this fashion have a statistically significant influence on weight gain (Christakis & Fowler, 2007). Once you have identified the type, number, and density of relationships through SNA, you can include these data in a hierarchical linear model as described below. Note this is a highly simplified explanation of the process. For more detailed information and resources on conducting SNA, see the additional resources listed at the end of this chapter. Table 5.2 outlines some of the key concepts and measures used in social network analyses.

Hierarchical Linear Modeling

The final type of analysis you may consider with a large sample that we will introduce here is hierarchical linear modeling (HLM). Public health researchers have recognized the importance of

Table 5.2   Selected definitions of the concepts and measures used in social network analyses

Concept	Definition
Actor	A person or social entity that engages with networks
Centrality	The position of the "most important" people within networks based on their relationships to others in the network
Cohesion	A measure of how tightly related multiple actors are to one another within networks
Density	Represents the proportion of relationships that an actor has compared to the total within a network
K-plex	Refers to the adjacency between actors—how closely they are tied to other actors in the network
Reciprocity	Denotes whether an actor's relationship with another in the network is reciprocal
Relational tie	The name for the linkage or relationships between actors

considering social, structural, and environmental influences on health outcomes (Bull, Eakin, Reeves, & Kimberly, 2006; Diez-Roux, 1998; Msisha, Kapiga, Earls, & Subramanian, 2008). However, in order to include consideration of these in our evaluation models, we do need larger samples so that we can account for intraclass correlation between individuals within groups that we are comparing (i.e., how much the similarities people share with each other as members of a group will influence other behaviors of interest in comparison with persons external to the group). This isn't often easy to accomplish, particularly at the stage of doing a program evaluation. However, when you do have the sample size adequate to this approach, you can consider HLM. As with the example above, one way your model could include multilevel variables is to include the SNA data from your data set. If you have information on an individual-level outcome, you could include information on that individual outcome along with the social influence of the individual's position in his or her network. Other examples of using multilevel variables in a statistical model include a geographic location (such as a zip code or census tract) or enrollment in a particular school. As with SNA, this description of HLM is limited to consider the types of scenarios in which you could use it for technology-based program evaluation. For more resources on the method, see the end of this chapter.

Dissemination of Findings Using Technology

The evidence on regular increases in Internet and mobile phone access and use across all demographics (Horrigan, 2004; Pew Internet and American Life Project, 2006) suggests that technology-based program evaluation will assist us in several important areas: (a) reaching our program populations, (b) standardizing our material, and (c) rapidly modifying our programs to facilitate sustainability over time. The RE-AIM framework is a framework for program evaluators to assess how well they are doing in each of these important elements. RE-AIM stands for reach, efficacy/effectiveness, adoption, implementation, and maintenance. Reach refers to the number of people eligible for your program who actually enroll. Efficacy is how well your program works for a pilot or small subset of the population; effectiveness is how well the program works when the participants are more diverse. Adoption is the rate at which different organizations will begin using or implementing a program. Implementation refers to the fidelity with which they adhere to program protocols once adopted. Maintenance is whether or not the program can be sustained over time. The framework was developed in response to a concern that our research in chronic illness prevention was focused too singularly on program efficacy—how well our interventions work for a specific study population (Glasgow, 2002; Glasgow, McKay, Piette, & Reynolds, 2001). Traditionally there has been little emphasis on how well our programs work for the general population, how often they are adopted for use by diverse organizations, how often they are implemented with fidelity, and how well they are sustained or maintained over time. Without these important considerations, we do not have elements in place that ensure we can outlay and support the resources needed to sustain effective programs that address public health over the long term.

Assessing each of the RE-AIM elements during our technology-based program evaluations can assist us in determining how well we are achieving the promise of technology to reach more people, reach more diverse audiences, and be able to sustain program effects consistently over time.

Table 5.3 illustrates each element of RE-AIM, considers limitations in standard program evaluation, and then offers suggestions for how technology can address these limitations.

Once your program evaluation has demonstrated that your technology-based health promotion efforts work well, you are well positioned to disseminate program results using technology. Certainly traditional mechanisms to disseminate findings from effective health promotion are still available (e.g., presentations at professional conferences, publication of findings in peer-reviewed journals, and offering information to local and national media). In addition, using the Internet and mobile phones can offer great opportunities to quickly disseminate information about a technology-based program. Consider using electronic mailing lists, websites targeting specific professionals who will be likely program adopters, and personal e-mail address lists. Consider posting information on professional social networking sites, and perhaps posting information about your program on popular video sites such as YouTube.

If you are in a position to be concerned about premature dissemination of information, for example, before important findings are published in a peer-reviewed journal, another option is to offer more detail than what is typically available in a print version of the journal by offering supplementary information about a program online. We are doing that with this book, allowing readers to access up-to-date information about technology-based health promotion and more detail on the programs we discuss in this book (www.sagepub.com/bull).

Table 5.3 Using the RE-AIM framework to consider the advantages of technology-based research

RE-AIM Element	Traditional Program Evaluation	Technology-Based Program Evaluation
Reach	Limited to populations that programs can access face-to-face, through the mail, or over the telephone; while it is possible to reach large numbers, it is difficult to do so quickly.	One of the primary advantages of technology-based program evaluation is that you can reach very large numbers of people quickly with electronic surveys and other data collection tools.
Efficacy/ Effectiveness	Focus is on efficacy; well-established standards for determining efficacy. Effectiveness in program evaluation is less common.	Several technology-based program evaluations have demonstrated efficacy; effectiveness is somewhat more elusive given digital divide and differences in patterns of access to technology across diverse groups.
Adoption and Implementation	Less research is done on what motivates adoption of health promotion programs with efficacy, but research suggests those that are simple, and do not require added staffing or infrastructure, are most likely to be adopted and implemented with fidelity.	Technology-oriented programs and innovations have the advantage of being easy to adopt; they are often self-directed, and do not require additional infrastructure if adopters have existing technology such as computers, Internet, and mobile phones. They also have the advantage of frequently being standardized, so they are delivered the same way each time, maximizing fidelity.
Maintenance	Less is known about maintenance of health promotion programs that have been adopted and implemented with fidelity, but issues such as simplicity, intervention standardization, and staff support appear important.	Technology-oriented health promotion programs are often low in cost once developed and tested, and don't require a lot of additional staff time or other infrastructural support, which can lend itself to facilitating maintenance and sustainability.

WHAT ARE CHALLENGES WE FACE WITH
TECHNOLOGY-BASED PROGRAM EVALUATION?

Conducting Evaluation and Technological Obsolescence

The primary challenge we face in technology-based health promotion is in conducting evaluation at all. Technological advances emerge rapidly and evolve quickly. In the face of new and different technological trends it is difficult to keep pace with programs and to evaluate them appropriately.

Typically it takes time to collect adequate amounts of data from program participants to learn about program effects on participant behaviors or other outcomes. Often program staff will have to follow participants for extended periods (e.g., 1 year) in order to see if program effects can be achieved and sustained. Our challenge is that we may not be able to make use of such learnings—it is possible that by the time we have evidence that a program can work to affect behavior change and that the change can be sustained over time, we will realize that the program itself is obsolete. An example of this has been mentioned earlier—by the time we learned that the Youthnet program could achieve effects—albeit quite small effects—in changing antecedents to risk behavior—the Web 1.0 features used to do so were no longer popular or embraced by the youth targeted for the program (Bull et al., 2008).

Traditional programs will often rely on rapid assessment and evaluation methods in order to make timely adjustments to programs and maximize effects within rapidly changing environments. This option (discussed in detail below) is certainly feasible—given our ability to quickly set up and administer surveys online, for example, we could very quickly make assessments about program effects in the short term. This, however, doesn't resolve the very real issue of obsolescence in the longer term. We still need to explore options for quickly translating useful findings into program practice and translating lessons learned into newly evolving technological strategies. The RE-AIM framework for evaluation described above is one tool that could help us achieve this. If we learn in the short term that a program has an effect, we should simultaneously be looking in the longer term to technological advances to learn if such a program is sustainable given the likely changing technological landscape. Recall that with the RE-AIM framework, we need to focus not only on efficacy but also on adoption—whether organizations would adopt the program, implementation—whether they can maintain fidelity to implementation of the program, and maintenance—whether the program can be sustained over time. In considering the challenge of potential technological obsolescence, we can (a) establish rapid assessment and evaluation procedures to evaluate program effects in the short term while (b) regularly assessing if technological advances or obsolescence will threaten program sustainability in the long run.

Retention of Program Participants

With technology-based programs on computer kiosks or desktops, you don't have a special advantage in terms of regular, always-on access to your participants. Unless you have obtained an e-mail address for them, you will most likely have to communicate with them as you would for any traditional program, either face-to-face when they come in to the program setting or perhaps via the telephone. If your program is delivered on the Internet or mobile phones, you may have the benefit of regular access to your program participants through e-mail, message boards, or text messages.

In both cases, you need to carefully balance your program retention efforts to ensure that you do not induce participant fatigue through excessive contact. If using electronic mechanisms for follow-up, we encourage regular enough contact to remind participants about new content for your program (if it is a multisession program or you wish for them to be engaged multiple times), but not so much as to annoy participants. This also holds true for reminders related to retaining participants in evaluation activities. You should explore in the formative development work devoted to your program the limits that your population identifies as too many reminders or contacts. For some it may be 10 or more; for others it may be no more than 3.

WHAT ARE THE CURRENT AND BEST PRACTICES IN TECHNOLOGY-BASED PROGRAM EVALUATION?

Utilizing Online Surveys

Figures 5.1a and 5.1b illustrate questions designed for a survey on Zoomerang, the data-tracking elements associated with these questions, and an example of the back-end database that houses data as they are collected. The added benefits the online survey programs offer are data storage, management, and transfer. These companies will include a back-end database that allows for storage of all data entered and for transfer of data. Persons using the service can pay for a subscription that allows them to create and post multiple surveys or post one survey for many people.

Utilizing ACASI

Figure 5.2 shows an example of an ACASI survey used in a clinic serving persons living with HIV. The survey was developed as part of the evaluation of a program to increase social support for persons with HIV by connecting them to others with HIV on the Internet. HIV Connect is the name of the website affiliated with The Positive Web project, intended to allow individuals to share strategies for medication adherence, discuss HIV status with friends and family, and connect to a wide array of medical information online about HIV. The Positive Web staff developed an ACASI assessment tool with audio to complete a pre- and postassessment of how well the program contributed to user medication adherence and status disclosure. In Figure 5.2 we include screenshots of the ACASI tool, with the first segment showing the programming needed to produce the questions in the second. The ACASI software is called QDS, developed by the NOVA Research Company.

(Text continues on page 140)

Figure 5.1a Creating a questionnaire in Zoomerang

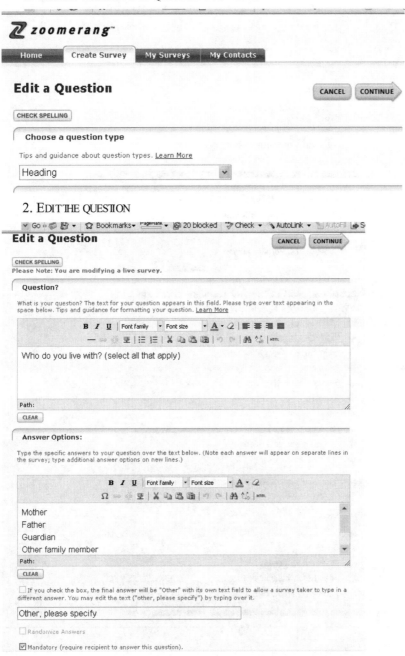

1. CHOOSE WHAT TYPE OF QUESTION YOU WANT.

2. EDIT THE QUESTION

(Continued)

3. The results within Zoomerang:

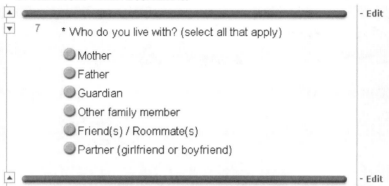

- Edit

7   * Who do you live with? (select all that apply)

- Mother
- Father
- Guardian
- Other family member
- Friend(s) / Roommate(s)
- Partner (girlfriend or boyfriend)

- Edit

4. What it looks like for the viewer:

Study Questionnaire

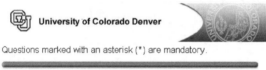 University of Colorado Denver

Questions marked with an asterisk (*) are mandatory.

6   * What is the highest grade level of education you completed?

- Eighth grade or less
- Ninth grade (HS freshman)
- Tenth grade (HS sophomore)
- Eleventh grade (HS junior)
- Twelfth grade (HS senior)
- Some college or technical school
- Associates degree or technical school degree
- College graduate or more
- Don't want to answer

7   * Who do you live with? (select all that apply)

- Mother
- Father
- Guardian
- Other family member
- Friend(s) / Roommate(s)
- Partner (girlfriend or boyfriend)

Figure 5.1b   An example of an online survey program

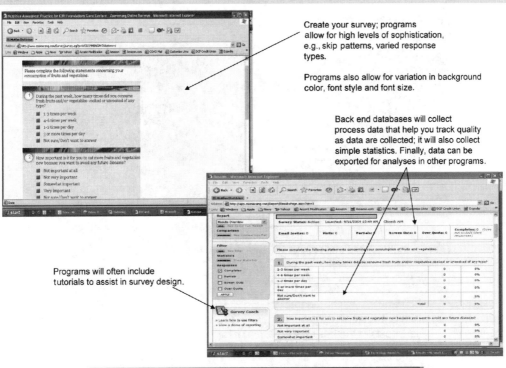

Create your survey; programs allow for high levels of sophistication, e.g., skip patterns, varied response types.

Programs also allow for variation in background color, font style and font size.

Back end databases will collect process data that help you track quality as data are collected; it will also collect simple statistics. Finally, data can be exported for analyses in other programs.

Programs will often include tutorials to assist in survey design.

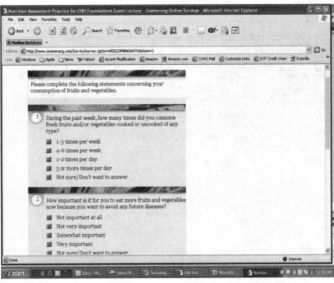

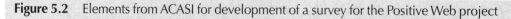

Figure 5.2   Elements from ACASI for development of a survey for the Positive Web project

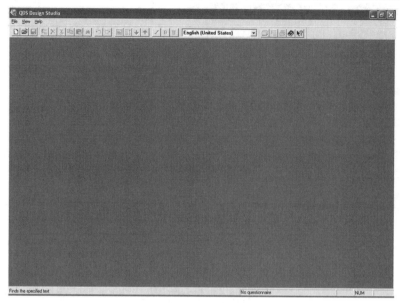

There are a few different environments users can work in, the two main ones being design and execution. This initial shot is of the design studio. From here, users design a brand new questionnaire or modify an existing one.

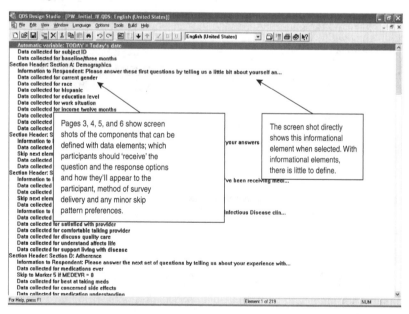

While in the design studio, once an existing questionnaire is selected – a question matrix appears. This is the Positive Web question matrix. In order to modify anything; data elements (actual questions), skip patterns, or informational elements (participant instructions) – users must select the item by double clicking it.

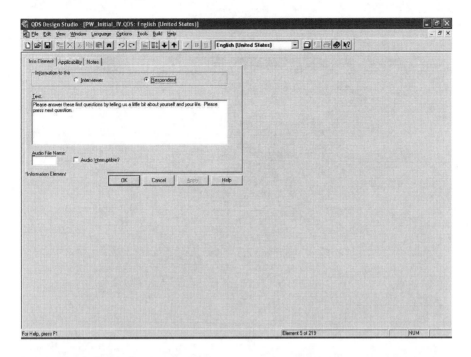

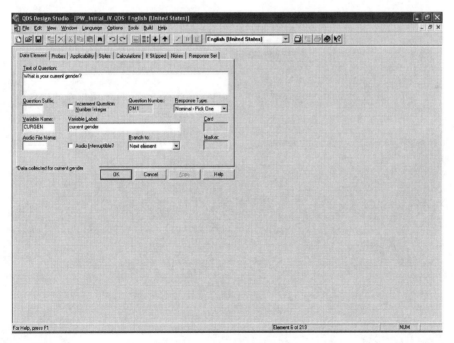

(Continued)

(Continued)

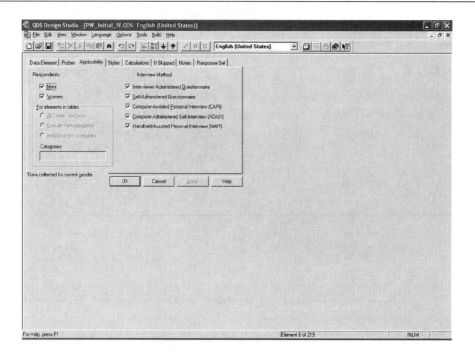

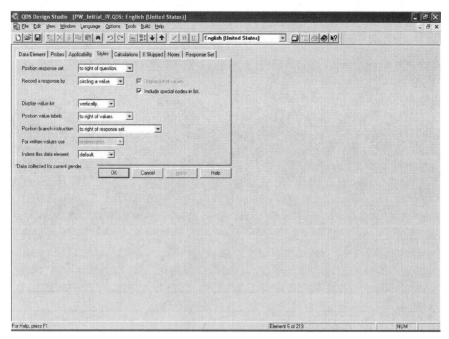

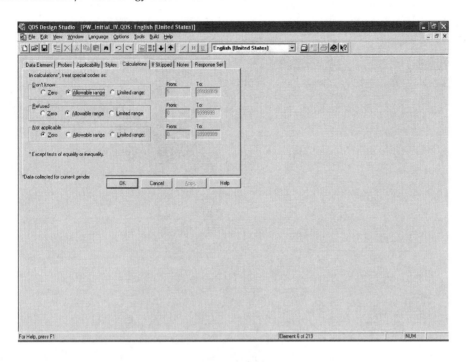

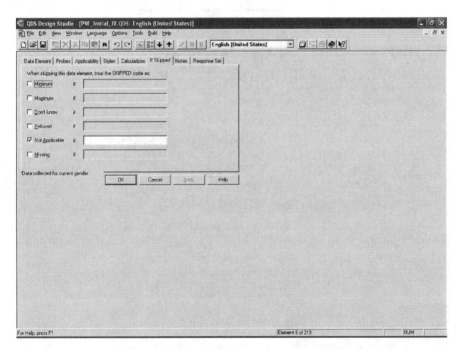

(Continued)

(Continued)

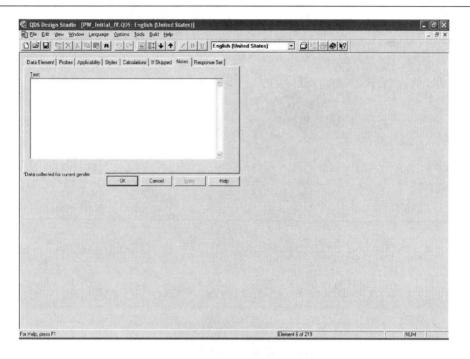

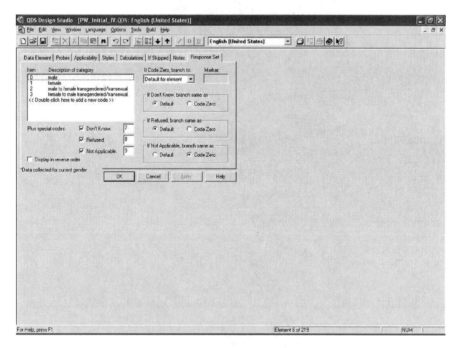

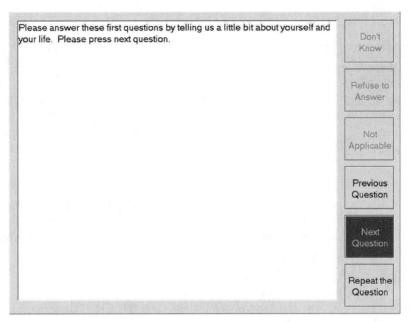

This screen shot shows how participants will see instructional elements. In order to give participants enough time to read the instructions, participants must select 'next question' in order to advance.

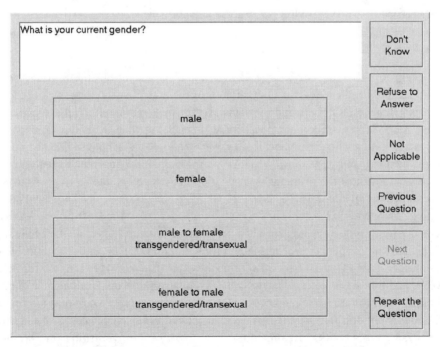

This screen shot shows how participants will see data elements and the response set. Once a response is selected, the program will automatically move on to the next question.

(Text continues from page 130)

As with web- or computer-based survey programs, there are multiple IVR programming systems available for purchase and use—a search online for "interactive voice response" software will reveal many. In Figure 5.3 we offer screenshots of the programming language used to develop the IVR program evaluation tool for the LUCHAR (Latinos Using Cardio Health Actions to Reduce Risk) project (described in detail in Chapter 6). In addition, we include a .wav audio file on the additional materials webpage that you can access as a purchaser of this book (www.sagepub.com/bull). This audio file is a short segment taken from that assessment offering an example of how the IVR system sounds once programmed. The segment was programmed in SurveyBuilder, the application you use to create surveys in SQL Server, and used Visual Studio using Tcl, or "tickle," scripts to run the system. This is a scripting language originally known as Tool Command Language. These Tcl scripts connect to the SQL Server database called "Surveyor_v2i2." The SQL Server database then has stored procedures that send specific information the Tcl scripts are requesting. Tcl scripts can also send information to a stored procedure so that data can be stored.

There are three stages to the Surveyor system:

1. SurveyBuilder is used to store questions, options, and so forth into the SQL database.

2. SQL Server is used to host the questions, options, question logic (e.g., after Question 2 go to Question 3), and question responses.

3. Amanda is used to fetch data from a SQL Server, store data to the SQL Server, and run scripts for logic.

Managing Rapidly Accruing Participants

In the Youthnet trials to use the Internet to promote HIV prevention among young people, we enrolled over 3,000 people in less than one month. At the time of enrollment, we needed to track the date of enrollment for all participants to ensure they were sent a reminder on the correct day to complete follow-up evaluation activities; we also needed to track when they completed their first program assessment to determine if they were eligible for a bonus. We had to monitor participants' activities and steps in the program or the evaluation, in order to determine if they had completed enough of the program or evaluation activity to be eligible to move to the next activity or to receive an incentive.

To achieve these ends, we established a tracking database in Microsoft Office Access™, and we collected a time and date stamp for each program activity and assessment. Thus, we could run queries on all participants who had completed enrollment and baseline evaluation activities on Day 1 and Day 2 of the program; these participants were eligible for a "bonus" incentive in addition to the initial incentive for completing the program evaluation baseline assessment. In addition, those logged on Days 1 and 2, respectively, were queried on Days 60 and 61, respectively, and sent the first of up to three reminders to return to the site for their follow-up evaluation activities. Again, those eligible on Day 60 returning on Day 60 or 61 were again eligible for a bonus incentive along with an incentive for completing the program evaluation follow-up; those eligible on Day 61 completing on Day 61 or 62 were offered the bonus along with the incentive. Figure 4.4 in Chapter 4 offers screenshots from this Access™ database showing sample queries and participant data.

Figure 5.3   Example of programming to develop an interactive voice response (IVR) program

```
# Universal Study for Department of Family Medicine for UCHSC
# 2005-2006, The Amanda Company, all rights reserved.

# This is a universal study application by doing the following:
# 1. It will allow the caller to login and list out what studies are available for them to take.
# 2. Each particular study will have a series of questions that will be TTS'ed to the caller
# 3. The caller will respond either via speech rec or the DTMF equivalent, with the answers stored away.

# The following are configuration settings for this application
#   default_speaker
#   spanish_speaker
#   sr_threshold_number_low
#   sr_threshold_yesno_low
#   sr_threshold_high
#   tmo_dtmf
#   tmo_menu
#   DFM_Universal_User
#   DFM_Universal_Password
#   DFM_Universal_Database
#   DFM_Universal_Facility_GUID
#   DFM_FreeForm_Mailbox
#   DFM_Error_Mailbox
#   DFM_EMPI_Database
#   DFM_Universal_Down_Box
#   DFM_Universal_Use_SR

# The following are the scripts for custom greetings/prompts. They need to be done for each
respective language
set english_prompt_list {
    1 {Sorry, there are currently no available studies to take.}
    2 {or, 9 to cancel this menu, and go back.}
    3 {will be available on,}
    7 {Press or say}
    8 {for}
    9 {If you would like to continue with this survey, press or say, one for yes, or two for no.}
    10 {Sorry, that was an invalid response for this question.}
    11 {For confirmation, did you say?}
    12 {You can come back, and resume this study at a later time.}
    13 {Selected}
    14 {Sorry, there are currently no available surveys to take.}
    15 {This survey is now complete.}
    16 {Sorry, but this survey is currently not available.}
}
```

(Continued)

(Continued)

```
set sr_prompt_list {
  ، 4 {I'm sorry, I did not understand you.}
    5 {I still did not understand you clearly.}
    6 {Did you say?}
}

set db_down_prompt_list {
    1 {I'm sorry, the survey is temporarily unavailable.  Please call back at a later time.}
}


proc load_universal_prompts { box lang list } {
    array set prompts $list

    set_universal_speaker $lang

    foreach grt [array names prompts] {
          set_tts_grt $box $grt $lang $prompts($grt)
    }
}

proc set_universal_speaker { {lang {} } } {
    global taaPriv config universal_speaker

    set universal_speaker $config(default_speaker)

    if [empty $lang] {
          if [info exist taaPriv(language)] {
              set lang $taaPriv(language)
          }
    }

    switch [string tolower $lang] {
          english {
          }
          spanish {
              set universal_speaker $config(spanish_speaker)
          }
    }
}

proc speak_language { text } {
    global universal_speaker
```

```
    if ![empty $text] {
        speak -speaker $universal_speaker $text
    }
}

proc set_tts_grt { box grt lang msg } {
    global universal_speaker

    create_mmo txt
    $txt set_text $msg
    set key "Grt Txt$grt $lang"
    store_mmo -box $box -mmo $txt -private world $key

    create_mmo m
    $m speak -speaker $universal_speaker -format mulaw $msg
    set key "Grt $grt $lang"
    store_mmo -box $box -mmo $m -private world $key
}

proc method_play_universal_tts_grt { box_token grt_token } {
    global %S$box_token %S$grt_token box_data g_has_played_error

    catch {unset g_has_played_error}

    if [empty $box_token] {
        set box $box_data(BOX)
    } else {
        set box [set %S$box_token]
    }

    if [empty $grt_token] {
        set grt $box_data(CUR_GRT)
    } else {
        set grt [set %S$grt_token]
    }

    if [catch {
        play_universal_tts_grt $grt $box
    }] {
        handle_universal_error "method_play_universal_tts_grt grt: $grt, box: $box"
    }
}
```

You can program your systems to flag those files where inconsistencies are found. Figure 5.4 shows some SAS programming to flag and identify inconsistencies related to participant identity, particularly for the circumstances when you are not enrolling participants face-to-face and are looking for an additional step in participant verification.

Maximizing Participant Retention

Tailoring Information at Welcome and Follow-Up

We have the capability of making information and communication tailored to individuals. If people enroll in your program, you can send them personalized letters, e-mails, newsletters, and other types of communication. You can tailor the communication to any number of individual factors—their name, their age, their city. You can also use information they offered at program enrollment about behaviors in tailoring material. A program targeting Spanish- and English-speaking Latinos for chronic illness self-management sent newsletters with

Figure 5.4   Sample programming language and queries to identify potential duplicates among potential program participants

*The following routine checks for possible exact duplicates of the name portion of an email address (any digits prior to the @) or a complete email address duplicate,
If the zip code for the email is also identical, a list of any potential duplicates
will be printed;
*/

```
Data Data;
 input UniqueID 1-2 emailtotal $ 3-21 zipcode 22-27;
cards;
    1   bobsmith@yahoo.com 90201
    2   bobsmith@yahoo.com 90201
    3   bobbysmi@gmail.com 90201
    4   bobbysmi@gmail.com 90301
    5   rsmith@gmail.com   90301
    6   rsmith@gmail.com   90201
    7   bsmith@msn.com     90201
    8   bobsmithe@msn.com  90201
    9   robsmith@gmail.com 90201
   10 robsmith@msn.com     90201
;
run;
        *separate name from the email system;
```

```
Data Data;
        set Data;
        emailname=scan(emailtotal,1,'@');
        emailsystem=scan(emailtotal,2,'@');
        run;


 *email beginning (email name) duplicates;
Proc freq data=Data noprint;
        table emailname/out=namedup;
        run;
Data namedup;
        set namedup;
        if count GT 1 then dupename='yes';
        else dupename='no';
        run;
Proc sort data=Data;   by emailname;run;
Proc sort data=namedup; by emailname;run;
Data namedupall;
        merge namedup Data;
        by emailname;
        run;


 *complete email duplicates;
Proc freq data=Data noprint;
        table emailtotal/out=emailtot;
        run;
Data emailtot;
        set emailtot;
        if count GT 1 then dupetot='yes';
        else dupetot='no';
        run;
Proc sort data=Data;    by emailtotal;run;
Proc sort data=emailtot; by emailtotal;run;
Data emailtotall;
        merge emailtot Data;
        by emailtotal;
        run;
        *merge duplicate files;
Proc sort data=namedupall; by uniqueID;run;
Proc sort data=emailtotall; by uniqueID;run;
Data MyDataDupes;
        merge emailtotall namedupall;
        by UniqueID;
        run;


Data MyDataDupes;
        set MyDataDupes;
        if dupename='yes' or dupetot='yes' then anydiscrep='yes';
```

(Continued)

```
        else anydiscrep='no';
        run;


        *Zip code duplicates if have any discrepancies;
Proc freq data=MyDataDupes noprint;
        table zipcode/out=check4dups;
        where anydiscrep='yes';
        run;
Data dupezip;
        set check4dups;
        if count GT 1 then dupezip='yes';
        else dupezip='no';
        run;
Proc sort data=Data;        by zipcode;run;
Proc sort data=dupezip; by zipcode;run;
Data dupezipall;
        merge dupezip Data;
        by zipcode;
        run;


Proc sort data=MyDataDupes;        by uniqueID;run;
Proc sort data=dupezipall;        by uniqueID;run;
Data DupesFinal;
        merge dupezipall MyDataDupes;
        by UniqueID;
        run;
ods rtf file='H:\MySpaceAnalysis.SRB\SASprgm\SheanaTestOutPut.rtf';
Proc print data=DupesFinal;
        var uniqueID emailtotal dupename dupetot dupezip;
        where dupezip='yes' and anydiscrep='yes';
        run;
ods rtf close;
run;
```
****

SAMPLE OUTPUT

****

Obs	UniqueID	emailtotal	dupename	dupetot	dupezip
1	1	bobsmith@yahoo.com	yes	yes	yes
2	2	bobsmith@yahoo.com	yes	yes	yes
5	5	rsmith@gmail.com	yes	yes	yes
6	6	rsmith@gmail.com	yes	yes	yes
9	9	robsmith@gmail.com	yes	no	yes
10	10	robsmith@msn.com	yes	no	yes

*This routine only checks for exact email matches. Any variations in names will be missed.

For further information on an algorithm to search for non-exact email duplicates please refer to:
'Using Edit-Distance Functions to Identify "Similar" E-Mail Addresses', Howard Schreier, US Department of Commerce, Washington DC, SUGI 29 Proceedings, Montréal, Canada, May 9-12, 2004.

information tailored to the specific dietary concerns they named (e.g., "Dear Senora Ortiz: This month this newsletter will focus on tips to replace lard with vegetable oil in cooking").

Facilitate Regular—but Not Overly Frequent—Communication

When using technology-based methods to communicate with program participants you should rely on information obtained directly from participants above all other sources on preferences for the types of communication and frequency of communication. Some audiences will feel comfortable with multiple reminders or even multiple reminders daily; others will not and may even report you as being in violation of terms of service if you do so, say, on an Internet site. Be sure to ask potential participants what their preferences would be for communication delivery and frequency.

Using Incentives to Facilitate Retention in Program Evaluation

Often, persons evaluating a program will offer participants in the evaluation a small incentive. This approach is common, although likely regulated by an institutional review board, or IRB, if you are under such jurisdiction. Incentives can be, but are not always, monetary. They are intended as a thank-you for the time involved in the evaluation effort and should not be coercive. IRBs regularly assess research programs to assess whether steps for enrollment and retention are coercive, so if you question if your incentive is, please contact a member of your local IRB or of an IRB from a nearby university or research institute.

Nonmonetary incentives can include small gifts (e.g., T-shirts, hats, key chains, coffee mugs). They are intended to acknowledge participation and offer gratitude. If you use these types of incentives in a technology-based program, you will have to include plans to obtain physical mailing addresses for all participants and budget for postage to mail them unless you are able to distribute them at the time of enrollment or during a face-to-face interaction.

Other nonmonetary incentives that have monetary value but are not cash that are popular and simple to deliver using technology include online gift cards. These are available from many vendors online and can often be purchased in bulk. Gift cards for sites where you can purchase books, music, videos, and other goods are popular. The advantages of using online gift cards as incentives are multiple. First, you can order a predetermined number for a predetermined amount (e.g., 500 cards valued at $5 each), and each gift has a unique serial number. This can be instantly transmitted to an eligible participant, and tracked to see if it has been redeemed. This limits the ability of participants to redeem multiple certificates or suggest that they lost or didn't receive it. It also removes security concerns you may have for your staff in handling cash or other gifts. Finally, you can tailor your gift card options for users based on their preferences. If you are working with a young audience, for example, participants may wish to receive online music; members of an older audience may prefer having access to a site where they can choose from a variety of items.

You can also use a third-party pay system such as PayPal to transfer cash for participants. This allows you to avoid direct contact with cash or information about participant bank accounts that could compromise security. However, this approach does have a drawback in that users of a third-party pay account will usually have to have a credit card or bank account that can be used to establish and utilize the account. This may limit opportunities for incentives if working with young people or people who may not have a checking account or credit card.

If you do use technology-based incentives as an approach to increase retention in program evaluation activities, one caution is to manage the expectations of participants. If you have hundreds or even thousands of program enrollees, you will likely need to verify that each person is indeed eligible for an incentive before you can release it. With a large volume of participants, this may mean notifying them that they can expect their incentive within 7 days or 5 days, or within a time frame you are comfortable will exceed the actual time it will take for you to process their data.

Finally, it is important to recognize that in many settings the use of incentives is not common, although it may be in U.S. settings, particularly for research-related evaluations. In settings or circumstances where incentives are not used or not possible, technology-based and traditional programs alike often utilize moral appeal, user agreements, and friendly reminders to encourage participation. Much on these strategies for traditional program evaluation has been detailed elsewhere and can be applied to the technology-based program context (Amthauer, Gaglio, Glasgow, & King, 2003; Ashing-Giwa, 1999; Brown, Long, Weitz, & Milliken, 2000; Brown, Fonad, Basen-Engquist, & Tortolero-Luna, 2000; Caban, 1995; Dancy, Wilbur, Talashek, Bonner, & Barnes-Boyd, 2004; Dennis & Neese, 2000; Ford et al., 2008; Gauthier & Clarke, 1999; Gilliss et al., 2001; Harachi, Catalano, & Hawkins, 1997; Lewis et al., 1998).

Retention strategies employed in one Internet-based HIV prevention program included a tailored welcome letter, short but informative e-mails at two times during the program, and no more than three e-mail reminders to complete a follow-up assessment. While these appeared acceptable to participants, perhaps the most effective strategy for retention in the program evaluation for this 18- to 24-year-old group of experienced Internet users was to offer a "bonus" incentive to persons who completed their follow-up evaluations within 48 hours of being eligible to do so. The majority of those completing the follow-up assessment did so within the 48-hour window (Bull, Pratte, Whitesell, Reitemeijer, & McFarlane, 2009).

WHAT ARE EMERGING TRENDS IN TECHNOLOGY-BASED PROGRAM EVALUATION?

Use of Geographic Information Systems (GIS)

Geographic information systems are more and more frequently integrated into evaluations of technology-based as well as traditional programs. We are just beginning to see a variety of applications of GIS to health-related programs, and we anticipate that new applications will be forthcoming in the next few years. For example, communities in South Africa used qualitative methods to describe their perceptions of how tuberculosis was concentrated in their communities; researchers were able to map "hot spots" for tuberculosis and quantify epidemiologic high-risk areas using GIS (Murray et al., 2009). Other investigators used GIS to identify community locations that could be ideal for delivery of prevention information related to breast cancer (Alcaraz, Kreuter, & Bryan, 2009).

GIS not only is used for technology-based programs but also represents a process of using technology to inform traditional research. Researchers from the University of Colorado did this in a project assessing the physical environment in a newly completed urban renewal effort. Their objective was to assess the opportunities for using the newly redesigned and renovated environment of the former Stapleton International Airport in Denver for physical activity and to access fresh fruits and vegetables. The urban communities surrounding the urban renewal project are lower-income communities, and quite diverse— they comprise new immigrant communities from Mexico, displaced refugee communities from Somalia and Sudan, long-term working-class African American communities, and long-term working-class Latino and Chicano communities. All these communities "ring" or surround the urban renewal project, and the University of Colorado assessed the physical environment of the project when completed to determine the barriers and facilitators in the physical environment to "ring" community member access to and use of the area for more physical activity and use of grocery stores and the farmers' market for accessing fresh fruits and vegetables.

To accomplish the project, researchers first collected data on the physical environment of all the ring communities and of the completed Stapleton area. Using the concept of physical incivilities and public courtesies, they documented housing conditions, visible signs of both positive (e.g., neighborhood watch, parks, trash cans, public invitations for social events) and negative elements (e.g., excessive graffiti, bars on windows, excessive numbers of liquor stores, check cashing stores) in each area. See Figure 5.5 for an example of their data collection sheet. They were able to document these physical incivilities and public courtesies and map them using GIS to indicate concentrations of areas where physical activity may be easier and more inviting and where fresh and healthy food was available. They could then share these maps in the community to encourage ring community members to avail themselves of the redesigned Stapleton environment (Caughy, O'Campo, & Patterson, 2001; Cohen et al., 2000, 2003; Edmonds, Baranowski, Baranowski, Cullen, & Myres, 2001; D. Main, personal communication, January 2008).

Persons delivering technology-based health promotion may wish to consider the influence of place on the effectiveness of their program. Do users living in one area benefit more from the program than users in another area, for example? Is there an association between living in a large city and program outcomes?

As with social network analyses, an in-depth discussion of GIS analysis for public health is beyond the scope of this book. However, in this section we can consider the typical types of assessments that have been done using GIS and consider how they could be used in program evaluation for your technology-based work. We also offer additional resources on GIS analyses for readers who wish to pursue this topic in greater depth.

Examples of Assessments Considering the Relationship Between Place and Health Outcomes

Multiple studies have shown a relationship between place and health (Graves, 2008). One example, from the Kaiser Family Foundation, examined the significance and the size of community impact on smoking, alcohol consumption, dietary fat consumption, and seat belt use. The researchers showed a small community effect on an individual's health behavior, with large differences in prevalence of these behaviors among communities. Investigators concluded

Figure 5.5 Data collection sheet for documentation of physical incivilities and public courtesies that can be used with GIS to document environmental supports for and barriers to physical activity and healthy eating

Auditor: ____________ NEIGHOBORHOOD ID:__________ Date:______________Time: _____am/pm

CENSUS TRACT#: ______BLOCK GRP#:________ BLOCK#: ________ DATA ENTRY: Date:__________ Rec # ____

# ______	# ______	# ______	# ______	# ______	# ______
name: ______	**name:** ______	**name:** ______	**name:** ______	**name:** ______	**name:** ______
H RH MO A HO MU	**H RH MO A HO MU**	**H RH MO A HO MU**	**H RH MO A HO MU**	**H RH MO A HO MU**	**H RH MO A HO MU**
Biz (type) ______	**Biz (type)** ______	**Biz (type)** ______	**Biz (type)** ______	**Biz (type)** ______	**Biz (type)** ______
NonRes^{oth} ______	**NonRes**^{oth} ______	**NonRes**^{oth} ______	**NonRes**^{oth} ______	**NonRes**^{oth} ______	**NonRes**^{oth} ______
BW Y / N	**BW** Y / N	**BW** Y / N	**BW** Y / N	**BW** Y / N	**BW** Y / N
Graf None / 1 tag / 2+tags	**Graf** None / 1 tag / 2+tags	**Graf** None / 1 tag / 2+tags	**Graf** None / 1 tag / 2+tags	**Graf** None / 1 tag / 2+tags	**Graf** None / 1 tag / 2+tags
Cond: E / F / P / D	**Cond:** E / F / P / D	**Cond:** E / F / P / D	**Cond:** E / F / P / D	**Cond:** E / F / P / D	**Cond:** E / F / P / D
Porch / Border high low	**Porch / Border** high low	**Porch / Border** high low	**Porch / Border** high low	**Porch / Border** high low	**Porch / Border** high low
Secur: WB / S / Dog	**Secur: WB / S / Dog**	**Secur: WB / S / Dog**	**Secur: WB / S / Dog**	**Secur: WB / S / Dog**	**Secur: WB / S / Dog**
FYD/ Grounds: Y / N	**FYD/ Grounds:** Y / N	**FYD/ Grounds:** Y / N	**FYD/ Grounds:** Y / N	**FYD/ Grounds:** Y / N	**FYD/ Grounds:** Y / N
Landscape / None	**Landscape / None**	**Landscape / None**	**Landscape / None**	**Landscape / None**	**Landscape / None**
Litter: Y / N	**Litter:** Y / N	**Litter:** Y / N	**Litter:** Y / N	**Litter:** Y / N	**Litter:** Y / N
YD Cond: E / F / P / D	**YD Cond:** E / F / P / D	**YD Cond:** E / F / P / D	**YD Cond:** E / F / P / D	**YD Cond:** E / F / P / D	**YD Cond:** E / F / P / D
rack: Y / N	**rack:** Y / N	**rack:** Y / N	**rack:** Y / N	**rack:** Y / N	**rack:** Y / N
parked: Y / N	**parked:** Y / N	**parked:** Y / N	**parked:** Y / N	**parked:** Y / N	**parked:** Y / N
Vac Lot Y / N	**Vac Lot** Y / N	**Vac Lot** Y / N	**Vac Lot** Y / N	**Vac Lot** Y / N	**Vac Lot** Y / N
VL Cond: E / F / P / D	**VL Cond**: E / F / P / D	**VL Cond**: E / F / P / D	**VL Cond**: E / F / P / D	**VL Cond**: E / F / P / D	**VL Cond**: E / F / P / D

Alleyways: Clean Y / N Condition: E/ F/ P **Ax:** None Stand/Sit/Parked Walk Play Oth work ________ Oth Social ________ Oth Illicit ________ ( )

Neigh Watch: ☐ Yes ☐ No **Lighting:** None Corners Mid-block **Threats:** None Scary dogs Loiter DisordYouth Gangs Drunk or Disord Adults (____________)

People: None Workers <12y Teens Adults Seniors **Ax:** None Stand/Sit/Parked Walk Run Bike Play Garden Oth work Oth Social Oth Illicit

Venue: Is ax performed in area designated for that ax? ☐ Yes ( ) ☐ No ( )

Opp PA: Off road Bike/walking trail Track Tennis Basketball Playing Field Pool Playground Golf Community Garden Other: ________

Park: Pocket Destination **Condition:** E / F / P / D

Park Amenities: Trails Track Tennis Basketball Playing Field Pool Playground Picnic Community Garden Lake Other: ____

Bus or Train stop: Y / N

Bench Y / N **Shelter** Y / N **Clean** Y / N

Condition: E / F / P

Street **Continuity of Walk:** Winding, disjointed / L-blocks, mostly direct routes / S-blocks, grid, direct routes

Curb Cuts 1) Y / N 2) Y / N 3) Y / N 4) Y / N

lane marked: Y / N **route:** Y / N

Traffic Posted Speed ___ **Volume** Light / Med / Heavy_

***Intersection:** Street Names ________/________/________ **Intersect. Geometry**: ╦ / ╬ / > 4way

Traff. Control: None / Yield / Stop (flashing red) / All-Ways / Light / Roundabout

Crosswalk Features: None / Marked Crosswalk / Pedestrian Overpass / Median / Refuge Island / Countdown / Audible sig.

 # Lanes to Cross: (widest leg): _____ **Time to Cross** (widest leg): # ____ seconds = + flashing

Do Curb Cuts connect at crossing? ☐ All corners ☐ Some corners ☐ None

Sidewalk None Intermittent Continuous **Cond.:** E / F / P / D **Width** <3 ft / 3-5 ft / >5 ft **Loc** Abuts Road ≤3 ft from curb >3 ft from curb **Perm Obstr** None / Part / Total

Walk Summary: **Safe Traff:** Safe / Caut / Unsafe **Safe Crime:** Secure/ Wary / Threatened **Aesthetics:** E F P **Challenges:** Easy / Mod / Diff

that there is potentially a strong likelihood that unique features in a community will influence health behaviors (Diehr et al., 1993). To accomplish these analyses, researchers can use hierarchical linear modeling, as with social networks, to consider location a variable external to the individual. Individuals are then nested within geographic locations, and the influence of place is taken into account. See more in the resources section below for references on conducting geospatial analyses and HLM.

These examples are of real-world settings rather than virtual settings. What we do not know is whether real-world location (e.g., zip code, city, region) has any influence on program participants who interact through technology-based programs. There are no studies published that explore these types of relationships. In a study delivered on the social networking site MySpace, researchers have completed a preliminary investigation to examine if there is an association between the zip code of the MySpace profiles they have viewed ($N = 44,836$) and characteristics of profiles; for example, are girls in Atlanta, Georgia, more likely to have privacy controls on their pages? Are boys in New York more likely to mention money and/or drugs on their profiles? (Breslin, 2010).

Analysis of Programs on Social Networking Sites Online

Readers may be familiar with literature that explicates the associations between real-world social networks and health outcomes. For example, Christakis and Fowler (2007) showed that the increase in obesity over time in members of the Framingham Heart Study was linked to their position in social networks; women were more likely to be obese if they had a sister who was also obese. Men were more likely to be obese if they had a good friend who was also obese. Similar research has been done on HIV and other sexually transmitted infection (STI) risk behaviors in social networks. Among injection drug users, persons who interacted with others in their social network who shared needles were more likely to also share needles. Persons in a network who had close ties to others with a high number of sex partners were more likely to have an STI than others whose ties were more distal (De, Jolly, Cox, & Boivin, 2006; Wylie, Shah, & Jolly, 2007).

To date, there are no known studies that have been published examining the relationship between online social networks and health outcomes. Of interest in social network analyses are both the overall properties of a network—for example, the number of members in a network, the types of ties, and the density of the network—and the individuals within the network and whether their position in a network and the types of relationships they have with others within networks is related to outcomes of interest. While this text is not intended to go into depth with regard to social network analyses, we will present some basic network concepts and consider how we can evaluate the relationship between various overall and individual network characteristics with regard to health.

The opportunities to explore the direct or indirect influences of social network characteristics within health promotion programs are numerous. If exploring overall network characteristics, you could use hierarchical linear modeling to nest individuals within networks, provided you have descriptors of overall network characteristics. For example, you may be interested in exploring whether being a part of a tightly cohesive network with many reciprocal ties has a positive association with self-reported sense of social support. If you are interested in exploring the relationship between overall network density and individual-level outcomes, then it would be necessary to nest each individual within his or her network; this assumes that you have individuals in your program who are members of varied and diverse networks.

When exploring influences of social networks on health, you may also look at individual network characteristics and consider these characteristics as independent variables in regression models. For example, you might examine the total number of ties individuals have, their position within the network (i.e., their "ranking" or k-plex score), or whether their ties are reciprocal, all as separate independent variables to consider your outcome of interest. This presentation of possible factors to study is an overview only; more resources on how to conduct social network analyses are identified at the end of the chapter.

In addition to the types of inquiries that can be pursued to analyze networks, program evaluators may be interested in the types of software available for analyzing networks. There are two that will be introduced and briefly described here: UCINET, which is a statistical program designed to define network characteristics; and Pajek, which is a software program intended to assist users in visualizing networks and network characteristics. UCINET is often used as the precursor to Pajek, where data on networks are run initially and then exported to Pajek for visualization. We include information on how to access more resources for conducting social network analyses, and for using UCINET and Pajek, at the end of this chapter.

SUMMARY

In this chapter we have covered details related to program evaluation for technology-based health promotion efforts. Most of the topics covered here are relevant to consider regardless of the type of modality you are using for your technology-based program. In the first part of the chapter we offered some considerations for the type of program evaluation design you might choose given the population you are working with, the modality you have chosen, and the circumstances of your program. Recall that technology-based approaches may allow you to collect data from much larger samples than previously possible for your program and may also allow you to collect data from persons not directly involved in your program, so as to facilitate the use of comparison groups for program evaluation.

When collecting data using technology-based methods, you have the opportunity to automate much if not all of the process. This will facilitate reduction or elimination of the need for cumbersome paper-and-pencil evaluation instruments in field settings; it can also reduce or eliminate the need for data entry if users are entering data directly into a program. Such an approach also offers the benefit of being able to build in data cleaning and verification procedures. When constructing automated data collection procedures you can automate skip patterns, and require persons to answer each question before proceeding to reduce or eliminate missing data (potentially allowing them to select "don't want to answer" as an option).

You can use technology-based methods to facilitate retention of program participants in your evaluation activities. During the formative process in which you develop your program, you should consult your potential audience members to ascertain their level of tolerance for electronic reminders related to program evaluation activities, delivered through mechanisms such as e-mail, instant messages, SMS, or posting on a social networking site. Other mechanisms to facilitate participant retention in program evaluation activities include the use of incentives— things such as online gift certificates, or cash through third-party payers.

While the advantages of technology-based program delivery may include the rapid accrual of large samples to your program, this also carries with it the challenges associated with management of large data sets. Automating this process where possible using databases for tracking participant activities will reduce errors in program delivery. In addition, taking time up front to make sure all program evaluation data collection activities are yielding data to a back-end database in the manner anticipated will save you challenges in data management once your evaluation begins.

While the discussion of analytic techniques is beyond the scope of this textbook, we offered several examples of analysis opportunities that have opened up given the larger samples that can be reached through technology-based health promotion. We closed the chapter with attention to the promise of technology-based health promotion to expand the reach, effectiveness, adoption, implementation, and maintenance of our health promotion efforts. Table 5.4 summarizes key terms associated with evaluation of technology-based health promotion presented in this chapter. Table 5.5 offers a summary of the unique opportunities and challenges related to program evaluation using technology.

Table 5.4 Key terms associated with evaluation of technology-based health promotion

Term	Definition
Automated data collection	Data collection for evaluation using computer-based technology.
Beta testing	Pretesting all automated data collection methods to ensure they are capturing and storing data as intended and they are easy for participants to use.
Experimental and quasi-experimental program evaluation	Program evaluation that uses a control group that is randomized (experimental) or not randomized but similar to the program participants (quasi-experimental)—called a nonequivalent comparison group.
Nonexperimental program evaluation	Program evaluation without a comparison group or randomization of participants. Can include a pre- and posttest design for program participants or a time-series design.
Online gift cards	Redeemable for purchase of items on the Internet at specific sites. You can purchase a bulk of gift certificates in a set denomination (e.g., $1, $5, $10) and then send participants the serial number for their use on that site.

(Continued)

(Continued)

Term	Definition
PayPal or third-party payer	Participants can be sent money through a third party using a secure server online. They will likely have to establish an account with the third-party payer, which often requires revealing their bank information and/or credit card number.
Rapidly accruing samples	When conducting technology-based health promotion it is possible to reach many more people than otherwise would be engaged in a program. Planning for and addressing issues that arise with rapidly accruing samples is key.
Technology-based program adoption	The rate at which different organizations will adopt and use your technology-based health promotion program.
Technology-based program efficacy and effectiveness	Efficacy—how well your program works (what impact it has) for an initial group (either a pilot group or one involved in an experimental or quasi experimental evaluation). Effectiveness—how well these outcomes are sustained when program participants are more numerous and diverse.
Technology-based program implementation	The degree of fidelity program adopters maintain to the originally evaluated program.
Technology-based program maintenance	How long the technology-based program can be sustained and continued over time.
Technology-based program reach	The number of people actually enrolled in your program divided by the total number likely eligible for your program.

In conclusion, evaluation of technology-based health promotion programs has great promise to streamline and facilitate our evaluation efforts. We have the potential to reach larger numbers of people with our technology-based programs, and can evaluate how well this contributes to improved health outcomes, provided we pay close attention to using rigorous evaluation methods. Many of our evaluation activities can be automated and standardized. This can greatly reduce human errors and costs for staff associated with evaluation activities.

Table 5.5 Unique opportunities and challenges related to program evaluation using technology

Issue	Opportunities to be realized when using technology	Challenges you may face when using technology
Beta testing	You can easily and quickly determine if data collection is going as intended and back-end data storage is working well through beta testing in-house.	Beta testing should occur with participants from your target audience, not only program staff, to ensure that intended participants understand all questions.
Data analysis	Having access to large samples means opportunities for more sophisticated analyses of measures through factor analysis; analyses of mediators and moderators through path analysis and SEM; analyses of nested data through HLM; and analysis of social networks.	Using these analyses requires advanced statistical training in social science that will likely require hiring outside experts for program evaluation.
Data cleaning/ coding	You can automate consistency checks, quickly identify missing data, and program data collection instruments to require responses to avoid missing data; you may be able to identify fraudulent responses or participants using these automated processes.	Participants may still be able to use deception when engaged with the evaluation; you may need to require proof of identity through verbal or visual inspection.
Data collection	You can automate your data collection processes; participants can access data collection tools online or on the phone using voice or text or touch screen surveys.	Digital divide means all participants may not have equal access to online tools; may need to work to establish rapport needed for participants to feel confident their data are secure; screens on phones are very small and difficult to read; participants may not appreciate automated voice accompanying IVR.
Data management	As with data cleaning and coding, having automated systems will facilitate data management from rapidly accruing samples; you can establish automated reminder systems to generate e-mail or phone reminders to participants to complete evaluation tasks as needed.	Without the opportunity to establish face-to-face rapport, you may face higher attrition from programs than is typical in traditional health promotion. You will need to identify and try out strategies to keep participants engaged and willing to complete your evaluation tasks.
Incentives	You can quickly link participants to online incentives such as gift cards; rewards are immediate; you can also use third-party payer systems to offer cash rewards and incentives.	Third-party payers may require users to have a credit card to establish an account, limiting access to persons without credit cards; incentives via gift certificates may not be of equal appeal to all audiences.
Participant confidentiality	Participant confidentiality can be maximized through data encryption; through Transport Layer Security; and by using firewalls and password protection.	Ongoing sophistication and evolution in hacking means you will have to continually ensure you are using the most up-to-date security measures to ensure protection of confidential information.

? CONCLUDING QUESTIONS

Following are questions to consider for your own technology-based program evaluation:

1. What type of design will be the most acceptable to my audience? Do I have access to a comparison group to consider any changes observed among program participants in contrast to persons not participating? Will I realistically be able to connect with, recruit, and follow-up with my participants multiple times in order to evaluate program outcomes?

2. Considering the modality I have chosen to deliver my technology-based health promotion program, is this the best modality to use to conduct an evaluation? If so, what limitations should I consider for length of program assessment?

3. What approaches can I realistically use to motivate participation in program evaluation activities? Are incentives appropriate? If delivering a program with little to no face-to-face interaction, what types of incentives would participants find appealing?

4. What types of systems do I need to develop to track evaluation activities, data collection, and data quality?

5. Are there new or different analytic techniques that are possible to employ in assessing evaluation outcomes?

6. How will my program use technology to (a) reach more and more diverse populations, (b) facilitate adoption of effective approaches for health promotion, (c) facilitate standardization and fidelity of program delivery, and (d) facilitate long-term program use?

CHAPTER EXERCISE

In this exercise, you will build on work done in previous chapters. Consider a simple pre- and posttest to evaluate program outcomes among those who participated.

1. What are the primary outcomes you expect from the program?
   a. What are the measures you will utilize to demonstrate these outcomes?

2. What are other important factors that will influence outcomes?
   a. Will you measure demographics?
   b. Are there any factors that you anticipate will mediate or moderate your outcomes?

3. Construct a survey using one of the software programs available—such as SurveyMonkey or Zoomerang.

4. Write your plan for evaluation, including information on what you plan to do, what your evaluation questions and measures are, and how you will recruit and engage participants in your evaluation.

ADDITIONAL RESOURCES

Listed here are additional resources related to software programs that are available for automated survey design, either for use on stand-alone computers or the Internet. We also offer resources for practice in analytic techniques identified in this chapter. Finally, we offer a resource for program evaluators interested in getting more information about RE-AIM and program evaluation using this framework.

Data Collection Resources

Resource	Description
Computer-based data collection http://www.snapsurveys.com/ http://www.freepatentsonline.com/4954699.html http://www.apian.com/index.php	These are resources that can be used to develop automated survey systems for use on the computer (although not exclusively—some can also assist in web-based surveys). They can include audio to assist participants as they self-administer a computer-based questionnaire or survey instrument.
IVR (interactive voice response) programs http://www.pronexus.com/english/view.asp?x=1	These are programs that can be purchased and used to develop an automated telephone-based survey for program participants.
http://www.coolsoftllc.com/articles/Interactive-Voice-Recognition.htm http://www.voiceguide.com/?gclid=CObW_NTcrJgCFQECGgodqnfHmA	
Online data collection systems http://www.surveymonkey.com/ http://www.questionpro.com/web-based-survey-software.html http://www.magicsurveytool.com/ http://zoomerang.com/online-surveys/ http://www.vovici.com/	These are resources that can be used to develop and self-administer an online survey or questionnaire. They often will include tools to assist in database design for storing data, and for sending data over the web using a secure server.

Data Analysis Resources

Books, Articles, and Other Peer-Reviewed Literature

Resource	Description
Structural equation modeling, factor analysis, and path analysis Bollen, K., & Long J. S. (Eds.). (1993). *Testing structural equation models.* Newbury Park, CA: Sage.	These are textbook resources to assist in learning about and becoming proficient in using SEM, FA, and path analysis for data analysis.

Resource	Description
Kline, R. (2004). *Principles and practice of structural equation modeling* (2nd ed.). New York: Guilford Press.	
Raudenbush S., Bryk, T., Cheong, Y. F., & Congdon, R. T., Jr. (2004). *Hierarchical linear and nonlinear modeling*. Lincolnwood, IL: Scientific Software International.	These are textbook resources to assist in learning about and becoming proficient in using HLM for data analysis.

 ## Websites

Resource	Description
http://www.statsoft.com/textbook/stsepath.html http://www.statmodel.com/	These are web resources to assist in learning about and becoming proficient in using SEM, FA, and path analysis for data analysis.
Social network analysis http://www.orgnet.com/sna.html http://www.analytictech.com/networks/ http://www.faculty.ucr.edu/~hanneman/nettext/ http://www.analytictech.com/ucinet/ucinet.htm http://vlado.fmf.uni-lj.si/pub/networks/pajek/	These are software programs to assist in learning about and becoming proficient in using SNA for data analysis.
Hierarchical linear modeling http://www.ssicentral.com/ http://pareonline.net/getvn.asp?v=7&n=1	These are software programs to assist in learning about and becoming proficient in using HLM for data analysis.

RE-AIM Evaluation Resource

Resource	Description
RE-AIM http://www.re-aim.org/	This website is a resource for professionals who use the RE-AIM framework in evaluation. It offers advice for how to incorporate RE-AIM into your evaluation and how to measure each element, and also offers links to articles on programs that have successfully used RE-AIM.

Note: The resources we identify here are selected from a large number that are available for you to consider, and by no means are they representative or exhaustive. Consider researching each option in more detail.

All websites noted here are hot-linked at www.sagepub.com/bull; at this site you will also find newer resources relevant to the material in this and other chapters.

REFERENCES

Albarracin, D., Fishbein, M., Johnson, B. T., & Muellerleile, P. A. (2001). Theories of reasoned action and planned behavior as models of condom use: A meta-analysis. *Psychological Bulletin, 127,* 142–161.

Albarracin, D., Gillette, J. C., Earl, A. N., Glasman, L. R., Durantini, M. R., & Ho, M. H. (2005). A test of major assumptions about behavior change: A comprehensive look at the effects of passive and active HIV-prevention interventions since the beginning of the epidemic. *Psychological Bulletin, 131,* 856–897.

Albarracin, D., Kumkale, G. T., & Johnson, B. T. (2004). Influences of social power and normative support on condom use decisions: A research synthesis. *AIDS Care, 16,* 700–723.

Albarracin, D., McNatt, P. S., Klein, C. T., Ho, R. M., Mitchell, A. L., & Kumkale, G. T. (2003). Persuasive communications to change actions: An analysis of behavioral and cognitive impact in HIV prevention. *Health Psychology, 22,* 166–177.

Alcaraz, K., Kreuter, M., & Bryan, R. (2009). Use of GIS to identify optimal settings for cancer prevention and control in African American communities. *Preventive Medicine, 49*(1), 54–57.

Amanda Enterprise (Version 3.1) [Computer software]. Sunnyvale, CA: Zmanda.

Amthauer, H., Gaglio, B., Glasgow, R. E., & King, D. K. (2003). Strategies and lessons learned in patient recruitment during a diabetes self-management program conducted in a primary care setting. *The Diabetes Educator, 29,* 673–681.

Ashing-Giwa, K. (1999). The recruitment of breast cancer survivors into cancer control studies: A focus on African-American women. *Journal of the National Medical Association, 91,* 255–260.

Azjen, I. (1991). The theory of planned behavior. *Organizational Behavior and Human Decision Processes, 50,* 179–211.

Breslin, L. (2010). *Profiles and risk display among social networks on MySpace.* Manuscript in preparation.

Brown, B. A., Long, H. L., Weitz, T. A., & Milliken, N. (2000). Challenges of recruitment: Focus groups with research study recruiters. *Women & Health, 31,* 153–166.

Brown, D. R., Fonad, M. N., Basen-Engquist, K., & Tortolero-Luna, G. (2000). Recruitment and retention of minority women in cancer screening, prevention, and treatment trials. *Annals of Epidemiology, 10,* S13–S21.

Bull, S. (2003). *The process of sex partner seeking online among men who have sex with men and related sexually transmitted disease risk.* Presentation to the 2003 STD/HIV Prevention and The Internet Conference: National Coalition of STD Directors and Centers for Disease Control and Prevention.

Bull, S., Eakin, E., Reeves, M., & Kimberly, R. (2006). Multi-level support for physical activity and healthy eating. *Journal of Advanced Nursing, 54,* 585–593.

Bull, S., Levine, D., Vallejos, D., & Ortiz, C. (2008). Improving recruitment and retention for an online randomized controlled trial: Experience from the Youthnet study. *AIDS Care, 20,* 887–889.

Bull, S., Pratte, K., Whitesell, N., Reitemeijer, C., & McFarlane, M. (2009). Effects of an Internet-based intervention for HIV prevention: The Youthnet trials. *AIDS and Behavior, 13*(3), 474–487.

Caban, C. E. (1995). Hispanic research: Implications of the National Institutes of Health guidelines on inclusion of women and minorities in clinical research. *Journal of the National Cancer Institute Monographs,* 165–169.

Caughy, M. O., O'Campo, P. J., & Patterson, J. (2001). A brief observational measure for urban neighborhoods. *Health & Place, 7,* 225–236.

Christakis, N., & Fowler, J. (2007). Change to obesity: The spread of obesity in a large social network over 32 years. *New England Journal of Medicine, 357,* 370–379.

Cohen, D., Spear, S., Scribner, R., Kissinger, P., Mason, K., & Wildgen, J. (2000). "Broken windows" and the risk of gonorrhea. *American Journal of Public Health, 90,* 230–236.

Cohen, D. A., Mason, K., Bedimo, A., Scribner, R., Basolo, V., & Farley, T. A. (2003). Neighborhood physical conditions and health. *American Journal of Public Health, 93,* 467–471.

Dancy, B. L., Wilbur, J., Talashek, M., Bonner, G., & Barnes-Boyd, C. (2004). Community-based research: Barriers to recruitment of African Americans. *Nursing Outlook, 52,* 234–240.

Dennis, B. P., & Neese, J. B. (2000). Recruitment and retention of African American elders into community-based research: Lessons learned. *Archives of Psychiatric Nursing, 14,* 3–11.

De, P., Jolly, A., Cox, J., & Boivin, J. F. (2006). Characterizing the drug-injecting networks of cocaine and heroin injectors in Montreal. *Canadian Journal of Public Health, 97*, 207–209.

Diehr, P., Koepsell, T., Cheadle, A., Psaty, B., Wagner, E., & Curry, S. (1993). Do communities differ in health behaviors? *Journal of Clinical Epidemiology, 46*, 1141–1149.

Diez-Roux, A. V. (1998). Bringing context back into epidemiology: Variables and fallacies in multilevel analysis. *American Journal of Public Health, 88*, 216–222.

DiIorio, C. (2005). *Measurement in health behavior: Methods for research and evaluation.* San Francisco, CA: Jossey-Bass.

Edmonds, J., Baranowski, T., Baranowski, J., Cullen, K. W., & Myres, D. (2001). Ecological and socioeconomic correlates of fruit, juice, and vegetable consumption among African-American boys. *Preventive Medicine, 32*, 476–481.

Ford, J. G., Howerton, M. W., Lai, G. Y., Gary, T. L., Bolen, S., Gibbons, M. C., et al. (2008). Barriers to recruiting underrepresented populations to cancer clinical trials: A systematic review. *Cancer, 112*, 228–242.

Gauthier, M. A., & Clarke, W. P. (1999). Gaining and sustaining minority participation in longitudinal research projects. *Alzheimer Disease & Associated Disorders, 13*(Supp. 1), S29–S33.

Gilliss, C. L., Lee, K. A., Gutierrez, Y., Taylor, D., Beyene, Y., Neuhaus, J., et al. (2001). Recruitment and retention of healthy minority women into community-based longitudinal research. *Journal of Women's Health & Gender-Based Medicine, 10*, 77–85.

Glasgow, R. E. (2002). Evaluation of theory-based interventions: The RE-AIM model. In *Health behavior and health education* (pp. 531–544). San Francisco: Wiley.

Glasgow, R. E., Klesges, L. M., Dzewaltowski, D. A., Estabrooks, P. A., & Vogt, T. M. (2006). Evaluating the impact of health promotion programs: Using the RE-AIM framework to form summary measures for decision making involving complex issues. *Health Education Research, 21*, 688–694.

Glasgow, R. E., McKay, H. G., Piette, J. D., & Reynolds, K. D. (2001). The RE-AIM framework for evaluating interventions: What can it tell us about approaches to chronic illness management? *Patient Education and Counseling, 44*, 119–127.

Glasgow, R. E., Vogt, T. M., & Boles, S. M. (1999). Evaluating the public health impact of health promotion interventions: The RE-AIM framework. *American Journal of Public Health, 89*, 1322–1327.

Graves, B. (2008). Integrative literature review: A review of literature related to geographical information systems, healthcare access, and health outcomes. *Perspectives in Health Information Management, 5*, 11.

Harachi, T. W., Catalano, R. F., & Hawkins, J. D. (1997). Effective recruitment for parenting programs within ethnic minority communities. *Child & Adolescent Social Work Journal, 14*, 23–39.

Horrigan, J. B. (2004). *Pew Internet project data memo.* Pew Internet & American Life Project. Retrieved from http://www.pewinternet.org/~/ media/Files/Reports/2004/ PIP_Wireless_Ready_Data_0504.pdf.pdf

Lewis, C. E., George, V., Fouad, M., Porter, V., Bowen, D., & Urban, N. (1998). Recruitment strategies in the women's health trial: Feasibility study in minority populations. *Controlled Clinical Trials, 19*, 461–476.

McKay, H. G., Feil, E. G., Glasgow, R. E., & Brown, J. E. (1998). Feasibility and use of an Internet support service for diabetes self-management. *Diabetes Education, 24*, 174–179.

Microsoft Office Access™ 2000 [Computer software]. Redmond, WA: Microsoft.

Moreno, M., Vanderstoep, A., Parks, M., Zimmerman, F., Kurth, A., & Christakis, D. (2009). Reducing at-risk adolescents' display of risk behavior on a social networking web site: A randomized controlled pilot intervention trial. *Archives of Pediatrics & Adolescent Medicine, 163*, 35–41.

Msisha, W. M., Kapiga, S. H., Earls, F. J., & Subramanian, S. V. (2008). Place matters: Multilevel investigation of HIV distribution in Tanzania. *AIDS, 22*, 741–748.

Murray, E., Marais, B., Mans, G., Beyers, N., Ayles, H., Godfrey-Faussett, P., et al. (2009). A multidisciplinary method to map potential tuberculosis transmission "hot spots" in high-burden communities. *International Journal of Tuberculosis and Lung Disease, 13*, 767–774.

Pajek [Graph drawing software]. Slovenia: University of Ljubljana.

Pew Internet & American Life Project. (2006). *Latest trends: February 15–April 6, 2006.* Retrieved from http://pewinternet.org/Shared-Content/Data-Sets/2006/February April-2006-Gadgets-and-Internet-Typology.aspx

Pew Internet & American Life Project. (2000). *The online health care revolution: How the web helps Americans take better care of themselves.* Retrieved from http://www.scribd.com/doc/219514/The-Online-Health-Care-Revolution-How-the-Web-helps-Americans-take-better-care-of-themselves

QDS ACASI [Computer software]. Bethesda, MD: NOVA Research.

SQL Server [Computer software]. Redmond, WA: Microsoft.

Steckler, A., & Linnan, L. (2002). *Process evaluation for public health interventions and research.* San Francisco: Jossey Bass.

UCINET 6 for Windows [Computer software]. Lexington, KY: Analytic Technologies.

Visual Studio [Computer software]. Redmond, WA: Microsoft.

Wylie, J. L., Shah, L., & Jolly, A. (2007). Incorporating geographic settings into a social network analysis of injection drug use and bloodborne pathogen prevalence. *Health & Place, 13,* 617–628.

6

Case Studies in Computer-Based Health Promotion

CHAPTER OVERVIEW

In this chapter, we use a case study format to highlight the beneficial aspects of, and challenges related to, using desktop computers and computer kiosks to deliver technology-based health promotion programs. The first study, called LUCHAR, is a computer kiosk program designed for delivery in community settings to improve nutrition behaviors and increase physical activity among Latinos. The second, an HIV prevention program called Project LIGHT, is adapted for use with a computer. We offer best practices associated with using this modality such as the use of theory for program development, development of relationships with community organizations for program delivery, specific considerations for location and delivery of the program, safety of the equipment, and data collection and storage. We consider emerging trends associated with computer- and kiosk-based programs and include information on key terms and additional resources.

CASE STUDIES OF LUCHAR AND PROJECT LIGHT

Case Study: The LUCHAR Program

Introduction

Cardiovascular (CV) disease remains the leading cause of death in the United States (Minino, Heron, & Smith, 2006), although it is preventable through improvements in

162

nutrition and physical activity (Greenland et al., 2003). Latinos are less likely to receive critical prevention messages than other racial/ethnic groups (Barbeau, Krieger, & Soobader, 2004; Glover, Greenlund, Ayala, & Croft, 2005; Hajjar & Kotchen, 2003; National Health Interview Survey, 2002) in part due to limited access to health services (Eakin et al., 2007).

Computer technology is rarely used to reduce CV disease risk among Latinos (Latino Issues Forum, 2004), although such technology might greatly extend the reach, fidelity, and sustainability of health promotion efforts (Glasgow & Bull, 2001). We developed a promising community-based computer program, encouraging healthy diet and increased physical activity, called the LUCHAR program (*Latinos Using Cardio Health Action to Reduce Risk*)—*luchar* means "to battle" in Spanish. The program was based in social-cognitive (Bandura, 1986, 1997) and social-ecological (Bronfenbrenner, 1979) theory.

Method

One of the first steps in the LUCHAR program was to establish partnerships to facilitate program development and delivery. When LUCHAR was in development, initial efforts were made to connect with the community both to define the specific "look and feel" of the program and to recruit organizations to partner in program delivery. Results of the program development are detailed elsewhere (Padilla et al., 2010), but in brief, developers obtained substantial information from this effort. They conducted 10 focus groups to inform program development, recruiting participants from six community sites, including churches, social service agencies, schools, and commercial establishments (i.e., a coffee shop). There were 110 participants in the groups, most of whom were female, younger than 40, and low-income with almost no computer access; all identified as Latino. Participants expressed four main themes in regard to website content, style, and design: (a) The Web site should be relevant for Latinos; (b) information presented on the website should be kept simple and easy to read; (c) the information should be useful; and (d) the website should be interactive and animated. Screenshots of the program developed based on this feedback can be seen in Figures 6.1 and 6.2, and the entire LUCHAR program can be reviewed online at our website accompanying this book (www.sagepub.com/bull).

Notice in Figure 6.1 the features include design elements created in response to specific focus group participant preferences. In Figure 6.2 there is an example of the type of personalized and tailored feedback a participant received after giving data and information on physical activity. The algorithm used to develop this particular graphic is shown in Chapter 3, Figure 3.2.

Table 6.1 outlines details on how LUCHAR program developers pursued partnership opportunities for the pilot project, and continue to pursue them as the project has now shifted to distribution and dissemination on a larger scale.

The LUCHAR program is self-administered, using a computer kiosk. Following are the specific steps involved in the program.

Figure 6.1   Features of the LUCHAR program

Participants are guided
through program
with role models
from a Latino family tailored to
participant gender and age

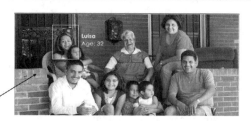

Steps in the Program

Step 1: Demographics. Users input demographic information (age, gender) and are matched to a computerized role model of the same gender and similar age (see Figure 3.1 in Chapter 3 for the algorithm employed for this outcome).

With pictorial, audio, and musical accompaniment, the role model and his or her family members introduce users to the program with a story about heart disease in their family. Pictures are shown of different members of a Latino family while the role model talks. There is instrumental guitar music in the background. Here is the story:

> My name is [here the role model is identified as Luisa—for female participants—or Jorge—for male participants] and I'm [46 or 28, depending on the age of the participant] years old. I'd like to share my story with you. Last month was a really stressful time for me. One day I woke up with awful chest pain—it was pretty scary. I went to Denver Health to get checked out. I didn't have a heart attack that day, but I do have high blood pressure and high cholesterol, so I'm at higher risk for heart disease. It made me remember my *tio* who died last year—he was only 68 and was sick for many months after his heart attack. We miss him a lot and are so sad he had to suffer.
>
> That day was so scary for my family and me—we decided it was time to start being healthy.

The model then invites users to answer questions and learn about their heart disease risk.

> If you're like me, I think it would help to know your own risk for heart disease and then think about ways to stay healthy.
>
> Here's what we'll do today. First, I'll help you see what your risk for heart disease is. Then, we'll take a look at the things you do now that are healthy and good for your heart—what kind of food you eat and how much activity you do every day. We'll also take a look at smoking—if you or people around you smoke.
>
> Next, we'll take some time to set a goal to improve your health. As a last step, we'll identify resources that you can use to help you meet your goal. This program will take about 20 minutes to complete—I'll stay with you to guide you through the entire process. You'll be answering some questions by using the kiosk. Go ahead—try it!

Step 2: Risk Assessment and Behavioral Goal Setting. Users answer questions about health status, diet, physical activity, and smoking. They are then offered graphical feedback

Figure 6.2   Screen shot of participant recommendations and goal setting

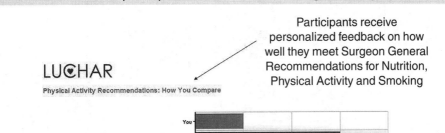

(see Figure 3.2) showing how close they are to meeting Surgeon General recommendations for each behavior. The role model then encourages users to set one goal for behavior change in physical activity, nutrition, or smoking.

Step 3: Identifying Barriers to Achieving a Goal and Strategies to Overcome Barriers. Users identify anticipated barriers to achieving their goal. They can select a barrier from a list or write in their own. Let's consider an example: Participant A chose to increase moderate physical activity by walking at least 15 minutes each day. When asked to identify barriers to achieving this goal, some options to choose from included "The weather is bad," "I have no one to walk with," "I walk very slowly," "I don't feel safe walking in my neighborhood," and "I have no time to walk." Participant A could choose from this list or write in his own barrier.

Once barriers are identified, users are asked to come up with strategies to overcome barriers. As with the barriers, users could choose from a list or write in their own. Continuing with the example of the participant who chose to increase walking, strategies to choose from include "Find a place to walk indoors, such as a recreation center or indoor track or shopping mall," "sign up for clubs that encourage walking," "volunteer with a community center to meet others who want to walk," "just keep moving, and don't worry about your speed," and "consider taking shorter walks of 5 minutes each on days when you cannot do a longer walk."

In closing, participants receive a printout that includes details on their health status, and graphical representation of how their own nutrition, physical activity, and smoking behaviors compare to the Surgeon General's recommendations. The printout also includes information on the behavioral goal they set along with referrals for local resources to support their goal. In the case of Participant A above, the resource list would include local recreation centers and community centers and the addresses for shopping malls open for indoor walking clubs.

The initial process yielded partnerships with six organizations: an elementary school, a Catholic church, a Catholic social service agency, a secular community-based social service agency, a café, and a community-based primary care clinic. Once the program was developed and partnerships were established, program developers worked with partners to house computers, printers, monitors, and kiosks in their organizations for program delivery. Each

Table 6.1 Applying considerations guided by the community-based participatory research framework in establishing partnerships to the LUCHAR project

Partnership consideration	Program not yet developed	Program developed and tested; needs wider distribution
What are the reasons you are seeking partnership(s) with this particular organization(s)?	Developers had a history of working on other health promotion efforts with most of these organizations; developers had received federal funding to pilot-test a new technology for health promotion.	LUCHAR has been shown to have promise but not yet established efficacy—developers need more partnerships to establish efficacy. The state health department in Colorado seeks to expand prevention services using settlement monies from tobacco companies. Expanding LUCHAR could be a practical use for these funds.
What will motivate the partner(s) to work with you?	Shared desire to address disparities in heart disease in Colorado; developers are well known in the Latino social service community.	Shared desire to address disparities in heart disease in Colorado; developers are well known in the Latino social service community; developers have maintained a strong partnership in the pilot, suggesting a future partnership in the pilot, suggesting a future effort will also be positive.
What benefit(s) will they derive from the partnership?	Computer and kiosk provide coverage of 20% of a full-time staff person to assist with project; participants get incentive and program benefit.	Computer and kiosk provide coverage of 20% of a full-time staff person to assist with project; participants get incentive and program benefit; developers will also recruit community members to serve on a permanent advisory board.
Are benefits equally distributed across partners?	Estimated distribution: 15% to community members, 85% to developers.	Estimated distribution: 40% to community members, 60% to developers.
What are potential limitations to the partnership?	Time involved for community staff members to engage people in project may be uncompensated.	Requires organizations to do something specific but potentially unplanned in response to heart disease.
How will you maintain the partnership after your project is completed?	By recruiting participants for the next phase of the project (dissemination and distribution of LUCHAR).	By working to identify from the start shared ideas for institutionalization of the program.

agency was offered these materials to keep in exchange for housing the program as part of the partnership agreement. LUCHAR utilized an infomediary; in this case, a Latina woman, completely bilingual in English and Spanish, was on hand at each site to recruit participants into the program at regular intervals. Partnering agency representatives could refer interested users to this recruiter when she was not on-site if they wanted to participate.

In the five community settings, LUCHAR screened 285 Latinos for program eligibility (i.e., English or Spanish speaking; residing in Denver; age 21 or older) and invited the 230 found eligible subjects to enroll, with 200 completing the program. In the clinic, LUCHAR screened 134 persons, of whom 103 were eligible and 99 completed the program. Two months after completing the program, 161 of the 200 community participants (81%) and 84 of the 99 clinic participants (84%) completed a telephone-based follow-up risk assessment.

Results

LUCHAR program users ($N = 200$ from community-based organizations, $N = 99$ from the clinic setting) were primarily between the ages of 31 and 50 (64%), and all self-identified as Latino. Just under half (47%) were exclusive Spanish speakers, and the same proportion were male. Just over half (54%) were married, and a third (35%) had not completed high school. Many were classified as obese (56%), and 48% indicated they had been diagnosed with one or more chronic conditions. Behavioral outcomes at 2 months are shown in Table 6.2. LUCHAR participation was associated with significant improvement in self-reported vegetable consumption, significant increases in overall nutrition scores, and significant increases in user-reported physical activity. There were no program effects on smoking behaviors.

Case Study: A Computerized Version of Project LIGHT

Introduction

Project LIGHT was a collaborative, multisite project developed to promote HIV prevention and funded by the National Institute of Mental Health. The original project was developed in response to the continuing threat of HIV infection in the United States. At the time of project development, HIV in the United States was especially high in African American populations, had particular impact among people during their reproductive years, and was growing among the younger population (National Institute of Mental Health [NIMH] Multisite HIV Prevention Trial Group, 1998). All these issues continue to be of serious concern today, and we remain in need of efficacious and effective interventions for young people and people of color in the United States. Dr. Marguerita Lightfoot and her colleagues recognized the potential of Project LIGHT, but wanted to extend the reach of the project using computers and targeting delinquent youth, noted to be at even higher risk than other young adults (Diclemente et al., 1996; Romero et al., 2007).

The original Project LIGHT (described in greater detail below) was a multisite small-group HIV prevention trial. Project LIGHT delivered HIV prevention content in seven 90- to 120-minute sessions delivered two times each week to gender-specific groups of 5 to 15 participants. Data from the randomized trial of over 3,700 participants showed that those in the intervention condition had

Table 6.2 Outcomes for LUCHAR pilot community and clinic samples

Goal	Outcomes	Community		Clinic	
		Baseline N = 200	2 months N = 161	Baseline N = 99	2 months N = 84
Nutrition	Latinos meeting national guidelines for fruit and vegetable consumption (≥5 daily servings)	14%	25%*	14%	30%*
	Latinos eating < 2 daily servings of fruits and vegetables	56%	46%*	68%	35%**
	Mean overall nutrition scores (higher scores = poorer nutrition)	5.1	4.6**	6.0	4.1**
Physical Activity (PA)	Latinos meeting PA guidelines (30 minutes/day, most days of the week)	33%	49%**	45%	65%**
	Latinos doing less than the recommended PA guidelines	52%	40%**	55%	35%**
Smoking	Current smokers	20%	19%	18%	16%

* $p < 0.05$

** $p < 0.01$.

fewer unprotected sex acts, more condom use, and more consistent condom use over time. In addition, men in the trial had a lower gonorrhea incidence compared to men in the control condition, and all intervention participants, male and female, had fewer sexually transmitted infection symptoms at 12-month follow-up compared to controls (NIMH Multisite HIV Prevention Trial Group, 1998).

Method

The computerized Project LIGHT was developed specifically for delinquent youth to be delivered via computer. The project developers delivered the computerized version of the program to 133 youth aged 14 to 18 years in three alternative school settings. These were settings for youth who had not been successful in mainstream schools, and they had already come in contact with or were at risk of becoming in contact with the juvenile justice system. The effects of the computerized Project LIGHT were tested with young people over a 3-month period.

Table 6.3 shows approaches the team used to adapt Project LIGHT in each session. Recall that the original program was delivered using small-group sessions with single genders, where activities included dialogue, role-playing, and other forms of social interaction. In the technology version described here, each session had adaptations to these approaches to reinforce messages and offer participants opportunities for practice.

The computerized Project LIGHT was delivered in six instead of seven sessions. This adaptation to the program was made after evaluations of the small-group Project LIGHT sessions showed redundancy between two of the sessions, which were then collapsed into one. Following is a description of the content for each session and examples of the types of activities youth would engage in for the computerized version. See Figures 6.3, 6.4, and 6.5 for examples of program screenshots.

Content in Computerized Project by Session

Session 1: HIV 101. This session covers basic facts about HIV in an effort to raise perception of HIV risk both at the individual level and in the community. The objective for this session also includes an effort to motivate young people to stay with the program and complete all six sessions.

The session includes information about HIV and then allows participants to interact with the computer and document their own motivations for staying healthy, future goals, reasons to care about HIV risk for themselves, and why HIV is a problem for the community. The session also offers basic transmission and prevention facts.

An activity central to this session is the "Myths and Facts" game, where participants can determine if a statement about HIV is a myth or a fact. Participants can also create their own "Myth or Fact" questions during this game. The session ends with a homework assignment: Notice anything you can about HIV—news, information, prevention, conversations, and so forth.

Session 2: Personalizing HIV Risk. In this session, participants are encouraged to personalize the information about HIV transmission and begin to consider their own behaviors that can place them at risk for infection. Prior to beginning the session, participants are asked to consider several topics as they view videos of people in their late teens and early 20s affected

Table 6.3 Approaches used to adapt Project LIGHT from small face-to-face group sessions to a computer-based kiosk program

Session number and content focus	Activities employed in Project LIGHT	Activities employed in technology-based adaptation of Project LIGHT
Session 1: HIV 101	Didactic presentation; group discussion	"Myths and Facts" game where participants get points for number of myths and facts identified; homework to discuss HIV with people over a weeklong period
Session 2: Personalizing HIV Risk	Didactic presentation; group discussion; role-play	Participants view a video of persons living with HIV; identify the risks those persons take and the ones they take in an online card game
Session 3: Antecedents to HIV and problem solving	Didactic presentation; group discussion; role-play	Participants view didactic material and then observe a "virtual" party to see who is present and what risks those at the party have; "Positive Self-Talk" is another game-based activity to reinforce healthy self-image
Session 4: Condom skills	Skills-building practice with condoms	Participants correctly identify steps in condom use and barriers to condom use in a game
Session 5: Communication	Didactic presentation; group discussion; role-play	Participants practice assertiveness for using condoms in a game called "Talk Tools" and can also practice specific language with a voice-recorded interaction with an avatar who can role-play a potential sex partner
Session 6: Wrap-up and relapse	Group discussion	Computer allows participants to revisit any game, element, or activity they choose to reinforce materials

by and infected with HIV. Topics include the following: What are risk behaviors that people engage in? What motivates people to get an HIV test? What is it like to live with HIV?

Participants then view role models telling their own stories about life with HIV in video clips: things they have done to place themselves at risk, how they learned their status, and why they were motivated to get tested. They also discuss what it is like to live with HIV.

Following the role model videos, participants are asked to read text on cards that are similar to playing cards; the text includes HIV-related risk behaviors. If a participant has engaged in this behavior, the card is kept in his or her hand. If not, it is discarded. The end result is the participant's "HIV risky hand."

Session 3: Antecedents to HIV and Problem Solving. In this session, participants are encouraged to identify the psychosocial and situational triggers that precede HIV-related risk behaviors. Triggers include substance use, types of people, types of places, and moods and feelings. Participants are first asked to document the types of circumstances that will trigger risk—do they drink or take drugs? Are they more vulnerable to risk behavior after they have been feeling lonely or isolated?

After participants document their own personal triggers, they play a game where they can observe avatars at a house party. They can move their cursor over any partygoer, and a text box above that partygoer will show what that individual's triggers are. Thus, participants get to see that others may have similar triggers to their own.

In addition to the computerized content, for this session, participants are given a workbook, and they are encouraged to elaborate on their triggers by detailing those they may have experienced the last time they had sex. Participants are notified that the workbook is private and that others won't see it. Participants cannot move forward in the computer program, however, unless they have had enough time elapse to allow them to write something down—the computer will not let them continue if they attempt to move along to Session 4 without adequate time passing.

In this session, participants are encouraged to set specific behavioral goals that will assist them in preventing HIV. For each goal they set, they are given opportunities to problem-solve triggers or barriers to achieving that goal. To do this, they interact with an avatar who has a preprogrammed set of goals and triggers and offers advice given the particular goal and set of triggers.

In this session, the participants also play a game called "Positive Self-Talk" in an effort to instill a more positive self-image as they are trying to adopt healthier behaviors. In this game, participants write down and then shoot positive thoughts into a character—like a video game—and then the character grows. Shooting negative thoughts into the character causes him or her to shrink.

Session 4: Condom Skills. In this session, participants watch a video clip of a group of kids talking about different condoms—different flavors, colors, sizes, and types (e.g., male and female, ribbed) and approaches for making condom use more fun and pleasurable. Participants can see instructions on condom use, with an animated condom demonstration for both male and female condoms. The activity associated with this session allows participants to correctly identify the steps and order for putting on and correctly using a condom.

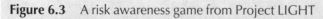

Figure 6.3   A risk awareness game from Project LIGHT

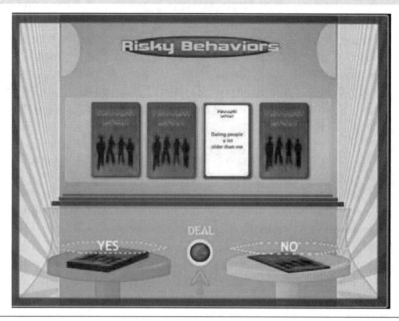

Figure 6.4   A skills-building game from Project LIGHT

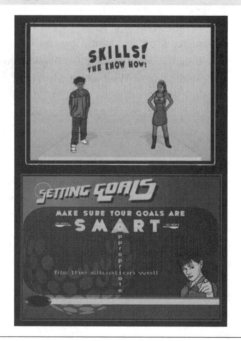

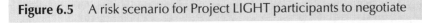

Figure 6.5   A risk scenario for Project LIGHT participants to negotiate

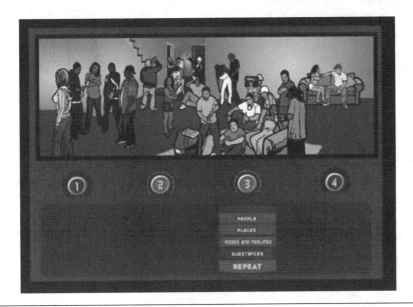

Session 5: Communication. In this session, participants focus on development of better communication skills, particularly for resisting pressure to take risks. They begin the session with a game allowing them to use their mouse like they would a can of spray paint. They spray over segments of a brick wall depicted on their screen, and doing so reveals situations and circumstances that can make having conversations around sex difficult.

This activity is followed by one that teaches participants the difference between aggressive, assertive, and passive talk. Called "Talk Tools," this game invites young people to play the role of a DJ in a computer game where they spin records—each record represents a type of talk (i.e., aggressive, assertive, or passive). Participants can also view video clips of young people talking assertively so they can learn from role models how to adopt this type of talk more consistently.

For practice, young people can practice talking assertively through an avatar. They meet an avatar, who pressures them for unsafe sex—they are then invited to respond, and their response is tape-recorded. The avatar offers a response, and participants can try to assert themselves to be safe again. After a few minutes, the computer will play back the tape-recorded conversation so they can hear the whole thing. The program isn't tailored to individual participants here, so participants are simply practicing different approaches for assertive talk despite multiple instances of pressure from the avatar.

Session 6: Wrap-Up and Relapse. In this final session, participants are asked to review their skills and knowledge—what are your current triggers, and how do you problem-solve them? They are offered an opportunity to reorient themselves with prior material—for example, when asked to consider that they have been successful in using condoms but slipped one time and couldn't do it, they are reminded to implement "Positive Self-Talk" to remind themselves to reinforce their positive self-image. At the end of the program, youth are reminded of all they have learned and are encouraged to serve as role models for others like them in their communities. They are given tips on how to start conversations about HIV prevention and how to begin sharing information about prevention in community settings.

Results

As reported in the *American Journal of Public Health*, when this adaptation of Project LIGHT for computers was tested and compared to the original program as well as a control group, the participants in the computerized version were significantly less likely than those in the group sessions from the original program to engage in sexual activity, and both those in the small-group sessions and those in the computerized sessions reported significantly fewer sex partners compared to control participants. Researchers observed differences that didn't reach statistical significance in reductions in unprotected sexual intercourse between those in the computerized Project LIGHT compared to both those in the original small-group session Project LIGHT and those in the control group, both of whom reported increases in unprotected sexual intercourse (Lightfoot, Comulada, & Stover, 2007).

It appears, then, that the computerized version of Project LIGHT functions equally well if not better than the original small-group session. What have we sacrificed by adapting this program to a computer and taking away the interaction of the group session? It isn't clear if some unmeasured factors are negatively impacted by this type of change. However, none of the behavioral outcomes assessed appear to be negatively impacted. Furthermore, there appear to be specific advantages to offering Project LIGHT on a computer. First, there were higher overall and session-specific completion rates with the computerized session compared to the group session. Investigators hypothesize this is due to the opportunity that participants had to complete sessions on their own time and at their own convenience. Second, participants completed sessions more than one time—if a game was fun and engaging, they could do it more than once. This could potentially contribute to improved effects due to dose response— something difficult to achieve in multisession small-group interventions (M. Lightfoot, personal communication, August 12, 2009).

UNIQUE AND BENEFICIAL ASPECTS OF LUCHAR AND PROJECT LIGHT

The case studies here illustrate several advantages that can be achieved through using desktop or computer kiosks for health promotion program delivery.

Computer-based programs (whether or not you are using a kiosk) are ideal to develop in the context of partnerships. This is true especially if you hope to have a program with extensive reach that can be made available in multiple community, clinic, or other organizational settings. It may not be likely or realistic to find an organization that simultaneously has the capacity to develop sophisticated technology-based health promotion *and* access to a wide network reaching diverse members of the intended audience for the program. Thus, considering development of partnerships that bring together technology experts with program developers and organizations that can deliver programs to members of the intended audience is important.

One approach to development of partnerships that is instructive, particularly in the development and delivery of effective health promotion interventions, is called community-based participatory research, or CBPR. CBPR is defined as "a collaborative process that equitably involves all partners in the research process and recognizes the unique strengths that each brings. CBPR begins with a research topic of importance to the community with the aim of combining knowledge and action for social change to improve community health and eliminate health disparities" (Minkler, 2005, p. 10). Although we are not discussing research per se in this textbook, we are considering the best practices for health promotion program development and delivery when using technology. While CBPR is research focused, it can offer useful perspectives in how to effectively form and sustain partners for program delivery as well. More than a decade of experience with CBPR has shown that research can be more relevant, culturally proficient, and effective when conducted through community-academic partnerships (Braithwaite, Bianchi, & Taylor, 1994; Braithwaite & Lythcott, 1989; Israel et al., 2005; Israel, Schulz, Parker, & Becker, 1998; Lasker & Weiss, 2003; Metzler et al., 2003; Puertas & Schlesser, 2001).

When developing a technology-based program, then, it can be important to consider from the start who your audience is, and whether representatives from that audience would endorse delivery of your program in their communities. It is important as well, as already mentioned in Chapter 3, to consider the types of technologies members of your intended audience currently use and what types they have access to. An ideal scenario informed by the CBPR perspective would include a program where members from a given community or from organizations serving that community identified technology-based health promotion as a priority and subsequently sought out technical program developers to help them realize this priority. Another viable CBPR approach would be to have a technical program developer seek out partnerships and collaborations with organizations serving a given community *before* developing a program to ensure the following:

1. There is support for such a program among leaders in the community.

2. There is an opportunity to gather evidence that community members would endorse a technology-based program, find it appealing and compelling, and use it.

3. Members from the intended audience can directly inform program development by offering opinions, critiques, and ideas about program content, delivery, and structure.

While it may seem somewhat counterintuitive to obtain buy-in from specific communities about program content and style when you hope to expand the reach of the program to diverse communities and large numbers of people, there are distinct advantages of doing so. By partnering *before* you develop your program for computer-based health promotion, you can not only do the work up front that is needed to ensure program content and design are appropriate (as discussed in Chapter 3), but you can identify specific locations and organizations where your program can be delivered. As mentioned for both case studies considered in this chapter, laying the groundwork for this ahead of time can be most helpful when you wish to expand and replicate your program.

The elements of a successful partnership for development and delivery of a computer-based health promotion program are likely dependent upon what stage of the program you are in. If you are just developing the program, you may want to place more emphasis on connecting with a small number of organizations you can partner with to obtain feedback on content and design. If you have done that and are now wishing to distribute your program more widely, then your partnership development may need to focus on developing relationships with organizations that have multiple sites or networks, such as school or hospital systems or professional and trade associations. In either case, consider some of the guidelines for partnership development within the CBPR framework that can facilitate your own work that are shown in Table 6.4.

Considerations for Program Location

Once you have established partnerships for your computer-based program, it is important to consider the exact placement of your equipment within the organizations where you will deliver the program. The placement should be in a location that has enough traffic so that people will be motivated to use it, but also in a place that affords quiet, so participants will not be distracted, and privacy, in the event you are asking personal, sensitive, or confidential questions (e.g., that need to be delivered in accordance with HIPAA regulations). Note you may wish to make your program mobile within your organization, and thus you may opt for a small mobile kiosk or the use of a portable mobile device such as an iPad™. Recall that choosing a portable device means additional attention to security to prevent or reduce theft, and to retrieve devices or limit access to data on devices that have been stolen or lost.

If you are using an infomediary for your program (described in detail in Chapter 4), this person will be working to recruit and ensure that program participants have access to and can use the program equipment. While you may have an initial idea of where to place the equipment, you can consult your infomediary after the program has been in place to ensure it is located advantageously.

If you are not using an infomediary, location of your program equipment may be vital to program success. You need to place it in an area where you know people will see it and be motivated to use it. Consider a few different scenarios: For example, if you have a kiosk at a grocery store, what will motivate people to stop—either on their way in, on their way out, or during shopping—to use your kiosk? If you have a desktop program in a clinic, what will entice and encourage people to use it? Once they have engaged with the equipment, you have to make sure that they can easily run the program. Make sure you have the program loaded and ready to launch. Consider loading only your program icon onto your monitor and hiding all other icons so users can click only on one thing that will launch your program. By hiding all other icons, there will be no confusion over what a user is to do to start.

Another approach used in the Health-e-Solutions project was to utilize a computer kiosk with a telephone that would link directly to a help line, so if users did encounter difficulty,

Table 6.4 Considerations guided by the CBPR framework in establishing partnerships for a computer-based health promotion effort

Partnership consideration	Program not yet developed	Program developed and tested; needs wider distribution
What are the reasons you are seeking partnership(s) with this particular organization(s)?	Person or organization works with the audience you wish to reach with your technology-based program; audience may not have good access to technology.	Person or organization works with much larger numbers of the audience you wish to reach with your technology-based program, and may be able to increase audience access to technology (e.g., schools, clinics).
What will motivate the partner(s) to work with you?	They recognize the health concern you are addressing is an issue for the community they serve.	They have identified addressing a health concern as a priority for their organization; they recognize the health concern you are addressing is an issue for the community they serve.
What benefit(s) will they derive from the partnership?	Consider offering technical equipment for them to keep as part of the partnership; consider hiring organizational staff or covering their time to participate in project development and delivery.	Consider offering technical equipment for them to keep as part of the partnership; consider hiring organizational staff or covering their time to participate in project delivery.
Are benefits equally distributed across partners?	What proportion of project funds are devoted to each partner? What is the net benefit to the community? To the technical partner?	What proportion of project funds are devoted to each partner? What is the net benefit to the community? To the technical partner?
What are potential limitations to the partnership?	If in development, a higher proportion of project funds may be required for the technical aspects of the program, making it appear less equitable.	If in distribution, working with larger numbers of partners may be challenging to maintain good communication and relationships.
How will you maintain the partnership after your project is completed?	Consider up-front issues such as where and how you can obtain funding to continue a successful project and what will be the involvement of current partners in sustaining a successful project.	Consider what it will take to institutionalize a successful project, allowing for regular evaluation to update and upgrade content, design, and technology as needed.

they could obtain technical support (Colorado Prevention Center, n.d.). While more costly than having stand-alone equipment, this is potentially less costly than an infomediary, especially when you have a number of kiosks distributed widely. Such an approach can also minimize frustrations with your program associated with technical difficulties.

Ways to ensure ideal placement can be facilitated through some simple data collection methods we have identified in previous chapters. You will recall that in Chapter 4, we presented information on time-space sampling using enumeration of venue-day-time increments. Such an approach is also useful for identifying high-traffic areas where your target audience may be likely to come in contact with your kiosk. Using the enumeration forms shown in Figure 4.5, you can identify various locations within an organization and document the number of people from your target audience who pass through these locations within a given time frame. If you have a kiosk, you can place it in these locations and observe and document the number of people who approach the kiosk. You can then compile these data to make an evidence-based decision on placement of your equipment (e.g. in high-traffic areas).

The other consideration you have with equipment location is safety from theft and vandalism. If in a public setting such as a grocery store or hospital emergency room, you may wish to maximize equipment security to avoid theft or vandalism. There are a number of different options for kiosks that can address these types of needs—we list some additional resources on computer kiosks at the end of the chapter. These include such options as having all your equipment completely enclosed in a kiosk, with only touch screen capability, and small windows that can print out paper so that all the equipment is accessible only with a key to the kiosk. This allows for greater assurance that someone cannot steal or vandalize specific parts (e.g., the mouse, keyboard, or printer).

Data Storage and Transfer

We discussed general strategies for data storage and transfer in more detail in Chapter 4 and encourage you to review those, particularly as they relate to database development and queries to ensure your data are being stored as intended. Additionally, for computer-based programs, a key consideration is the location for your data. Do you plan to store data on participants gathered at the computer or kiosk on each machine individually? If so, consider developing a detailed protocol on how often you will download data for storage in a central location, what protections of protected health information mandated by the Health Insurance Portability and Accountability Act (HIPAA) you will have in place, and what you will do with data on the hard drive of the equipment once these data are downloaded elsewhere. You need to program your computer for administrators or program personnel to perform these functions and include information in the protocol about who they are and how they will obtain data from the hard drive (e.g., through password-protected folders on the hard drive).

In many, if not all, cases, you will find it will be safer to write and store data directly to a central location and *not* on the hard drive of a computer or kiosk. However, this requires "always on" Internet access that is reliable, and there may be firewall concerns that prevent transfer of data from community settings to a secure server behind an institutional firewall.

Another option is to regularly transfer data over a secure connection to a central location. One of the easiest ways to achieve this is through file transfer protocol (FTP) across a secure server using a Transport Layer Security (TLS) procedure described in detail in Chapter 2. Using this procedure requires that there be a reliable Internet connection so data can be automatically routed on a regular basis (e.g., daily) to avoid loss or damage. This may also be challenging when attempting to send data to a secure server behind an institutional firewall. Consult with information technology experts in your institution or organization to determine what will work the best for you as you deliver your own program.

Finally, if you do use a portable device you may be able to access wireless mobile networks, circumventing the need for always-on Internet access by using 3G networks. Recall that relying on this method for data collection and storage will require additional attention to security protocols for access to and retrieval of data from portable devices.

WHAT ARE EMERGING TRENDS IN COMPUTER-BASED HEALTH PROMOTION?

Newer Kiosks, Portable Notepads

Use of Technology as Adjunctive and Hybrid

We have showcased two studies here that have demonstrated the potential for using computer kiosks in community settings for health promotion. Others include commercial ventures, including a program similar to LUCHAR called "Cardio Pharm," which allows consumers to utilize kiosks in pharmacy settings to obtain information on cardiovascular risk. They complete an interactive program with questions about nutrition and physical activity, can review pamphlets near the computer, and can then obtain more information directly from their pharmacist (Hariri, Goodyer, Anderson, & Meyer, 1997). In Australia, investigators have experimented with putting health promotion computer kiosks in diverse health and non-health-related public settings—such as movie theaters, shopping malls, and clubs licensed to sell liquor. The intent was to observe whether users would engage with the kiosks and would seek information on or obtain feedback regarding their specific behaviors in numerous areas (e.g., skin cancer prevention, smoking, heart health, seat belt use, violence prevention; Radvan, Wiggers, & Hazel, 2010).

As mentioned in this and other chapters, there is substantial potential to utilize kiosks in health or other community settings to reinforce, extend, or expand clinical services. As seen from the examples above, they can also be used to promote health more globally, and it may not be necessary to have a computer kiosk tied to a specific clinic or hospital. We anticipate proliferation of programs in care and community settings that can engage users in a way that goes beyond the unidirectional message of advertising or social marketing so they can personalize information, seek tailored advice, and make health promotion individually relevant. We also anticipate that these programs could well remain as kiosks or will evolve to include portable devices.

SUMMARY

Using computer-based approaches for health promotion, be they CD-ROM or computer kiosk, has substantial promise and is likely a growth area for this field. When considering whether these modalities are appropriate for the type of health promotion you wish to undertake, you should consider your partners as well as your target audience.

The CD-ROM is a modality that will be ideal if you are already working with a network of institutions that has ample access to hardware such as computers and monitors. You need to be confident that developing and distributing a CD-ROM will ultimately result in having the CD-ROM used. If you are working with a school system, for example, and there are computer labs, the CD-ROM can be loaded onto existing machines and your program implemented with fidelity. Recall, however, that this modality is relatively more expensive to produce given the extra programming costs that go into a CD-ROM. If you are confident that your program will not need changes and upgrades in a short time, then this modality may be ideal. If you do think you will need minor upgrades but still want to use a CD-ROM, then you can consider using the Ruby on Rails modular programming concept discussed in earlier chapters that will allow you to update one module without having to reprogram the entire project.

The computer kiosk is a modality that can be used with or without the CD-ROM—you can deliver a CD-ROM on a kiosk, certainly. However, if you want more flexibility and greater opportunity to upgrade and update content, you may wish to develop a program using XHTML and deliver it on a kiosk. The advantages of doing this are that you can expand the reach of your health promotion project, often to populations that may not have adequate access to computers and technology. While we regularly hear of the shrinking digital divide, we also hear that access to computers and technology doesn't translate directly into regular or habitual use (Latino Issues Forum, 2004). Placing computer kiosks in settings that can reach populations disproportionately and negatively impacted by health outcomes can allow us to both expand health promotion reach and contribute to a shrinking digital divide.

Using CD-ROM and computer kiosk modalities is an ideal way to integrate technology-based health promotion with important principles for CBPR. These modalities can be expanded into multiple settings, and allow program planners to partner effectively with communities and organizations that serve target audiences and groups at elevated risk. Consider the opportunities you have when developing your program to enlist the support and partnership of organizations with direct and ongoing relationships with those you wish to reach.

Consider the location for your program—while you obviously should place your equipment in locations where there will be high traffic to reach more of your target audience, you will need to balance this with the needs and flexibility of the partnering organizations, the privacy needs of participants, and the safety of your equipment. If you plan to use an infomediary to assist you in recruiting participants for your program, you may be able to place your equipment in a quieter location and ask the infomediary to alert participants to the location. You can use methods such as enumeration from time-space sampling to identify the best locations for maximum exposure to your program.

Data storage is important to consider in locations without live and regular Internet access to upload and transfer files. You will need to plan for the best approach to download or upload and transfer data and will need to employ state-of-the-art security procedures to protect any project data as they are transferred. See Chapter 2 for more detail on data security.

? CONCLUDING QUESTIONS

1. If you are considering using a CD-ROM, do you have a relationship with an institution or a set of organizations that will distribute your product and ensure that it will be played and utilized?

2. If you are considering using kiosks, do you have relationships with organizations serving the target audience you wish to reach with your program, and are they willing to host a kiosk?

3. Who are your program partners, and what steps have you taken to adhere to accepted CBPR principles for your computer-based program?

4. What are your plans for determining the best location for your program?

5. Will you use an infomediary to recruit and enroll program participants? How will you store and transfer program data?

CHAPTER EXERCISE

In this exercise, your task is to identify a potential opportunity to create a hybrid health promotion program using computer kiosks or tablets or an iPad™.

1. Identify an opportunity in your community. What is the health behavior or condition that you would like to address?

2. Are there clinical organizations that could champion this effort (e.g., primary care clinics)? Interview a representative from a clinical care services organization.
   a. Identify how the organization's health promotion priorities could be operationalized through computer kiosks.
   b. Do you want your program to be primarily informative? What interactive activities will you employ?

3. What community organizations might you partner with to address this health behavior or condition?
   a. How can the clinical providers partner with the community organizations?
   b. How will you determine the best locations for a kiosk?
   c. How will you engage people in community settings to use a kiosk or tablet?

4. Based on your answers to the questions listed here, write a preliminary proposal (up to 5 pages single-spaced) that describes your plan.

ADDITIONAL RESOURCES

More information on various computer kiosk initiatives for health can be found through the following links shown here.

Information on Selected Health-Related Computer Programs in Development or With Demonstrated Efficacy

Resource	Description
http://www.changemakers.net/node/1192	A project linking multiple large inner-city church congregations to computerized health programs on kiosks—programs are tailored for specific churches
http://www.bluejayconsulting.com/PDF/09BJC_Kiosk_Technology_0218.pdf	Using computer kiosks in emergency rooms to offer information to patients on seat belts, smoke alarms, poison storage, and prevention of other hazardous outcomes
http://www.goodsamhosp.org/cgi-bin/news_room.pl?action=show_article&article_id=13	The kiosk offers medical information about illnesses, treatments, prevention, wellness, and other health care issues
http://www.changemakers.net/node/148	Delivery of an educational program on prevention of domestic violence for patients in emergency rooms

Note: All websites noted here are hot-linked at www.sagepub.com/bull; at this site you will also find newer resources relevant to the material in this and other chapters.

REFERENCES

Bandura, A. (1986). *Social foundations of thought and action: A social cognitive theory.* Englewood Cliffs, NJ: Prentice Hall.

Bandura, A. (1997). *Self-efficacy: The exercise of control.* New York: Freeman.

Barbeau, E. M., Krieger, N., & Soobader, M. (2004). Working class matters: Socioeconomic disadvantage, race/ethnicity, gender, and smoking in NHIS 2000. *American Journal of Public Health, 94,* 269–278.

Braithwaite, R., Bianchi, C., & Taylor, S. E. (1994). Ethnographic approach to community organization and health empowerment. *Health Education Quarterly, 21,* 407–416.

Braithwaite, R. L., & Lythcott, N. (1989). Community empowerment as a strategy for health promotion for black and other minority populations. *JAMA, 261,* 282–283.

Bronfenbrenner, U. (1979). *The ecology of human development: Experiments by nature and design.* Cambridge, MA: Harvard University Press.

Colorado Prevention Center. (n.d.). *Colorado heart healthy solutions.* Retrieved from tp://cpcmed.org/prevention/chhs.html be an acceptable substitute

Diclemente, R. J., Lodico, M., Grinstead, O. A., Harper, G., Rickman, R. L., Evans, P. E., et al. (1996). African American adolescents residing in high-risk urban environments do use condoms: Correlates and predictors of condom use among adolescents in public housing developments. *Pediatrics, 8,* 269–278.

Eakin, E. G., Bull, S. S., Riley, K., Reeves, M. M., Gutierrez, S., & McLaughlin, P. (2007). Recruitment and retention of Latinos in a primary care-based physical activity and diet trial: The Resources for Health study. *Health Education Research, 22,* 361–371.

Glasgow, R., & Bull, S. S. (2001). Making a difference with interactive technology: Considerations in using and evaluating computerized aid for diabetes self-management education. *Diabetes Spectrum, 14*(2), 99–106.

Glover, M. J., Greenlund, K. J., Ayala, C., & Croft, J. B. (2005). Racial/ethnic disparities in prevalence, treatment, and control of hypertension. *Morbidity & Mortality Weekly Report, 54,* 7–9.

Greenland, P., Knoll, M. D., Stamler, J., Neaton, J. D., Dyer, A. R., Garside, D. B., et al. (2003). Major risk factors as antecedents of fatal and nonfatal coronary heart disease events. *JAMA, 290,* 891–897.

Hajjar, I., & Kotchen, T. A. (2003). Trends in prevalence, awareness, treatment, and control of hypertension in the United States, 1988–2000 [Comment]. *JAMA, 290,* 199–206.

Hariri, S., Goodyer, L., Anderson, C., & Meyer, J. (1997). Cardio: Interactive multimedia health promotion software for community pharmacy. *Nutrition & Food Science, 97,* 71–75.

Israel, B., Parker, E. A., Rowe, Z., Salvatore, A., Minkler, M., Lopez, J., et al. (2005). Community-based participatory research: Lessons learned from the Centers for Children's Environmental Health and Disease Prevention Research. *Environmental Health Perspectives, 113,* 1463–1471.

Israel, B. A., Schulz, A. J., Parker, E. A., & Becker, A. B. (1998). Review of community-based research: Assessing partnership approaches to improve public health. *Annual Review of Public Health, 19,* 173–202.

Lasker, R. D., & Weiss, E. S. (2003). Broadening participation in community problem solving: A multidisciplinary model to support collaborative practice and research. *Journal of Urban Health, 80,* 14–47.

Latino Issues Forum. (2004). *Latinos, computers and the Internet: How Congress and the current administration's framing of the digital divide has negatively impacted policy initiative established to close the significant technology gap that remains.* Retrieved from http://www.lif.org/download/ digitaldivbrief.pdf

Lightfoot, M., Comulada, W., & Stover, G. (2007). Computerized HIV preventive intervention for adolescents: Indications of efficacy. *American Journal of Public Health, 97,* 1027–1030.

Metzler, M., Higgins, D., Beeker, C., Freudenberg, N., Lantz, P., Senturia, K., et al. (2003). Addressing urban health in Detroit, New York City and Seattle through community-based participatory research partnerships. *American Journal of Public Health, 93,* 803–811.

Minino, A. M., Heron, M. P., & Smith, B. L. (2006). Deaths: Preliminary data for 2004. *National Vital Statistics Reports, 54,* 1–49.

Minkler, M. (2005). Community-based research partnerships: Challenges and opportunities. *Journal of Urban Health, 82,* ii3–ii12.

National Health Interview Survey. (2002). State-specific trends in self-reported blood pressure screening and high blood pressure—United States, 1991–1999. *Morbidity & Mortality Weekly Report, 51,* 456–460.

National Institute of Mental Health Multisite HIV Prevention Trial Group. (1998). The NIMH Multisite HIV Prevention Trial: Reducing HIV sexual risk behavior. *Science, 280,* 1889–1894.

Padilla, R., Bull, S., Raghunath, S. G., Fernald, D., Havranek, E. P., & Steiner, J. F. (2010). Designing a cardiovascular disease prevention web site for Latinos: Qualitative community feedback. *Health Promotion Practice, 11*(1), 140–147.

Puertas, B., & Schlesser, M. (2001). Assessing community health among indigenous populations in Ecuador with a participatory approach: Implications for health reform. *Journal of Community Health, 26,* 133–147.

Radvan, D., Wiggers, T., & Hazel, T. (2010). HEALTH C.H.I.P.s: Opportunistic community use of computerized health information programs. *Health Education Research, 19,* 581–590.

Romero, E. G., Teplin, L. A., McClelland, G. M., Abram, K. M., Welty, L. J., & Washburn, J. J. (2007). A longitudinal study of the prevalence, development and persistence of HIV/sexually transmitted infection risk behaviors in delinquent youth: Implications for health care in the community. *Pediatrics, 119,* e1126–e1141.

7 ▪▪

Case Studies in Internet-Based Health Promotion

CHAPTER OVERVIEW

This chapter covers issues that are unique to the Internet for technology-based health promotion interventions. The chapter includes two case studies of Internet-based programs that illustrate some successes with efficacy in health promotion. The first, called WRAPP (the Wyoming Rural AIDS Prevention Project), is an HIV prevention program designed for delivery exclusively on the Internet to gay men in rural Wyoming. The second, a diabetes self-management program called D-Net, is designed for delivery online to persons with diabetes. We consider the unique and beneficial aspects of each of these cases, along with considering challenges these programs faced. We offer examples of what we know to be the best practices for Internet-based health promotion, and look to emerging trends in using the Internet for promoting health. As with other chapters, we offer information on key terms and additional resources.

CASE STUDIES OF WRAPP AND D-NET

Case Study: The Wyoming Rural AIDS Prevention Project (WRAPP)

Introduction

The Wyoming Rural AIDS Prevention Project, or WRAPP, was developed and evaluated by a team affiliated with the University of Wyoming, including Drs. Anne Bowen and Mark Williams. The audience for the project included gay men living in rural Wyoming, but the product the researchers produced is applicable to gay men in other rural or urban settings with access to the Internet. The program offers HIV prevention, including awareness and knowledge of HIV, prevention strategies with male partners, and the context in which HIV risk behaviors are most likely to occur.

Program users would interact with the program on the Internet—recruitment for the program happens online, and people complete all program elements on the Internet. Thus, it is available to anyone who has Internet access in diverse settings. Each of the three WRAPP topics is covered in two sessions, for a total of six sessions interacting with the computer.

WRAPP is designed to have the feel of a group session for HIV prevention. Group-level interventions for HIV prevention with gay men have been documented as having a high level of efficacy for behavior change, particularly in areas of condom use and partner reduction (Centers for Disease Control and Prevention, 1999). Users who log on to the program are shown pairs of men or a group of diverse men depicted in realistic cartoon figures. Theoretically, the program is designed to allow users to identify with the men, as one would a role model, consistent with concepts supported by the diffusion of innovations theory and social cognitive theory (Bandura, 1986; Rogers, 1995). The program aims to convey the theoretical concept of social support, as shown by the group of men, as well (DiMatteo, 2004). Users are guided through the program and given different content based on their responses to questions. The content and questions were developed using a gain-and-loss framing perspective (Block & Keller, 1995), which suggests that under certain circumstances and for certain health conditions, it is more beneficial to emphasize the negative outcomes associated with performing a behavior rather than the positive ones. While the use of gain-and-loss framing as an effective method in this program hasn't been evaluated per se, results from a randomized trial of effects of the intervention on condom attitudes and self-efficacy were positive at 1 week postintervention. This trial didn't include a long-enough follow-up of participants to demonstrate an impact on HIV prevention behaviors (Bowen, Horvath, & Williams, 2007). Each module is described more fully here. Screenshots from the program are available in Figure 7.1.

Program Content

Module 1, Session A: HIV Knowledge. The goals of this module were first to raise awareness of and support for persons with HIV and second to consider prevention options—not only condoms, but HIV testing and monogamy. Participants in this module were shown a conversation between two gay men who are discussing risk behaviors. One man calls up his friend, who is HIV positive, and tells him he has had a one-night stand. The friend is a role model—he is HIV positive, and has the opportunity to share what he knows about HIV and risk with his friend. The first man presents his worries and concerns about having had sex with an unknown partner without a condom. His friend is able to reassure him that such behavior doesn't translate into a death sentence or even necessarily into being HIV positive, but that the only way to know is to go get tested for HIV. He stresses to his friend the importance of thinking about what might happen if he were to acquire HIV, mentioning how his own life has been affected by having to take numerous drugs, worry about paying for medications, and experience side effects associated with HIV medication. At the end of this and all other sessions, the

Figure 7.1   WRAPP screenshots

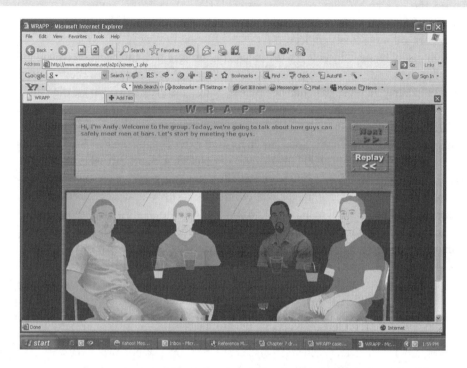

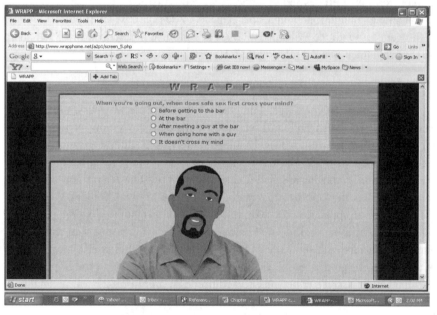

user is invited to print out a summary of the conversation so he can keep it on hand or easily accessible.

Module 1, Session B: HIV Knowledge. At the second session associated with HIV knowledge, the first man returns with a negative HIV test result. His friend talks to him about prevention options, including condom use. At this stage of the program, the user is presented with a quiz, allowing him to pick the right condom for HIV protection (i.e., latex or polyurethane). He is also shown a map of how HIV is distributed in the United States. This element allows the rural gay man to realize how concentrated HIV is in larger urban areas, and to consider that when traveling to these areas, he may want to take extra precautions for HIV prevention, knowing he may have greater chance of exposure. The session also includes a slot machine game—users can "spin" the wheel of a slot machine and ascertain their level of protection from HIV—if the result is three condoms, they are fully protected. Finally, the session ends with step-by-step instructions and illustrations on how to use a condom.

Module 2, Session A: Partner Skills. The goal of this session is to develop and practice planning skills with partners for prevention. The user is introduced to a group of diverse men depicted in cartoon sitting in a circle, simultaneously underscoring role models and social support. The focus of this module is also to emphasize the concept of motivations from the information, motivation, and behavior change model of Fisher and Fisher (2002) to emphasize motivations for staying safe. Specifically, participants are asked to think of their long-term goals and then consider short-term behaviors that would help them achieve those goals. Assessment of life goals is stressed here—where participants want to be in 10 years, for example. With new partners, participants are asked to consider these long-term goals—and to specifically identify what long-term relationship goals they have (e.g., monogamy, family, strong friendships but no intimate relational ties)—so these are clarified for them when they do initiate sexual behaviors with a new partner. Participants are asked to role-play a sexual encounter with a new partner, and consider these goals within the context of that encounter. If they were reluctant to use a condom or do other things to stay safe, they are asked why they made that choice—and then shown why short-term "excuses" (e.g., lack of trust if condoms are brought up) are inconsistent with long-term life and relationship goals. The users can then go back and amend the role-play to incorporate intentions for safer sexual behavior.

Module 2, Session B: Condom Use With Partners. The emphasis in this module is on building awareness and skills regarding condom use when monogamy is not certain. The theoretical concept of self-efficacy from Bandura's social cognitive theory is emphasized here—skills building and confidence in skills to apply them in varying and sometimes challenging circumstances (Bandura, 1997). Participants again interact with the computer using a role-play, and it is carried out with cartoons of diverse men in a group setting. Users observe the group conversation and are asked to choose conversation prompts to bring up condoms—"I want to stay safe," "I do trust you, but this is something I've chosen for myself," and so forth. The participants role-play the conversation about condom use, and then assess their own level of self-efficacy for condom negotiation. If they are less than satisfied with their self-efficacy, they can go back and review the conversation. In addition to the role-play, participants are introduced to the "red flags," or potential triggers they have experienced that could keep them from condom use. This activity can be tailored to individuals in as much as they choose from among common triggers those that apply to them.

Module 3, Session A: Safer Sex in Context. This module was developed with substantial input from formative work with rural gay men, who described the process of partner seeking and risk behaviors in the context of the rural environment. The first session asks the participants to consider the process of getting ready to go to a gay bar—either in a rural environment or in a more distant urban one. The session focuses on approaches to establish intentions to stay safe and steps that they will take to ensure this can happen. Participants are asked to consider potentially challenging issues: "What if you drove all the way to an urban area, and then weren't able to find a partner or 'hook up' for sex? How would you feel?" and "How often do you consider plans for safer sex when you are planning to go to a gay bar?" Participants are asked to choose specific steps to facilitate preparation—buying condoms, carrying them with them, and having them on hand. They are then asked to consider challenges that may arise when they are actually at the bar—what are the "red flags," or triggers that could impede their intention to use condoms? Once they identify these triggers, they can consider a scenario at a bar and develop their skills in negotiating and using condoms with a casual sex partner.

Module 3, Session B: The Internet as a Context for Sexual Risk. Gay men and men who are not iden- tified as gay but who have sex with other men (MSM) are among those who have had sex with people they first met online, an activity that has been established as conveying a risk for transmis- sion of sexually transmitted infection (STI; McFarlane, Bull, & Rietmeijer, 2000). In this second session of Module 3, men are asked to consider the naïve Internet user who has interest in meeting a sex partner over the Internet. The module focuses on opportunities MSM and gay men have to reduce risk in these circumstances. Specifically, the module introduces users to various profile tem- plates from sex solicitation sites that can signal potential risk. Profiles that are risky include those that explicitly state that "condoms are optional," or they want to "party and play" or "P&P" (meaning they want to mix sex and drugs in an encounter), or they are seeking "bareback" sex (i.e., anal sex without condoms). The emphasis here is on how to be selective on Internet sites to avoid those who are explicitly unsafe. Users then are given information and shown data on Internet and STI risk. Finally, they are asked to consider their physical safety if they do decide to have sex with someone after meeting online. Where will they meet? Who will know they are going there? Users are advised to bring their cell phone and give someone their number. The module also includes a self-efficacy component to gauge skills in preparing for an Internet-initiated encounter.

At the end of the program, men are offered printouts with referrals for additional prevention ser- vices. The program concludes with a summary of the content, and users are invited to repeat program use as often as they wish.

Results

To date, WRAPP remains one of only two published trials on the efficacy of an Internet-based rather than a computerized HIV prevention delivered via kiosk. Research on the efficacy of WRAPP shows that participants exposed to the program have significantly improved condom attitudes and self-efficacy for condom use at 1 week postintervention. This research didn't include a long-enough follow-up of participants to demonstrate an impact on HIV prevention behaviors (Bowen et al., 2007).

Case Study: Diabetes-Network Internet-Based Physical Activity Intervention (D-Net)

Introduction

D-Net was a program designed and rigorously tested to determine whether using the Internet could improve physical activity and biomedical outcomes for persons living with diabetes. D-Net, like other computer-based programs studied in this book, included many features of the Web 1.0 environment: tailoring messages and offering individualized feedback and using updated content and graphics to make information more appealing. What is of particular interest is the addition of social support features to the D-Net program. In addition to the tailored messages, participants had access to an online coach and to each other for peer support related to behavioral change and self-management. Following is a detailed description of the program and the results of formal research evaluations of the program, which are also offered in publications on the results of initial D-Net pilot studies (McKay, King, Eakin, Seeley, & Glasgow, 2001).

Program Content

The D-Net intervention was designed to be delivered over an 8-week time frame. Participants initially completed an assessment of their current levels of physical activity (PA) and got tailored feedback on how well their activity matched national guidelines for moderate levels. Participants then completed "5 Steps to Action," which was a planning process to facilitate increased PA. First, they identified the benefits they perceived as being associated with PA. Then they selected a PA goal—this was intended to help them increase both activity level and frequency. They could then choose the activities they liked best from a list and schedule the days of the week and times of the day when they would do these activities. They would further identify potential barriers to completing their activities and strategies for overcoming these barriers. They could print out their plan, and they could also log on to the website to review it. Also available on the site was a resource library of PA tips, how-to articles, and testimonials about success with PA from others. On the site participants could log in and input total minutes of PA daily and generate graphs to track their PA progress.

Unique to D-Net among scientifically evaluated Internet-based interventions was the aspect of social support. While social networking, peer-to-peer communication, and user-generated content are ubiquitous online now and central to the Web 2.0 world, these features have yet to be consistently included in and evaluated in Internet-based health promotion programs. Social support on D-Net came in two forms. First, participants had access to a personal coach for counseling and support. The coach offered comments on their PA action plan and encouraged participants to communicate by posting in the personal coach conference area regarding questions, problems, or successes as the program continued. The coach would remind participants to review their goals and offer encouragement every 2 weeks over the life of the program.

The second type of support was through peer-to-peer contact both in an asynchronous discussion forum and in focused group chat on specific topics that were peer or program staff generated. All topics related to self-management and issues related to support for self-management.

Results

In long-term program evaluation, program participants who used the D-Net site on three or more occasions experienced significantly higher levels of moderate to vigorous physical activity. Users engaged with D-Net more intensively in the first 2 weeks, and then use dropped off. Participants largely agreed that the online coach was helpful (88% of users), and only about a third (35%) felt the peer support was helpful (Glasgow, Boles, McKay, Feil, & Barrera, 2003).

UNIQUE AND BENEFICIAL ASPECTS OF THE WRAPP AND D-NET PROGRAMS

Access in Rural Settings

For the WRAPP program in particular, the benefit of the Internet is that it allows users access to important health-related information in a rural setting. WRAPP addresses HIV-related risk; in rural areas, issues of stigma regarding homosexuality in general and HIV disease in particular continue to be identified as contributors to HIV risk (Galvan, Davis, Banks, & Bing, 2008). Having access to information and interactive computer programming that can help rural men understand and address risk is a benefit.

Rural access to the Internet is a benefit that will continue to facilitate health promotion for other conditions as well. While rural communities will likely continue to face issues of bandwidth that can limit access to high-speed interactive and graphic-heavy programs, even with dial-up connections they can still access information and some low-bandwidth interactive activities that will allow them to benefit from Internet-based programs.

Access to Elderly and Naïve Users

The D-Net program described here illustrates the potential for Internet health promotion for diverse users, including the elderly. D-Net illustrates that even naïve users or persons reluctant to try new technologies will engage with the Internet and use health promotion programs online. We should not assume that the elderly will not engage with the Internet; rather, we can acknowledge that within the elderly population there is likely a continuum of people, ranging from persons eager to adopt and try new technological approaches to health promotion, to those who may try reluctantly, to those who will never try an Internet-based program. This underscores the need for appropriate program development discussed in Chapter 3.

CHALLENGES IN WRAPP AND D-NET AND OTHER INTERNET-BASED HEALTH PROMOTION PROGRAMS

Considering If the Internet Is the *Best* Technological Modality for Your Population

The latest trend data on Internet access by the Pew Internet & American Life Project (Carter-Sykes, 2010) show that 73% of American men and 75% of American women aged 18 and older have used the Internet. Close to 90% of those under 30 have, and between 72% and 82% of those aged 30–64 have, with 41% of those over 65 having done so as well. The highest proportion of users by ethnicity includes Whites (77%) followed by Blacks (64%) and Hispanics (58%). A full 93% of teens are reported to use the Internet. We expect that trends like this will continue, with Internet use becoming more common, particularly as young people age.

The question used by Pew in assessing these trends is "Do you ever go online to use the Internet or to send or receive e-mail?" It is important not to infer that *ever* using the Internet is equivalent to widespread access and consistent use. Pew also reports that those who have Internet access *in their homes* and *regularly use* the Internet are fewer. Just over half (55%) of adults aged 18 and older have broadband and higher-speed Internet access at home, and poor Americans haven't seen increases in broadband access.

It is also important not to infer that if a person uses the Internet once he or she will automatically use it daily or even weekly. Although Internet use may be nearly universal in workplace settings and among middle-income and/or wealthier individuals and families, it is not a regular source of information and communication for many. Importantly, these groups may be overrepresented among persons with health disparities—for example, the poor, the elderly, and/or communities of color.

It is helpful to ascertain what people do when they connect to the Internet—for example, although young people are the largest group online, recall (as seen in Chapter 3) they aren't online to use e-mail—rather they send instant messages to friends, go to online gaming sites, and use social networking sites.

Be sure to investigate how well the population you wish to serve is connected to the Internet—investigate the extent to which members of this population have access—through broadband or other high-speed connections at home or in other locations—what they do online, and how often they access the Internet. This information will assist you in determining whether Internet is indeed the correct modality, and, if so, what are the best approaches to use to capitalize on the potential for reaching large numbers of your target audience. Figure 7.2 shows an algorithm to determine whether this technological modality will be the most appropriate for you to use.

Participant Retention and Dropout

In previous chapters we have covered strategies to recruit participants for health promotion programs online such as banner advertising and instant messages. We have also covered issues related to verifying that participants are who they say they are, and using mechanisms such as electronic reminders, incentives, and bonuses to retain participants in programs and/or for retention of participants for program evaluation activities.

Figure 7.2 Algorithm for determining appropriateness of Internet-based intervention for your target audience

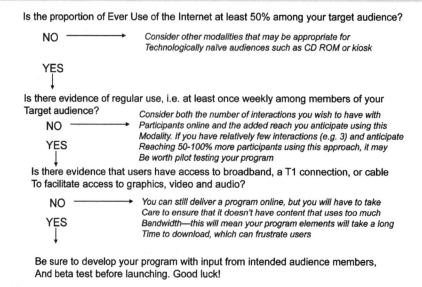

Be sure to develop your program with input from intended audience members,
And beta test before launching. Good luck!

Sustainability Without Incentives

Each program showcased in this chapter was developed and tested in the context of research, and as is common in such endeavors, participants were offered incentives (e.g., cash or gift cards) to participate and complete program elements.

Because technology-based health promotion is still a relatively new field, we do not have strong evidence that people will continue to engage with programs in the absence of any financial incentive. People may stay engaged with a particular site as long as they suffer from a given condition, such as chronic pain (Lorig et al., 2002). They may not be willing to engage or stay connected with a site that encourages primary prevention (e.g., to prevent onset of smoking). We need further exploration and study of the motivations people have for initial and ongoing engagement with health promotion websites, and we need an understanding of the variability of initial and ongoing engagement across different health conditions and stages of disease.

BEST PRACTICES EMPLOYED IN INTERNET-BASED PROGRAMS

Participant Retention

In this segment the focus is on how to keep the interest of your participants once they have enrolled—consider the length of your program and how many sessions you want participants to complete; consider how often you will be able to refresh and update content so users sense it is current; and consider how you can integrate Web 2.0 elements that link participants to each other.

Program Length and Number of Sessions

While the interest in development and delivery of health promotion programs on the Internet continues to grow, we have also seen challenges associated with retention of participants in program implementation. One challenge is participant drop-off. Several studies—including those we showcase here—show that participants lose interest in programs over time and will drop out. Data suggest that programs requiring participants to log on regularly will experience a precipitous drop-off at 3 months (Gustafson et al., 2001; McKay, Feil, Glasgow, & Brown, 1998). Some program planners have adapted materials with this information to ensure that retention of program participants will be strong, only to see disappointing levels of program efficacy (Bull, Pratte, Whitesell, Reitemeijer, & McFarlane, 2009). We don't have enough consistent data from multiple research studies to specify an optimal time period for delivery of online health promotion messages. We also do not know from current research whether there is an ideal number of sessions and amount of time to spend on a health promotion intervention that will generate adequate effects before users burn out or lose interest. Current data suggest that more than one session is needed to ensure larger program effects (Noar, Black, & Pierce, 2009) but that we also need to pay attention to participant tendency to lose interest over time (e.g., 3 months). The issue of program length and intensity may also vary by condition addressed. If working on programs associated with relief of chronic back pain, for example, precipitous drop-off in participation may not be as great an issue— these participants have ample motivation to stay engaged in the program as long as it helps alleviate pain (Lorig et al., 2002). On the other hand, maintaining attention among persons without a history of STI may be more challenging when trying to deliver messages designed to motivate safer sexual behaviors (Bull, McFarlane, & Rietmeijer, 2001).

Consider that the primary focus of the case studies in this chapter is on programs that were designed as stand-alone Internet-based interventions, not tied to any clinic or other face-to-face health promotion program. We urge readers to consider the opportunities that likely exist in utilizing the Internet as a tool to enhance, support, and extend face-to-face health promotion interventions. We have seen relatively few programs that have taken full advantage of the Internet in this manner. Issues of recruitment and retention may be circumvented if you can initially connect with people face-to-face through a clinic or community-based program, and then follow up with them online. This may reduce the reach of programs, but could have potential for helping with critical aspects of health promotion such as maintenance of behavior change over time.

Program Updates

An approach that program planners using the Internet will employ includes regularly updating information, material, and activities online. Internet users have become accustomed to frequent changes to the material and information they access online. Some sites not only refresh content daily, but can do so multiple times each day, up to hourly. The frequent user may become accustomed to regular new content and expect it. This may add substantial challenges for health promotion online—if you intend to make your program one with multiple sessions but want users to come back several times, consider the approaches you may be familiar with on websites: a "what's new" link on the home page and/or a "this week on the site" link to activities or sessions for the week. Figure 1.2 shown in Chapter 1 shows an example of a diabetes-related website highlighting its "what's new" content. You should consider polling potential users to ascertain how frequently they expect updates—a more technologically connected group that uses the Internet frequently will expect more frequent updates.

Employing Web 2.0 Elements

As mentioned in Chapter 1, we are now operating online in a Web 2.0 world (i.e., one that incorporates not only interactive features and graphics, but also opportunities for participant communication. To stay current within the Web 2.0 environment, many sites offer users opportunities to connect with program staff or each other through Web logs or blogs, through threaded discussions on various topics, through instant messaging to other users, or through chat. Figure 7.3 shows an example of an online blog about smoking cessation—other options are threaded discussions, auditorium chat, and chat by instant messaging. The efficacy of using these strategies as part of a health promotion intervention hasn't been established in the current research—however, it is likely that with the growth of social networking and other Web 2.0 technologies emphasizing user-driven content, we will see these approaches employed more consistently in technology-based health promotion.

WHAT ARE EMERGING TRENDS IN INTERNET-BASED HEALTH PROMOTION?

Efforts to Meet People Where They Are Online

Social Networking Sites

Social networks have been with us since the formation of societies; as described in more detail below, research of "real-world" social networks has offered support to the intuitive hypothesis that the people we engage with regularly in social circumstances have an influence on our health.

As explained in Chapter 1, the advent of Web 2.0 applications on the Internet fundamentally altered the way people engage with the World Wide Web. *Web 2.0* is the term given to those applications that facilitate networking online. Recall that initially, the Internet offered opportunities for individuals to interact with computers and receive tailored and personally relevant information and content. Web 2.0 now allows individuals not only to maintain these activities but also to interact with others while they are interacting with the Internet. Social networking sites such as MySpace, Facebook, and LinkedIn are all examples of sites where this happens. People use these sites to share information about their lives or other topics of interest with other people they select from their real-world networks and/or with people they have only engaged with online. The key activities people engage in on social networking sites online are outlined in Table 7.1. These are not the only activities people engage in online; rather they are those that they utilize to connect with or share information with other people in their networks.

Figure 7.3 Examples of threaded discussions, blogs, and chat on health-related topics

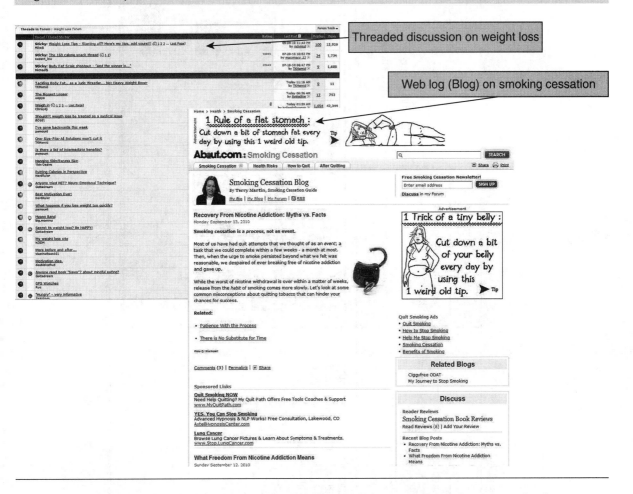

Figures 7.4 and 7.5 show examples of social networking sites and how they are used online. Figure 7.4 shows an example from Facebook and Twitter. Internet Sexuality Information Services (ISIS), a public health organization, uses these social networking sites to engage communities and begin conversations about health and wellness, prevention, and access to care.

Figure 7.5 shows a page from LinkedIn, a social networking site developed for professional networking, as opposed to exclusively social networking; it also includes a screen shot from STD Prevention Online, a site devoted to professional networking and information sharing for infectious disease professionals. These sites have features that are primarily intended to connect professionals working in a field or an area with one another. The first, LinkedIn, is a global professional networking site that allows people to interact across a multitude of fields, sharing networking advice, tips on creating résumés and curricula vitae, ideas for landing and

Table 7.1 Typical social networking activities online

Activity	Definition	Examples or other resources for more information
Blogs or Blogging	An online diary or journal written by a person about a given topic or topics; not limited to social networking sites, these can be popular online versions of regular columns by journalists.	A resource on the health care system in the United States: http://www.thehealthcareblog.com/ A blog about nutrition: http://www.thehealthblog.com/ A blog about new technological developments in health: http://blogs.msdn.com/healthblog/
Posting Pictures	People can post pictures of themselves or other people and places and share them with others—consider this like a personal photo album that is available to people within networks.	

196

Activity	Definition	Examples or other resources for more information
Testimonial	This offers people an opportunity to share their story or experience with a particular topic so that others can be inspired or informed.	Testimonials to support a given weight loss approach: http://www.scribd.com/groups/discussion/926–6-tips-to-maintain-weight-loss A testimonial about HIV and prevention: http://www.abanet.org/AIDS/testimonials/mthembu.html
Threaded Discussion	An asynchronous conversation about any topic. Threaded discussions are often used to help people find out more information or to get advice from others about something they are interested in. It could be something they want to purchase, or something they need information about. Discussions show multiple user postings related to the topic; people can add their own posting at the end of the series of other postings.	A threaded discussion on ways to quit smoking: http://www scribd.com/groups/discussion/831-what-are-some-great-ways-to-quit-smoking A threaded discussion on weight loss: http://www.scribd.com/groups/discussion/926–6-tips-to-maintain-weight-loss
Twitter	This activity links people online to mobile phones. People can register on Twitter.com and create a list of mobile phone numbers that they wish to "tweet" with. Then, they can create a text message on their phone and have it automatically sent to everyone on their list. The term twitter is intended to represent the notion that messages are generally very brief allowing for people to get an up-to-the-moment briefing on what an individual is up to.	http://twitter.com/
Yelp	This activity is not embedded in social networking sites but, like Twitter, is rather a site in and of itself online. It is designed to be an online consumer review site, and includes user reviews of restaurants, movies, and other commercial and service establishments.	www.yelp.com

Figure 7.4 Examples of Facebook and Twitter sites used by ISIS

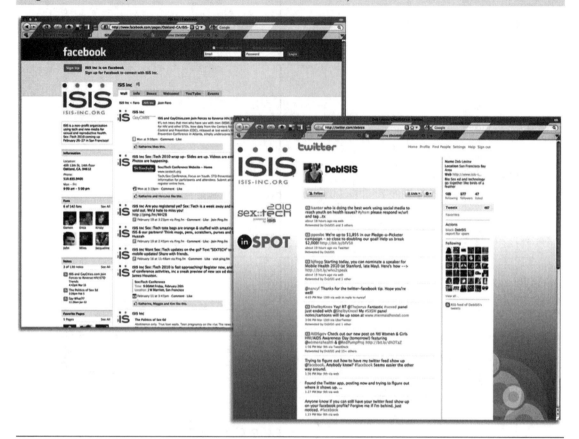

performing well in job interviews, and so forth. The second, STD Prevention Online, is a social networking site designed for providers engaged in prevention, diagnosis, and treatment of sexually transmitted diseases. The site offers weekly updates and information about current practices, emerging strategies for care and prevention, information on conferences and publications, and opportunities to blog and participate in threaded discussions.

These are tools that people use, all to convey information to their online networks. People often set up networks online to facilitate connections with people they already know in the real world; for example, Facebook can be used to connect all the members of one family. Rather than getting on the telephone 12 times to report a momentous event, users can post the information to their Facebook page, and then others within their network can see the information when they log on to the site. Users can choose to use the sites for more pragmatic purposes as well. Imagine you want to plan a family vacation. You can use your social networking page to post ideas for destinations and hotels, links to reviews about vacation packages, or information about airline availability and cost.

Young people use social networking sites to offer their real-world friends up-to-the-minute information about themselves. They also use the telephone to do the same thing en masse. The

Figure 7.5 Example of a LinkedIn social networking page and a page from STD Prevention Online, a social networking site for health professionals

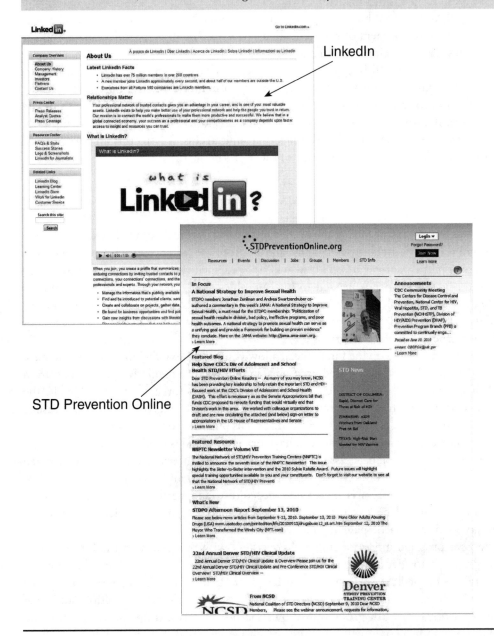

website called Twitter does this and has grown tremendously in popularity since its debut in 2006 as a platform that can be accessed online or via the telephone and text messaging to send single messages to large groups of people (Malik, 2010). We have yet to see people utilizing Twitter for health promotion, but anticipate that the approach of giving regular updates in a simple manner to large numbers of people (called "tweeting") will be perceived as useful for program updates, message reinforcement, and simple information sharing.

In previous generations, this type of communication across networks may have been accomplished through long hours on the telephone with multiple friends. Social networking sites allow the users to create and personalize a profile that will then become visible to others who use the site. A profile will be accessible to every user of the site, essentially completely public, unless the user engages privacy settings that limit access only to certain people (e.g., those who are specifically invited to be a part of the user's network).

SUMMARY

The Internet can be a very promising modality for delivery of a technology-based health promotion program. It is particularly appealing and appropriate when you wish to reach very large numbers of participants who you know will have adequate access to both computers and the minimum broadband speeds needed to load graphics that you include in your program content. Similar to other technology-based programs, the Internet can tailor information to individual users based on responses they give to surveys, and you can include a high degree of branching and structure in your programs.

In addition, programming on the Internet can allow you more flexibility than you would have for CD-ROM or strictly computer-based programs, in that you can regularly update and refresh content to maintain users' interest and meet their expectations for new content. Finally, the Internet offers many opportunities to enhance social support and connectivity—this isn't feasible in computer-based kiosk programs or programs that focus on Web 1.0 technologies exclusively.

Remember, however, that the Internet can have drawbacks and isn't always the ideal choice. If your population has limited access to computers and the Internet, especially high-speed broadband or cable access, you limit the reach to your intended audience using this modality. Furthermore, even when access is increased, the culture and patterns of use among your intended audience should be explored to ensure members of your intended audience are inclined to go online and participate in your program.

To make your program more enticing and consistent with the trends on the Internet, you should be prepared to give regular updates to the materials you post—depending on the audience, updates needed may be more or less frequent. At the same time, consider that your program will likely have a short life span for unique users. Evidence across multiple studies of Internet-based work for health promotion shows that user interest drops off over time, and that by about 3 months people will leave the site altogether (Bull, Levine, Vallejos, & Ortiz, 2008).

The programs considered here, WRAPP and D-Net, are examples of Web 1.0 and Web 2.0 applications for reaching large numbers of individuals for interventions in HIV prevention and diabetes self-management. They employ tailoring and personalized feedback, personal coaching, goal setting, and peer support. As interest in the field grows it will be likely that we will begin to see more evidence about the relative efficacy of each of these approaches for health promotion programs. As of now we can say they work to affect factors that influence behavior change such as norms and attitudes and intentions, and they have effects on short-term behavior change with repeated program exposure (i.e., three or more times).

? CONCLUDING QUESTIONS

1. What evidence do you have that the population you wish to work with has access to the Internet? Do you know where members of this population use the Internet most often? Do you know how often they use it? Do they have broadband, cable, or T1 (high-speed cable) connections to access the Internet?

2. What resources do you have to provide active and dynamic content with your program? How often can you update it? Is this consistent with the frequency and type of updates that are on sites popular with your target audience?

3. How much exposure will your participants have to your content? How often will you expect them to participate, and how many times through the life of your program?

4. What strategies will you use to deliver content?

   a. Tailoring and personalized feedback?

   b. Goal setting?

   c. Testimonials, blogs, or other user-driven content?

   d. Coaching or contact with a care provider?

   e. Videos?

CHAPTER EXERCISE

Your task in this exercise is to come up with a plan for translating all or selected elements of a successful technology-based health promotion intervention to a social networking site, or to design a social networking site that would incorporate these elements.

You may choose any of the interventions showcased in Chapter 1, or any of the case studies highlighted in this chapter, or Chapter 6, or the Appendix. Follow these steps to complete this exercise:

1. Select an intervention and identify those elements that will be most amenable for use on a social networking site.

2. Consider which social networking site you will use or if you will create a new social networking site.

3. Whether you are using an existing or a new site, describe the strategies you will employ to engage people in the intervention material. The strategies should be plausible, and match the types of engagement strategies common to social networking sites.

   a. How will you identify and recruit persons to engage with your content?

   b. How will you utilize networks to share or exchange ideas about your content?

   c. How will you monitor who sees your content? How will you measure the impact of exposure to your content?

ADDITIONAL RESOURCES

There are resources for multiple health conditions online, and existing online programs to assist persons living with chronic and infectious conditions. Consider if there is an association affiliated with a health topic you are interested in. The below associations have websites and regular updates in information and content on their sites. In addition, theses sites offer elements of interventions such as quizzes to determine your level of risk for heart disease, cancer, lung disease, and so forth.

Websites

Resource	Description
http://www.cancer.org/docroot/home/index.asp	American Cancer Society website
http://www.diabetes.org	American Diabetes Association website
www.americanheart.org	American Heart Association website
http://www.lungusa.org	American Lung Association website

You may also wish to search for sites online that cater to a specific audience, such as AARP.org. Sites such as MTV.com target young people, and BET.com targets African Americans. Both of these sites have had numerous campaigns that offer information and helpful program information for health considerations.

Resource	Description
http://www.aarp.org	AARP website
http://www.BET.com	BET website
http://www.MTV.com	MTV website

Currently there isn't a clearinghouse for online sites that are specifically designed for health promotion interventions.

Resource	Description
http://www.STDPreventiononline.org	Serves as a clearinghouse for information on Internet- and computer-based approaches for sexually transmitted disease prevention
http://www.re-aim.org/	A resource for professionals who use the RE-AIM framework in evaluation; offers advice for how to incorporate RE-AIM into your evaluation and how to measure each element, and also offers links to articles on programs that have successfully used RE-AIM

Look in the future for portals, where sites can be established as clearinghouses to access information about effective health promotion programs using the Internet.

Note: All websites noted here are hot-linked at www.sagepub.com/bull; at this site you will also find newer resources relevant to the material in this and other chapters.

REFERENCES

Bandura, A. (1986). *Social foundations of thought and action: A social cognitive theory.* Englewood Cliffs, NJ: Prentice Hall.

Bandura, A. (1997). *Self-efficacy: The exercise of control.* New York: Freeman.

Block, L. G., & Keller, P. A. (1995). When to accentuate the negative: The effects of perceived efficacy and message framing on intentions to perform a health-related behavior. *Journal of Marketing Research, 32,* 192–203.

Bowen, A., Horvath, K., & Williams, M. (2007). A randomized controlled trial of Internet-delivered HIV prevention targeting rural MSM. *Health Education Research, 22,* 120–127.

Bull, S., Levine, D., Vallejos, D., & Ortiz, C. (2008). Improving recruitment and retention for an online randomized controlled trial: Experience from the Youthnet study. *AIDS Care, 20,* 889.

Bull, S., Pratte, K., Whitesell, N., Reitemeijer, C., & McFarlane, M. (2009). Effects of an Internet-based intervention for HIV Prevention: The Youthnet trials. *AIDS and Behavior, 13*(3), 474–487.

Bull, S. S., McFarlane, M., & Rietmeijer, C. (2001). HIV and sexually transmitted infection risk behaviors among men seeking sex with men on-line. *American Journal of Public Health, 91,* 988–989.

Carter-Sykes, C. (2010). *Get the latest statistics.* Pew Internet & American Life Project. Retrieved from http://www.pewinternet.org/Data-Tools/Get-The-Latest-Statistics.aspx

Centers for Disease Control and Prevention. (1999, November). *Compendium of HIV prevention interventions with evidence of effectiveness.* Atlanta, GA: Author.

DiMatteo, M. R. (2004). Social support and patient adherence to medical treatment: A meta-analysis. *Journal of Health Psychology, 23,* 207–218.

Fisher, J., & Fisher, W. (2002). The information-motivation-behavioral skills model. In R. DiClemente, R. Crosby, & M. Kegler (Eds.), *Emerging theories in health promotion and research: Strategies for improving public health* (pp. 21–64). New York: Jossey-Bass.

Galvan, F. H., Davis, E. M., Banks, D., & Bing, E. G. (2008). HIV stigma and social support among African Americans. *AIDS Patient Care and STDs, 22,* 423–436.

Glasgow, R. E., Boles, S. M., McKay, H. G., Feil, E. G., & Barrera, M. (2003). The D-Net diabetes self-management program: Long-term implementation, outcomes, and generalization results. *Preventive Medicine, 36,* 410–419.

Gustafson, D. H., Hawkins, R., Pingree, S., McTavish, F., Arora, N. K., Mendenhall, J., et al. (2001). Effect of computer support on younger women with breast cancer. *Journal of General Internet Medicine, 16,* 435–445.

Lorig, K. R., Laurent, D. D., Deyo, R. A., Marnell, M. E., Minor, M. A., & Ritter, P. L. (2002). Can a back pain e-mail discussion group improve health status and lower health care costs? A randomized study. *Archives of Internal Medicine, 162,* 792–796.

Malik, O. (2010). *A brief history of Twitter.* Retrieved from http://gigaom.com/ 2009/02/01/a-brief-history-of-twitter/

McFarlane, M., Bull, S. S., & Rietmeijer, C. A. (2000). The Internet as a newly emerging risk environment for sexually transmitted diseases [Comment]. *JAMA, 284,* 443–446.

McKay, H. G., Feil, E. G., Glasgow, R. E., & Brown, J. E. (1998). Feasibility and use of an Internet support service for diabetes self-management. *Diabetes Education, 24,* 174–179.

McKay, H. G., King, D., Eakin, E. G., Seeley, J. R., & Glasgow, R. E. (2001). The diabetes network Internet-based physical activity intervention: A randomized pilot study. *Diabetes Care, 24,* 1328–1334.

Noar, S. M., Black, H. G., & Pierce, L. B. (2009). Efficacy of computer technology-based HIV prevention interventions: A meta-analysis. *AIDS, 23,* 107–115.

Rogers, E. M. (1995). *Diffusion of innovations theory.* New York: Free Press.

8 ▪▪

Case Studies in Mobile Phone-Based Health Promotion

CHAPTER OVERVIEW

Perhaps the newest type of technology-based approach for health promotion being used today is the mobile phone. Mobile phones can be very simple, with only voice capabilities for making and receiving telephone calls. However, mobile phones can also be highly sophisticated, allowing for calls, short message service (SMS, also known as text messaging), access to the Internet, and storage of files, photos, and music. Mobile phones are distinct from handheld computers and devices such as the Palm Pilot™ and others that allow for users to access word processing, accounting, databases, scheduling, address books, and other software features on a small handheld computer. Because of rapid evolution in handheld computing, we have seen the rise of "smart phones" (i.e., universal devices that incorporate all the features of a handheld computer and telephone). Given the current state of the field, the examples and considerations offered in this chapter allow the reader to consider program possibilities primarily using phones and smart phones. The advantages of using mobile phones are numerous: As with other technologies, they offer substantially greater reach to populations heretofore isolated from health promotion. In addition, they may offer new opportunities to bridge digital divides in access to technology. Unlike other technologies, they can offer constant access to users. Disadvantages of mobile phones include limited opportunities for extensive, detailed, and exhaustive messaging and education.

While some digital divide issues can be overcome using mobile devices, we still face challenges in inequitable access to the Internet and other advanced features on mobile phones. Let us consider these advantages and disadvantages in greater detail.

This chapter covers issues that are unique to the mobile phones for technology-based health promotion interventions. As with other chapters, we offer two case studies of health promotion using mobile phones. The first, called STop Smoking Over Mobile Phone, or STOMP, has strong evidence of effectiveness for smoking cessation. The second, called EpiSurveyor, is one of multiple efforts transpiring in developing country settings to improve the delivery of public health messages and services. We consider some challenges associated with mobile phone-based health promotion, and consider best practices that are related to the use of this modality including considerations for choosing a phone or mobile computer for your technology-based project and suggestions for what is feasible and shows promise with mobile computing. Of particular importance is the shift from using a technology that requires large equipment and a place to operate it to the ubiquitous and "always on" nature of the mobile phone. Another important consideration is the substantially expanded reach offered by mobile technologies. The chapter also includes key terms and additional resources.

CASE STUDIES OF STOMP AND EPISURVEYOR

Case Study: STop Smoking Over Mobile Phone— The STOMP Program

Introduction and Methods

The STOMP program was first developed and evaluated for efficacy in a randomized trial with over 1,700 smokers with mobile phones in New Zealand. Those in the intervention group received materials and information via text messages that were designed to promote smoking cessation. They were encouraged to set a quit date. Participants could text back information about their goals to quit, and, once a date for cessation was established, participants would receive five messages each day for the 5 days leading up to the quit date. On the quit day, participants received 1 month of free outgoing text messages. They were encouraged to communicate with all their friends and family members about their intentions to quit. This was designed to link them into existing networks to facilitate support. During the subsequent 4 weeks following the quit date, they continued to receive five messages each day (Rodgers et al., 2005).

STOMP recognized that smokers have strong cravings during cessation attempts, and organized the multiple messages and texting opportunities specifically as a distraction and to offer users something to do with their hands during their quit attempt. Other features of the program included "quit buddies" (i.e., people with similar characteristics and quit dates with whom the user could communicate); a library of strategies that users could access for tips on craving management; polls, sent to all intervention participants on a current topic; and quizzes on health and smoking issues.

At the end of the intensive text messaging period lasting 4 weeks after the quit date, messages tapered off to three per week for the remaining 5 months of the program. These messages focused on maintenance for those who had quit. Messages were tailored to individual user stages of quitting throughout the program.

Results

STOMP was shown to be successful; almost a third of those enrolled in the intervention quit compared to 13% in the control group (Rodgers et al., 2005). STOMP is licensed exclusively by HSAGlobal from the University of Auckland Clinical Trials Research Unit and is the first program to be supported by its HealthMessagingEngine (HME; http://www.hsaglobal.net/ node/63). The New Zealand government has branded the program nationally as "Txt2Quit" and offers the service through the national quit line. STOMP can be licensed in the United States through i.e. healthcare (www.iehealthcare.com) where it is branded as Kick Buts™. Current users of the program include The Quit Group, New Zealand's national quit line (www.txt2quit.co.nz), and TELUS as part of its corporate employee wellness program. As a result of working with The Quit Group and real-world user feedback, the licensed program has been modified somewhat to reduce the daily messages prior to the quit date and the daily messages during the 4 months following the quit date. The current program messaging plan is outlined in Table 8.1, reprinted from hsaglobal.net.

STOMP is now being tested in other countries, including Turkey, where it is being rolled out as part of a randomized trial to determine fidelity in replication (M. Ybarra, personal communication, September 25, 2009). The original program was developed with substantial community input from the Maori in New Zealand; Maori community members crafted messages that were culturally relevant and acceptable within their community (Rodgers et al., 2005). Thus, program replication requires adherence to a similar process of crafting messages with community input to ensure relevance and appropriateness. Figure 8.1 shows screenshots of the messages in the STOMP program along with an image of the back-end database that stores program messages and incoming text content from participants.

Case Study: EpiSurveyor—Expanding Program Evaluation and Delivery Through Handheld Computers

Introduction

Many of the programs showcased in this book consider the application of technology for direct-to-consumer programs on health. While these are certainly appropriate, and do underscore our ability to increase program reach, we have not yet considered programs for health promotion that target providers of care. Making provider tasks easier and increasing capacity to collect, store, and transfer data using handheld devices means there is substantial promise for increasing the reach of services beyond clinics to community settings, including rural settings where primary care may be severely limited.

Table 8.1 Message type, frequency, and tailoring used in the STOMP program

The STOMP Program				
The Program	*Stage*	*Period*	*Message Rate*	*Message Type*
	Prequit	14–1 Days Prior to Quitting	1–2 daily	Cessation
	Quit Day	1 day	3 on day	Cessation
	Intensive	Quit Day–4 Weeks	3 per day	Cessation
	Maintenance	Week 5–end	1 every 3 days	Cessation
Relapse	Relapse (Early or Late)	4 Weeks–After Quit Day Only	3 per day	Relapse
Craving and Slip-Ups	Anytime	Anytime	Up to 50	Craving/Slip-Up

Source: HSAGlobal (2009).

EpiSurveyor is a simple and easy-to-use software program, designed initially for personal digital assistants (PDAs) and handheld computers such as the Palm Pilot™. As PDAs have gradually transformed into, and been replaced by, mobile phones, DataDyne (creator of EpiSurveyor) has now created a version of its software program that is compatible with mobile phones and with smart phones.

The primary goal of EpiSurveyor is to allow providers to collect important health information from patients and community members in rural and hard-to-reach areas that are remote and may lack electricity and/or other computing equipment. These data can be collected to inform and evaluate programs. Epidemiologic data are useful in understanding distribution and patterns of disease, although this approach can be limited when data are not available in hard-to-reach areas for lack of opportunity to carry and access desktop computers, databases, and electricity.

Providers using EpiSurveyor can easily create a survey online, transfer it to their phone, and then transfer it to their phone in order to administer the form in diverse field settings. A fundamental advantage of EpiSurveyor is the free access to the software that allows for simple database and

Figure 8.1   Screenshots of messages from STOMP

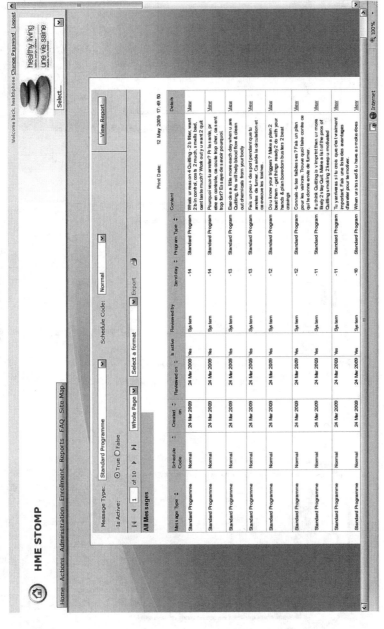

(Continued)

(Continued)

Example Text Messages

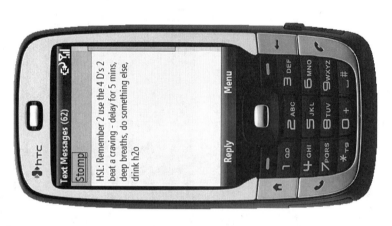

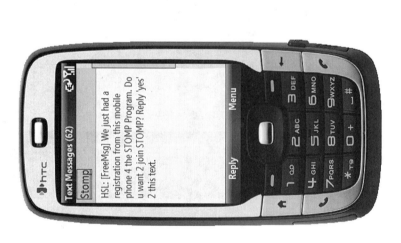

survey design by nonprogrammers; typically, using software programmers can be an expensive endeavor that is less accessible to persons in low-resource areas, particularly in developing country settings. As a result, people in these areas typically continue to rely on paper-and-pencil data collection; such an approach requires resources to copy surveys, transport them, and complete data entry after having completed forms by hand. By having a handheld computer device in the field, all of these steps are eliminated—surveys are stored on the handheld device, data can be uploaded via satellite or to a desktop or laptop computer as soon as one is available, and data entry occurs as the interview takes place, limiting chances of potentially problematic data entry errors.

The creators of EpiSurveyor consider that the tool has important potential for improving quality of care in resource-poor settings. They anticipate that persons who create a survey using the program could share it electronically and, in so doing, reduce the need for re-creating an entire new survey locally on the same topic. For example, if there can be a centralized database of surveys, practitioners interested in completing a needs assessment on maternal and child health could access this database rather than beginning from scratch to create a new tool. Furthermore, EpiSurveyor makes it easy to modify surveys, so you can adapt such a tool for local relevance, changing language and adding or deleting questions as needed.

Product Use

Figure 8.2 shows sample elements of the EpiSurveyor program, including information on how to develop and customize a survey. The process is similar to using Microsoft Office Access™ to create a database. Figure 8.2 shows screenshots from the finished product—how a survey would appear on paper and how it appears on a mobile phone device (Selanikio, 2010). Text Box 8.1 illustrates the steps involved in designing a handheld interface for data collection and data transfer.

EpiSurveyor has been used to improve the delivery of care through assessments and evaluations with organizations such as the Centers for Disease Control and Prevention, the American Red Cross, and the U.S. Army. EpiSurveyor has been used in many resource-poor settings such as Ghana and Sumatra, but is also currently used in the United States, Canada, and Europe. Since the online version (www.episurveyor.org) was introduced in July 2009, more than 1,400 users have registered and begun collecting data on mobile phones. By March 2010, more than 25,000 forms had been uploaded from phones to the EpiSurveyor website.

The creators of EpiSurveyor, DataDyne, say in their own words,

> By creating simple yet powerful software, making it affordable to all, actively disseminating it, and providing technical support, we can overcome the most important current barriers to a data-driven model of developing country public health. (Selanikio, 2010)

CHALLENGES IN STOMP AND EPISURVEYOR AND OTHER MOBILE PHONE-BASED PROGRAMS

Limited Opportunities for In-Depth Programs

With mobile phones one of the major drawbacks is the limited opportunity for going into depth with program content. Screen size of the device is usually very small, and larger screens, while

Figure 8.2 Examples of a questionnaire on paper and handheld device

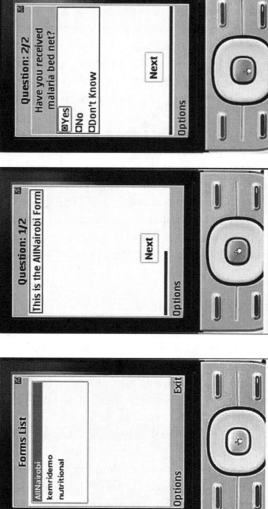

Survey Name: AllNairobi
No of Questions: 4

1: **This is the AllNairobi Form (label)**

2: **Have you received malaria bed net (multi)**

Data Field Name: Malarial
Possible responses:
- Yes
- No
- Dont Know

3. **How many have received bed net? (free)**

- Data Field Name: howmany

4. **Data (date)**

- Date Field Name: Date

appealing, limit the advantage of portability desired by consumers. With smaller screens it is difficult to communicate detailed content through text—having more text may mean smaller font, making things very difficult to read. Additionally, if considering a text messaging program, the limits to SMS in the United States are 160 characters, including spaces, so messages must be short. The ability to use a variety of content delivery strategies such as video, audio, and graphics can be limited because of the viewing space on the device.

Limited Access to Advanced Features of the Mobile Device

While an advantage offered by mobile devices is access to populations previously affected by the digital divide, there remain concerns that the types of features available on mobile phones, such as Internet and e-mail access, text messaging, and other nonvoice capabilities, are not accessible equally across socioeconomic groups. In the United States, the costs associated with data packages on mobile phones can be prohibitive—users have to pay for each incoming and outgoing call and text message or buy expensive packages to cover costs for unlimited text messaging and voice plans; access to the Internet to check e-mail or surf the web adds cost also. A recent report suggests that even when consumers have the capability to access e-mail and the Internet and use text messaging on their phone, they are not taking advantage of it—a survey of U.S. mobile phone users aged 13 and older showed that almost half (45%) of phone users preferred to use the device solely for voice communication and didn't take advantage of other nonvoice capabilities (Graham, 2009). It isn't clear whether the trends in computing that are historical and constant of smaller, more portable, and cheaper devices will translate into greater use of ubiquitous computing worldwide.

Device Sharing and Associated Lack of Confidentiality

Mobile phones are much easier to share with family and friends. This could actually be an advantage, particularly if you have a program that you are eager to disseminate to anyone and everyone. However, if your program participants need to meet specific eligibility criteria and if they are receiving content that is sensitive or personal, then you may be at a disadvantage using a mobile phone. Maintaining security on mobile phones will be a challenge—you cannot be completely sure that the person you are communicating with is indeed the person enrolled in your program.

BEST PRACTICES EMPLOYED IN STOMP AND EPISURVEYOR AND OTHER MOBILE PHONE-BASED PROGRAMS

Reaching Audiences With Mobile Devices

As with other modalities, one of the primary advantages of using mobile phones for health promotion is the potential to have greater reach with your programs to a much larger audience than would typically be seen for more traditional programs. Mobile phones continue to grow in popularity; in the United States, estimates are that 75% of adults have a cell phone and 62% use the device for activities such as text messaging, e-mail, taking pictures, recording video,

TEXT BOX 8.1

1. Register with the EpiSurveyor site, at http://episurveyor.org/user/ index, by clicking on "Create an Account" under "New to EpiSurveyor?":

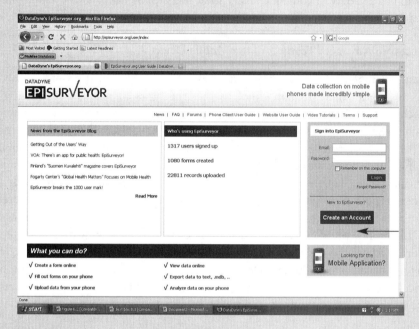

2. Create a new survey in EpiSurveyor by clicking "New":

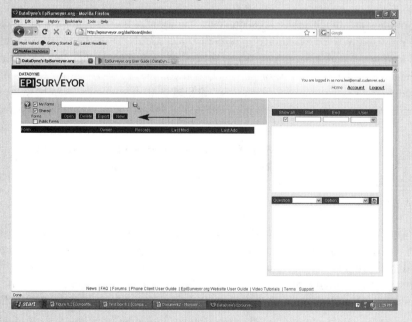

- Add these 5 parts:

  Label indicating the purpose of the form

  Date of interview (Make this a date question.)

  Number of children (Make this free input numeric, and required.)

  Number of people living in the house (Make this multiple choice.)

  Sex of respondent (Make this multiple choice [M or F], and radio.)

3. Install EpiSurveyor to your mobile device:
   - If the GPRS/EDGE/3G connection on your phone is not activated, activate according to user manual.
   - Go to http://www.episurveyor.org/m.
   - Select your phone make and model.
   - Follow the prompt to save the application; select the folder where you want to save the EpiSurveyor .jar file.
   - Once the download is complete, you can either (a) copy the EpiSurveyor installation file to the phone's memory card or (b) transfer the file via Bluetooth to the phone.

4. Download a form to your mobile device:
   - Go to "Forms List" and select "Options" and then "Get New Forms"; click on the form you want to download.
   - Collect data.
   - Basic analysis can be performed on the mobile device.

5. Transfer data from your mobile phone to the server (one or all unsent forms):
   - Highlight the form on the "Forms List" screen from which you want to send records.
     - Select the "Options" menu; highlight the "View Saved" menu option.
     - Sent records are marked with a check.
   - Check the boxes of all the records you want to send.
     - Press the "Options" button; scroll to "Send Data to Server."
     - Once records are sent, a confirmation message will appear.
     - At the top of the screen, you will see the form name, total number of records, and in parentheses how many records are unsent.
     - All data that have been sent are accessible for view and analysis by logging into the online account.
   - To go back to the "Forms List" screen press the "Options" button.
   - Scroll down to "Back" and press "Enter."

Source: http://datadyne.org/episurveyor/webguide; http://datadyne.org/episurveyor/phoneguide

and looking up information (Horrigan, 2008). In addition, there is evidence that populations previously disadvantaged by the digital divide have better access to mobile computers. For English-speaking Latinos and African Americans, use of mobile phones is equal to or surpasses that of White Americans and is almost universal among teens and young adults. Note, however, that these data are from surveys conducted in English—disparities in access to mobile phones remain in the United States for Spanish-speaking Latinos (Horrigan, 2008).

Other sources indicate that as many as 1 in 7 adults in the United States use only a mobile phone, and 20% have given up their landlines altogether (Harris Interactive, 2008). Industry trends on the use of smart phones show continuing increases in proportions of cell phone users who intend to purchase a smart phone as their next mobile device. There is a high degree of competition between the BlackBerry™ from Research in Motion (RIM), which holds the highest market share, and the iPhone™ from Apple, with the second highest share. Data suggest that the iPhone™ will continue to grow in popularity as Apple continues to make the device more affordable—there are units available costing between $99 and $299 (Carton & Woods, 2009). Furthermore, Apple has developed a mechanism whereby independent computer programmers can create applications ("apps")—also called "widgets"—that are simple, easy-to-use programs that can be very lifestyle oriented. Widgets or apps can allow for such health-related activities as identifying the caloric and nutrition content of fast food meals, monitoring blood pressure, reminding users to take medications, accessing healthy recipes, and monitoring physical activity—and many are free to iPhone™ users or available for very low cost (e.g., 99¢). The introduction of these apps has meant that the iPhone™ has become the handheld device most used for accessing the Internet (M:Metrics, 2008). Google has developed the Android (Open Handset Alliance) program, which is a free, open-source platform for creating widgets and applications that can be run on smart phones. With Android (http://source.android.com/), the capability for applications and widgets can now extend beyond the iPhone™ to other smart phones. Figure 8.3 shows the screen of an iPhone™ and selected health applications. The user can touch any icon on the screen and be directed to the application.

Outside the United States, there has also been a proliferation of cell phone access and use. Reports indicate that as many as 60% of adults worldwide have signed up for mobile phone service or handsets (Daily Mail Reporter, 2009) and that there are as many as 3 billion mobile phone users globally (Ridley, 2007). Some suggest the promise of mobile technologies for health promotion in the developing world has surpassed the potential of computers, the Internet, and kiosks—the low cost, limited need for equipment, and wireless capability all point to portability and access that mean far greater reach than could be achieved with desktop or even laptop computing equipment (Selanikio & Donna, 2005).

Constant Access and "Always On" Features of the Mobile Device

Another opportunity programs take advantage of with mobile devices is their portability, making users much more accessible. Because people can carry and have access to their phones and handheld computers much more consistently than they can to their desktop or laptop computers, we as health professionals can have access to them more frequently. This becomes important when considering health promotion approaches that are time-sensitive—reminders to take medications, to make appointments, and to check blood pressure or blood sugar levels can all be delivered through text messages at predetermined times of the day and days of the week. It may be much more likely to reach people with a text message to remember their hypertension medication on their phone at 7 a.m. than via e-mail on the computer. The other advantage that portability lends is the ability to conduct health promotion in remote, hard-to-reach, or potentially dangerous areas. Collecting data for a program evaluation using a handheld device allows for the program evaluator to access more remote areas; it may also allow for access to areas where higher crime levels thwart attempts to carry obviously expensive computing equipment such as laptop computers.

Figure 8.3 The iPhone™ and opportunities for health-related applications

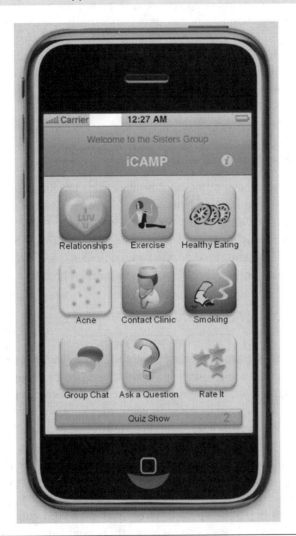

WHAT ARE EMERGING TRENDS IN MOBILE PHONE-BASED HEALTH PROMOTION?

Efforts to Incorporate Streaming Video and Other Smart Phone Applications

There is a growing interest in the use of smart phones for the delivery of content via cell phone. In particular, people are experimenting with the use of video delivery and delivery of data such as e-mail.

We face challenges in attempting to utilize smart phone features such as video and e-mail. In the United States, such phones are still expensive, often require a costly monthly service plan, and are not universally popular among cell phone users. It is critical to revisit the considerations for program development outlined in Chapter 3 in planning to utilize such features in your program. If your target audience doesn't access or utilize smart phones, then you may be making inappropriate plans to incorporate these features in your program. While the cost of phones and plans may diminish over time, we still do not have good evidence that smart phones and their advanced features are in use among the audiences we should reach with technology-based health promotion.

Linking Phones to Face-to-Face Clinic-Based Services

We are beginning to see strategies employed by clinics that can facilitate linkage to care via cell phones. Using phones to encourage patients to take medication has been employed with some promising success (Connelly, Faber, Rogers, Siek, & Toscos, 2006; Logan et al., 2007). Using cell phone text messages to remind patients of appointments or to advise them that test results are available is another approach with promise. As with computer kiosk and Internet programs, cell phones have ample promise for increasing clinic services outside clinic walls.

SUMMARY

We are in the very early stages of using mobile phones to deliver health promotion—either as stand-alone programs or to enhance existing programs. While we have yet to amass substantial data on the efficacy of this modality for health promotion, the field continues to yield important and compelling information that handheld devices have enormous potential.

As considered in other chapters, the decision to use mobile phones in your health promotion program should be based on a number of different factors. If you are working with a population that readily and consistently uses mobile phones, you may consider this ideal to reach larger numbers of your target audience. Consider carefully the program features you wish to provide; what mobile phones offer in terms of "always on" or ubiquitous computing may be diminished by an inability to deliver sophisticated or detailed content. If you seek to have a program that can be scaled up to different states or even countries, you should pay close attention to the hardware and wireless program components to ensure compatibility in technology across different settings. Finally, it may be shortsighted to consider the mobile device as a tool only for stand-alone health promotion efforts. Ultimately, the devices could be used to enhance existing programs by reinforcing messages users have received in a clinic setting, or reminding patients to take medications, or offering detailed directions on how and when to access services.

Table 8.2 offers definitions for terms you may come across in considering a promotion program using a mobile device. Below the table are some key concluding questions for this chapter.

Table 8.2   Key terms and definitions related to mobile phones

Term	Definition	Additional Resources
3G, or Third Generation	The term given to the newly emerging, faster wireless systems currently available on the market; the popular iPhone™ and BlackBerry Curve™ use the 3G system	http://www.itu.int/home/ imt.html
IMT 2000, or International Mobile Telecommunications	The term developed by the International Telecommunication Union and used to describe the systems intended to link all the newly developing wireless communication systems; systems can be linked through a combination of land-based wired technologies and satellites	http://www.itu.int/home/imt.html
Java Virtual Machine	Computer software that allows for a virtual machine to execute computer programs	http://en.wikipedia.org/wiki/Java_Virtual_Machine
NGN, or Next-Generation Networking	A name given to the anticipated advancements we will see in the coming 5–10 years in telecommunications and technology-based networks	http://en.wikipedia.org/wiki/Next_Generation_Networking
Open Systems	The name given to a system that allows for interoperability and portability of programs	http://en.wikipedia.org/wiki/Open_system_(computing)
WiMax	Worldwide Interoperability for Microwave Access; the wireless transmission of data across devices	http://en.wikipedia.org/wiki/WiMAX

? CONCLUDING QUESTIONS

1. Does your intended program audience use mobile phones or handheld computers?

2. Which is more commonly owned? How often is the device used?

3. If you intend to use a mobile phone, will you use your program to communicate via voice and/or SMS? Why? Do you have evidence that your intended audience has a preference for one over the other?

4. If using SMS, how will you develop program messages? How will you incorporate best practices for health promotion (e.g., use of theory for behavior change) into your SMS messages?

5. Will you incorporate other nonvoice elements into your program such as video or links to the Internet? If so, what do you know about the wireless connection capabilities of your users? If their device has the capacity to download videos and access the Internet, will they be willing to utilize their device to do this? Will they have to pay extra to do this?

6. How do you intend to collect evaluation data for your program? Can you use the mobile phone or handheld computer to collect data? If so, how will you program your data collection instruments to collect information feasibly via the handheld device?

7. How will you store and subsequently transmit your program evaluation data?

 ## CHAPTER EXERCISE

We know from literature in health promotion that there are multiple theoretical factors that contribute to behavior change at the individual level. Several of these have been shown to consistently impact behaviors (see Chapter 1):

Outcome expectancies (also called positive outcome expectancies and negative outcome expectancies) are the outcomes that an individual anticipates will happen if he or she performs a given behavior. For example, if a person quits smoking, he can expect improved health in the long term and improved breath in the short term (positive outcome expectancies). He may also anticipate experiencing weight gain (negative outcome expectancy).

Norms are beliefs related to what peers "normally" believe, accept, or do. For example, individuals may believe that their peers consider consistent helmet use during bike riding to be important, and an individual may also believe that others like her will consistently use a helmet for bike riding.

Self-efficacy is the belief that an individual has that he or she has both the capacity (skill) to perform a behavior and the confidence to do it, even when circumstances make it challenging to do so. For example, a person can develop self-efficacy to avoid drinking sugary sodas by successfully practicing refusal and making substitutions.

Your task is to identify a behavior or behaviors that you would like to impact with your text messaging program. Design several messages (between three and five) that are crafted to address outcome expectancies, norms, and self-efficacy related to your selected behavior. Remember that your text messages cannot exceed 160 characters.

 ## ADDITIONAL RESOURCES

The use of mobile phones is only beginning, and we anticipate that in the coming decade there will be substantial growth in this area. Of particular interest to observe in the coming decade will be the proliferation of use in developing country settings. The United Nations Foundation in conjunction with Vodafone has written a report on various programs in developing country settings that are employing this technology for health promotion—they range from HIV prevention to tuberculosis treatment adherence to training health care providers (Baron & Ling, 2007; Vital Wave Consulting, 2009). As mentioned above, the STOMP program is being scaled up for use in multiple countries and across multiple populations, and we anticipate that this could be one of the earliest with data on effective dissemination strategies for mobile phone interventions (HSAGlobal, 2009). However, with such little evidence of intervention efficacy using these modalities, there remain few resources as of yet that can offer detailed information on best practices for health promotion for ubiquitous computing.

 ## Websites

Resource	Description
http://www.hsaglobal.net/node/34	STOMP program
http://www.unfoundation.org/global-issues/technology/mhealth-report.html	United Nations Foundation report written in conjunction with Vodafone
http://www.unfoundation.org	United Nations Foundation website
http://www.vodafone.com/index.VF.html	Vodafone website

Note: All websites noted here are hot-linked at www.sagepub.com/bull; at this site you will also find newer resources relevant to the material in this and other chapters.

REFERENCES

Baron, N. S., & Ling, R. (2007). Emerging patterns of American mobile phone use: Electronically-mediated communication in transition. In G. Goggin & L. Hjorth (Eds.), *Mobile Media 2007: Proceedings of an International Conference on Social and Cultural Aspects of Mobile Phones, Convergent Media and Wireless Technologies* (pp. 218–230). Sydney, Australia: University of Sydney.

Carton, P., & Woods, J. (2009). *Smart phone survey findings: 90 day outlook.* Retrieved from http://blog.changewave.com/2009/04/smartphone_iphone_blackberry_pre.html

Connelly K. H., Faber, A. M., Rogers, Y., Siek, K. A., & Toscos, T. (2006). Mobile applications that empower people to monitor their personal health. *Springer E&I, 4,* 123–124.

Daily Mail Reporter. (2009, March 3). *Mobile phone use explodes as 60% of the world's population signs up for a handset.* Retrieved from http://www.dailymail.co.uk/ sciencetech/article-1158758/Mobile-phone-use-explodes-60-worlds-population-signs-handset.html

Graham, L. (2009). *The NPD Group: Nearly half of mobile phone users eschew multi media features and use handsets solely to make calls.* Retrieved from http://www.npd.com/press/releases/press_090106.html

Harris Interactive. (2008). *Cell phone usage continues to increase* (The Harris Poll, #36). New York: Author.

Horrigan, J. (2008). *Info on the go: Mobile access to data and information.* Retrieved from http://pewresearch.org/pubs/753/mobile-access-data- information

HSAGlobal. (2009). *STOMP (STop Smoking Over Mobile Phone)*. Retrieved from http://hsaglobal.net/node/34

Logan, A. G., McIsaac, W. J., Tisler, A., Irvine, M. J., Saunders, A., Dunai, A., et al. (2007). Mobile phone-based remote patient monitoring system for management of hypertension in diabetic patients. *American Journal of Hypertension, 20*, 942–948.

M:Metrics. (2008). *M:Metrics: iPhone hype holds up*. Retrieved from http:// mmetrics.com/Press_Events/Press_Releases/2008/03/iPhone_Hype_ Holds_Up/

Ridley, K. (2007, June 27). Global mobile phone use to pass 3 billion. *Reuters UK*. Retrieved from http://uk.reuters.com/article/idUKL27121 99720070627

Rodgers, A., Corbett, T., Bramley, D., Riddell, T., Wills, M., Lin, R. B., et al. (2005). Do u smoke after txt? Results of a randomised trial of smoking cessation using mobile phone text messaging. *Tobacco Control, 14*, 255–261.

Selanikio, J. (2010). *DataDyne*. Retrieved from http://www.datadyne.org/

Selanikio, J., & Donna, R. (2005). EpiSurveyor [Computer software]. Washington, DC: DataDyne.

Vital Wave Consulting. (2009). *mHealth for development: The opportunity of mobile technology for healthcare in the developing world*. Washington, DC: UN Foundation-Vodafone Foundation Partnership.

9 ▪▪

Epilogue

OVERVIEW

In this epilogue we review and briefly summarize the main points of this book. We then consider emerging trends in the field of technology-based health promotion and offer advice and thoughts on ways to embrace new innovations.

REVIEW OF THE UNIQUE AND BENEFICIAL ELEMENTS OF ALL TECHNOLOGY-BASED HEALTH PROMOTION PROGRAMS

Technology-based health promotion has tremendous promise, as could be inferred from the tremendous growth in the field over the past decade. Consider how quickly we have adopted computers, the Internet, and mobile phones—and you can imagine how much opportunity there is to integrate health promotion into our daily lives through technology.

In Chapter 1 we offered specific detail on ways in which technology-based health promotion offers advantages over standard face-to-face health promotion. We reiterate these advantages, in summary, in Table 9.1.

Table 9.1   Relative advantages offered by technology-based health promotion

Advantage of technology-based health promotion	Definition	Related references
Reach	Because technology is available in so many places, via computer, Internet, and cell phone, there is opportunity to reach many more people with a health promotion program than you otherwise may be able to through clinical or institutional sites (e.g., schools).	Bull, Gaglio, McKay, & Glasgow, 2005; Glasgow, Klesges, Dzewaltowski, Estabrooks, & Vogt, 2006; Glasgow et al., 2006, 2007
Impact	With greater reach, it is possible to see greater impact of program efficacy, even when effects are small—programs with small effects delivered to large numbers of people will have greater impact on disease outcomes than those with large effects that can reach only small numbers of people.	Estabrooks & Gyurcsik, 2003; Glasgow et al., 2006; Gustafson et al., 2005; Heller & Dobson, 2000 Ironson et al., 2005; Joffe & Mindell, 2002
Standardized program delivery	Technology allows for uniformity in program delivery—for example, the same message, delivered in the same order using the same content, means programs aren't dependent on an individual staff member for program success.	Glasgow et al., 1997; Prochaska, DiClemente, Velicer, & Rossi, 1993; Strecher et al., 1994; Taylor, Houston-Miller, Killen, & DeBusk, 1990
Tailoring	Responses and messages can be tailored to individual needs using algorithms that generate preprogrammed responses. Tailoring can help make program messages more personally relevant (e.g., when a message is delivered by a role model that matches participant age, gender, or race) and more clinically relevant (e.g., by focusing on a behavior directly relevant for an individual).	Clark et al., 2004; Etter, 2005; Gore-Felton et al., 2005; Kukafka, Lussier, Eng, Patel, & Cimino, 2002; Scholes et al., 2003; Smeets, Brug, & De, 2008; Strecher, Shiffman, & West, 2005
Interactive	Participants can respond to questions, post their own opinions, play games, and get engaged with technology.	Booth, Nowson, & Matters, 2008; Glasgow, Bull, Piette, & Steiner, 2004; Glasgow, Christiansen, Smith, Stevens, & Toobert, 2008; King et al., 2004; Leeman-Castillo et al., 2007; Linke, Murray, Butler, & Wallace, 2007; Noar, Clark, Cole & Lustria, 2006; Rotondi, Sinkule, & Spring, 2005

Advantage of technology-based health promotion	Definition	Related references
Private	For health promotion that is sensitive or personal (e.g., sexual health, addiction intervention) users can engage with program content without having to disclose sensitive information to a health educator or clinician.	Bull, Pratte, Whitesell, & Rietmeijer, 2009; Turner et al., 1998
Autonomy	Users in technology-based health promotion may be able to move around at will to various program elements and choose to engage with those they find most interesting or relevant.	Pew Internet & American Life Project, 2000
Portability	Technology is ubiquitous, and programs can be as well. Using cell phones and the Internet, it is possible to reach people in places and at times that haven't been possible before.	Brendryen & Kraft, 2008 ; Cellular News, n.d.; Curioso & Kurth, 2007; Krishna, Boren, & Balas, 2009; Logan et al., 2007; Harris Interactive, 2008; Hurling et al., 2007; Ybarra & Bull, 2007
Cost-effectiveness	If we can achieve all the other advantages described here, it may result in a substantial cost savings— by making programs reach more people, standardized and relevant, we could cut delivery costs.	Boase, Horrigan, Wellman, & Rainie, 2006; Booth et al., 2008; Brendryen & Kraft, 2008; Bull et al., 2005; Cassell, Jackson, & Cheuvront, 1998; Feil, Glasgow, Boles, & McKay, 2000; Formica, Kabbara, Clark, & McAlindon, 2004; Glasgow et al., 2007

REVIEW OF THE CHALLENGES OF TECHNOLOGY-BASED HEALTH PROMOTION PROGRAMS

It is critical to consider the challenges inherent in technology-based health promotion programs *before* implementing them. Just because you *can* use technology doesn't mean you *should* use it. Indeed, it may be argued that the seduction of technological advances that are intriguing, fun, or captivating may overshadow program decisions, and health promoters may make errors in developing programs without careful attention to the needs, desires, and practices of their target audience vis-à-vis technology.

Although technology does offer many advantages in health promotion, there remain fundamental challenges to technology-based programs. These are also detailed in Chapter 1, and summarized here in Table 9.2.

Table 9.2 Relative advantages offered by technology-based health promotion

Challenge	Definition	Related references
Sampling	There is no good sampling frame for users of the Internet or cell phones, so finding ways to generalize positive effects from a program to a larger population may be difficult.	Pequegnat et al., 2007
Confidentiality/security	Concerns abound related to computer security and data transfers over the Internet. While security systems are very sophisticated and can be employed in ways to substantially reduce breaches in confidentiality, this requires a level of technical expertise and oversight from information systems experts on projects.	King & Miles, 1995
Attention span	Users may be accustomed to shorter periods of engagement with technology, so programs may need to achieve effects with less contact time.	Ross, 2002
Competing attention	As the Internet continues to grow and the use of technology becomes more ubiquitous, we face ongoing challenges to competition for the attention of participants. Why would they want to participate in your health promotion program if they can be playing a fun game online?	Lavoie & Pychyl, 2001
Digital divide	While shrinking, the digital divide still exists and persists. Program planners need to pay careful attention to delivering content using technology that is accessible, affordable, and familiar to their audience.	Bernhardt, 2000
Obsolescence	Computer technology will continue to evolve, and may do so rapidly. We need methods to quickly develop and test interventions so that our findings aren't obsolete by the time we generate them.	Pequegnat et al., 2007

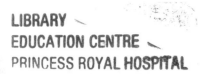

REVIEW OF THE EMERGING TRENDS AND FUTURE DIRECTIONS IN TECHNOLOGY-BASED HEALTH PROMOTION PROGRAMS

There are multiple technological advances that are regularly identified in the media and through peer-reviewed literature that have potential for advancing the field of health promotion. Trying to predict the next waves of technology is difficult at best, and to some extent, it is a questionable practice for public health interventions. Given that there is a digital divide between high- and low-income individuals, and considering that the majority of public health messages are aimed at people of reduced income, it is not likely that the target audience for many messages will be the early adopters of new technology. The exception to this rule is adolescents, who are the primary target audience of most new communications technology and advertising. Even in this case, however, it is difficult to predict which technologies will "catch on" and which will be less successful. When trying to decide on a modality or innovation to use for a research study, it seems a risky gamble to use the newest, most cutting-edge device. There is, however, a concern that it takes so long to study new technologies that the results of the studies are available only when the technology is obsolete, or at least no longer new. Clearly there are benefits and downsides to predicting the future of communications innovations. There are, however, several categories in which innovations are emerging or are currently developing, and these emergent technologies may prove extremely helpful to moving forward the field of health communications. We will enumerate them here, with the caveat that this is a snapshot in time, and one that must be revisited often to provide the nearest view of the future.

Gathering Information Online

Gathering Data Across the Internet

In previous chapters, we have discussed online surveys, interviews, focus group–type chats, and similar methods for gathering data from study participants or potential participants. What if, on the other hand, we want to gather data about a broader group of people or about the Internet itself? For example, let us suppose that a new treatment becomes available for malaria, a widespread and deadly disease in many parts of the world. As health communications researchers, we may be interested in the way in which Internet users discuss the new treatment. Are users outside of the developed world aware of it? Do they know the risks and implications? Are the people who are most at risk for malaria aware of the treatment, or is it simply being discussed on medical sites? Are there concerns about side effects or misuse of the treatment? Are there socioeconomic impacts being discussed (e.g., the potential for reduced infant mortality and the effects of a healthier population on world economic development)? All of these bits of information would probably be discussed in various parts of the online world. How can we learn about these conversations without having to spend days and weeks online? The answer involves a *web crawler* (also called *web robot* or *web bot, web spider,* or combinations of these terms). The purpose of a web crawler is to search the web for pages on which a particular word or topic is discussed. Think of the web crawler finding all of the possible pages with *malaria* mentioned, creating a copy of those pages, and storing those copies in a folder. Once the pages are stored, the crawler can then search through the folder for pages that are similar to each other, pages that contain particular messages about malaria, or pages with other attributes determined by the crawler or its programmer. The amount of effort it takes to program a useful web crawler is considerable, because the goals of the user are often complex and require the crawler to process language found on websites. Detecting a particular word on a website is easy; deciphering the language to determine whether the site discusses the issue positively or negatively, for example, is difficult. Despite the complexity involved in programming a crawler, there are several in existence at this time, and no doubt there are more to come. One example of a web crawler can be found at http://www.epispider.org and is aimed at public health researchers. The crawler searches for medical events mentioned on news sites and on sites where doctors post questions and answers for one another. Based on the data gathered from the "crawl," EpiSpider can generate maps and reports describing medical events occurring all over the world. Each image generated, of course, is a snapshot of the time period over which the data were gathered. Still, the system is valuable for detecting possible outbreaks or emerging disease situations.

Gathering Data About Your Website

In nearly every case, the owners of a website are interested in knowing the number, demographics, and interests of people who view their site. Are teens viewing their page? What do they click on most often? How much time do older women spend reading their blog? Where are men going on their site, and what information do they seek out? Does anyone click on the advertisements? How many pages "deep" do people get into the website before abandoning it? This kind of information is called *web analytics* or *web metrics* and is key to the evaluation of a website or communications tool. Generally, acquiring this information requires installing a program that counts the visitors to the websites and records "click streams" (the paths followed by the users as they navigate the site) and time spent on the site. The most popular of the web analytics software programs is currently Google Analytics, which also links to Google Website Optimizer, a program that uses Google Analytics to determine what combination of layouts, content, and so forth are likely to provide the most successful viewing experience (as measured by the time spent on the site, the number of people who buy a product, or other metric). To assess the characteristics of the people who visit your website and to gauge which users are most likely to achieve what goals, a web analytics program is highly recommended.

Virtual Experiences

As the ability to play long videos and interact quickly with the computer becomes more pervasive, many organizations will be developing online, interactive simulations of real-life experiences. Online "virtual worlds" are websites in which users can create simulated structures, tools, clothing, food, creatures, and any number of other objects. In Second Life (Linden Lab), for example, people create avatars (graphical representations of themselves), purchase virtual buildings or islands or other properties, and create their own environments in which to interact. Virtual worlds of this type easily accommodate the enterprising health communicator who may wish to build, for instance, a virtual clinic. The virtual clinic can demonstrate the process of a physical exam, or perhaps a counseling session or another health-related experience. Such virtual experiences can mitigate the anxiety that patients often experience before a medical procedure. Of course, the inhabitants of virtual worlds are only a tiny fraction of the people who need assistance with potential health care visits. How can such simulated experiences be made available to a wider, more general audience?

The answer lies in the application of this innovation to more general websites where people search for information about the health conditions or procedures they are experiencing. Consider a hypothetical teenager who is diagnosed with diabetes. Much information is available regarding diabetes, but how can the adolescent sort through it? How can he learn about the various medical excursions he will be required to embark upon? Perhaps a website that shows an avatar (a virtual patient) learning to measure his own blood sugar, monitor his diet, exercise appropriately, carry requisite supplies with him, go to school and explain his condition to friends and teachers, and attend regular medical visits would help such a patient. To add interactivity to the program, the teen could make choices for his avatar and see the consequences of those choices. Small subprograms could require the user to interactively move the virtual glucose monitor into position to perform sugar tests, pack a bag of supplies to take on vacation, or keep track of symptoms and activities. Adolescents may be an ideal target audience for such an innovation due to their comfort and familiarity with technological products and because they may face anxieties that they are not comfortable expressing to peers or parents. This makes a virtual environment that can be experienced privately even more valuable to the patient.

Mobile phones can be a part of a virtual medical excursion and can help with the in-person medical care as well. Reminders to attend the virtual (and real-life) clinic can appear via text messages. Video or audio notes (short video or audio recordings that can be sent to mobile phones in a manner similar to text messaging) and related features can help ensure that insulin shots are administered properly, or diet and exercise are recorded, by providing brief video reminders of the process. Ideally, such a program would also be supported by the doctor's office at some level; perhaps the teenager could have regular question-and-answer contact with an office nurse or other staff member. Finally, blood sugar measurements can be entered into a mobile device and sent to the doctor's office so that a regular record of blood sugar is kept and periodically examined by the practitioner. If the readings are not submitted, or if the readings are indicative of problems, the office staff can contact the patient immediately.

The benefits of virtual excursions are not limited to patients. Rather, such virtual environments are useful for a whole range of communications and training. Clinician education programs can assist student nurses with learning the layout of hospital rooms, performing basic operations with the various monitors and machines that are at the patient's bedside, or learning the order of instruments on a surgical tray. A student nurse may be able to use software to learn to assist the clinician with an exam, take medical history and physical information from an unyielding patient, or learn a whole host of scenarios that can occur in medical settings. Virtual experience cannot, of course, take the place of in-person experience, but can provide the health worker with some basic tools to assist in training and education.

Telemedicine

Telemedicine is a field of medical practice that relies on high-speed communications devices and software, and often video equipment, to allow medical personnel to conduct examinations or even perform some procedures from a distance. Both synchronous (real-time) and asynchronous versions of telemedicine exist. In the asynchronous form of telemedicine, information about a patient or medical situation is stored and sent to a distant expert; for example, a mammogram may be saved by a technician in Botswana and forwarded to a radiologist in New Jersey for assessment. Similarly, a nurse practitioner may send case files to a specialist for review and consultation. The patient need not be present when the information is transmitted.

Synchronous telemedicine is far more complex. In one example, a counselor may consult with a patient who is physically inaccessible, perhaps on a ship in the middle of the ocean, or in a prison or another facility. Simple videoconferencing can allow such an encounter to proceed. More complex is a procedure in which an onsite clinician examines the patient with medical tools that transmit the data to a distant consultant. For example, imagine an endoscope examining a patient's sinuses in one location, while a doctor in another location sees the video from the endoscope and studies the anatomy while talking to both the patient and the onsite staff. Further, imagine that a distant doctor controls a robot as it performs surgery on a patient.

These forms of telemedicine are obviously incredibly high-tech and are evolving rapidly. For health communications and intervention purposes, however, there are obvious implications of this technology. Interventions that are begun in a doctor's office can be extended using mobile video notes, text messages, or online virtual excursions. Various drug dependency interventions can be supported by monitors that detect and transmit the physical symptoms of drug cravings and allow "sponsors" or counselors to immediately contact the patient to provide support.

Hybrid Programs—Technology as an Adjunct to
Clinical and Community Health Promotion

This book has focused largely on the endeavor of delivering health promotion through technology, and we have assumed many if not most of these efforts to be stand-alone technology-based programs.

It is overly simplistic to think about technology-based programs as stand-alone efforts, however. It may also be misguided to do so. Hospitals, clinics, schools, employers, and other institutions that regularly come in contact with large segments of the population are well positioned to consider the delivery of technology-based health promotion through their institutional channels to large numbers of people. Thus, we anticipate that hybrid efforts to connect technology to existing organizations and programs are an important focus for future program development. Indeed, linking technology to existing programs may be a way to overcome the fundamental challenge of getting and holding people's attention. With an ever-crowded Internet and technology-dominated environment, people may need to have a credible referral in order to engage with a technology-based program. We certainly cannot expect people to stumble onto the latest evidence-based smoking cessation or weight loss program on their own.

Hybrid programs have the potential to take many forms. They can serve as extensions of existing programs—say, for example, a busy clinic is trying to offer "booster" sessions for a group-level diabetes self-management program. Offering adjunctive and enhancing activities online to persons enrolled in the program has the potential for reinforcing and expanding program exposure. Such activities can be a way to offer social support and/or a "buddy" system, linking people engaged in a face-to-face program in a virtual world where they can offer testimonials or real-life personal stories, for example, to encourage and support others in behavior change efforts. We anticipate such uses of technology will be forthcoming and of interest for clinical and institutional providers of care.

Systems-Level Efforts—Using Technology to Improve Care Delivery at the Provider and Systems Level

The field of health promotion has been criticized for an overemphasis on individual-level behavior change, and policymakers have made urgent calls for interventions that go beyond the individual to affect social, organizational, and environmental factors contributing to healthy behaviors (Hardy, 2004; McCormack, Laska, Larson, & Story, 2010; Piot, Bartos, Larson, Zewdie, & Mane, 2008).

How can technologies be utilized to facilitate interventions operating beyond the individual? We have considered one here—STD Prevention Online, which seeks to establish networks of care providers to facilitate more timely adoption and sharing of best practices for sexually transmitted infection prevention and care. STD Prevention Online operates at the provider level. Changing community and social norms to facilitate behavior change may be augmented via the telephone—consider following an individual on Twitter as he or she attempts to lose weight through improved nutrition and physical activity—can the individual's "tweets" to his or her social network have an impact the behaviors of others? Using Internet blogs and camera phones could facilitate policy change—imagine asking people to take and post pictures online of areas in their physical environment that limit or represent a barrier to physical activity—for example, lack of sidewalks, or no bike lanes, or few curb cuts. Collective action to document physical barriers in the environment may be a powerful tool to influence policymakers to assist in creating a physical environment more conducive to physical activity. These are just a few of the ways we can utilize technology to go beyond the individual and facilitate health promotion.

CONCLUDING THOUGHTS

Use of Technology as Adjunctive and Hybrid

While much of this book focuses on the use of technology for health promotion programs that are intended to be stand-alone efforts, this overlooks the fundamental opportunities to utilize technology to enhance and expand programs. We look forward in coming years to the integration of technology more consistently into primary care and other health promotion programs; we are confident that there are multiple opportunities to streamline and standardize care delivery for primary prevention and general health promotion within care settings (Glasgow, Bull, Piette, & Steiner, 2004).

In addition to the use of hybrid programming within clinic settings, we also anticipate development of strategic partnerships between community-based agencies serving persons at risk of negative health outcomes and clinical delivery systems. Primary care providers could potentially greatly expand their reach by partnering with communities to access their clients through technologies such as kiosks, the Internet, and cell phones.

Use of Theory

While we have outlined a theoretical framework in Chapter 1, we still lack a cohesive theoretical understanding of linkages between technology and health promotion generally. There are opportunities to develop theoretical perspectives that can better elucidate how to capitalize on technological reach, how to engage and retain people's participation in programs, and how to incorporate rapidly evolving technologies into health promotion programs. We look forward to contributions from social scientists and other theorists in theory development for technology-based health promotion in coming years.

REFERENCES

Bernhardt, J. M. (2000). Health education and the digital divide: Building bridges and filling chasms. *Health Education Research, 15*, 527–531.

Boase, J., Horrigan, J., Wellman, B., & Rainie, L. (2006). *The strength of Internet ties: The Internet and email aid users in maintaining their social networks and provide pathways to help when people face big decisions.* Pew Internet & American Life Project. Retrieved from http://www.pewinternet.org/~/media//Files/Reports/2006/PIP_Internet_ties.pdf.pdf

Booth, A. O., Nowson, C. A., & Matters, H. (2008). Evaluation of an interactive, Internet-based weight loss program: A pilot study. *Health Education Research, 23*, 371–381.

Brendryen, H., & Kraft, P. (2008). Happy ending: A randomized controlled trial of a digital multi-media smoking cessation intervention. *Addiction, 103*, 478–484.

Bull, S., Gaglio, B., McKay, G., & Glasgow, R. E. (2005). Harnessing the potential of the Internet to promote chronic illness self-management: Diabetes as an example of how well are we doing. *Chronic Illness, 1*, 143–155.

Bull, S., Pratte, K., Whitesell, N., Rietmeijer, C., & McFarlane, M. (2009). Effects of an Internet-based intervention for HIV prevention: The Youthnet trials. *AIDS and Behavior, 13*(3), 474–487.

Cassell, M. M., Jackson, C., & Cheuvront, B. (1998). Health communication on the Internet: An effective channel for health behavior change? *Journal of Health Communication, 3*, 71–79.

Cellular News. (n.d.). *Latest news stories.* Retrieved from http://www.cellularnews.com

Clark, M. M., Cox, L. S., Jett, J. R., Patten, C. A., Schroeder, D. R., Nirelli, L. M., et al. (2004). Effectiveness of smoking cessation self-help materials in a lung cancer screening population. *Lung Cancer, 44*, 13–21.

Curioso, W. H. & Kurth, A. (2007). Access, use and perceptions regarding Internet, cell phones and PDAs as a means for health promotion for people living with HIV in Peru. *BMC Medical Informatics and Decision Making 7*(24), 1–7.

Estabrooks, P. A., & Gyurcsik, N. C. (2003). Evaluating the public health impact of physical activity interventions. *Psychology of Sport and Exercise, 4*, 41–55.

Etter, J. F. (2005). Comparing the efficacy of two Internet-based, computer-tailored smoking cessation programs: A randomized trial. *Journal of Medical Internet Research, 7*, e2. doi:10.2196/jmir.7.1.e2

Feil, E. G., Glasgow, R. E., Boles, S. M., & McKay, H. G. (2000). Who participates in Internet-based self-management programs? A study among novice computer users in a primary care setting. *Diabetes Educator, 26,* 806–811.

Formica, M., Kabbara, K., Clark, R., & McAlindon, T. (2004). Can clinical trials requiring frequent participant contact be conducted over the Internet? Results from an online randomized controlled trial evaluating a topical ointment for herpes labialis. *Journal of Medical Internet Research, 6,* e6.

Glasgow, R., Nelson, C., Kearney, K., Reid, R., Ritzwoller, D., Strecher, V., et al. (2007). Reach, engagement and retention in an Internet-based weight loss program in a multi-site randomized controlled trial. *Journal of Medical Internet Research, 9,* e11.

Glasgow, R. E., Bull, S. S., Piette, J. D., & Steiner, J. F. (2004). Interactive behavior change technology: A partial solution to the competing demands of primary care. *American Journal of Preventive Medicine, 27,* 80–87.

Glasgow, R. E., Christiansen, S., Smith, S., Stevens, V. J., & Toobert, D. (2008). Development and implementation of an integrated, multi-modality, user-centered interactive dietary change program [Electronic version published ahead of print]. *Health Education Research.* doi:10.1093/her/cyn042

Glasgow, R. E., Klesges, L. M., Dzewaltowski, D. A., Estabrooks, P. A., & Vogt, T. M. (2006). Evaluating the impact of health promotion programs: Using the RE-AIM framework to form summary measures for decision making involving complex issues. *Health Education Research, 21,* 688–694.

Glasgow, R. E., La Chance, P. A., Toobert, D. J., Brown, J., Hampson, S. E., & Riddle, M. C. (1997). Long-term effects and costs of brief behavioural dietary intervention for patients with diabetes delivered from the medical office. *Patient Education Counseling, 32,* 175–184.

Glasgow, R. E., Strycker, L. A., King, D., Toobert, D., Kulchak Rahm, A., Jex, M., et al. (2006). Robustness of a computer-assisted diabetes self-management intervention across patient characteristics, healthcare settings, and intervention staff. *American Journal of Managed Care, 12*(3), 137–145.

Gore-Felton, C., Rotheram-Borus, M. J., Weinhardt, L. S., Kelly, J. A., Lightfoot, M., Kirshenbaum, S. B., et al. (2005). The Healthy Living Project: An individually tailored, multidimensional intervention for HIV-infected persons. *AIDS Education and Prevention, 17,* 21–39.

Gustafson, D. H., McTavish, F. M., Stengle, W., Ballard, D., Hawkins, R., Shaw, B. R., et al. (2005). Use and impact of eHealth system by low-income women with breast cancer. *Journal of Health Communication, 10*(Suppl. 1), 195–218.

Hardy, G. E., Jr. (2004). The burden of chronic disease: The future is prevention. Introduction to Dr. James Marks's presentation, "The Burden of Chronic Disease and the Future of Public Health." *Preventing Chronic Disease, 1,* A04.

Harris Interactive. (2008). *Cell phone usage continues to increase* (The Harris Poll, #36). New York: Author.

Heller, R. F., & Dobson, A. J. (2000). Disease impact number and population impact number: Population perspectives to measures of risk and benefit. *British Medical Journal, 321,* 950–953.

Hurling, R., Catt, M., De Boni, M., Fairley, B. W., Hurst, T., Murray, P., et al. (2007). Using internet and mobile phone technology to deliver an automated physical activity program: randomized controlled trial. *Journal of Medical Internet Research, 9*(2), 1–12.

Ironson, G., Weiss, S., Lydston, D., Ishii, M., Jones, D., Asthana, D., et al. (2005). The impact of improved self-efficacy on HIV viral load and distress in culturally diverse women living with AIDS: The SMART/EST Women's Project. *AIDS Care, 17,* 222–236.

Joffe, M., & Mindell, J. (2002). A framework for the evidence base to support health impact assessment. *Journal of Epidemiology and Community Health, 56,* 132–138.

King, D., Bull, S., Christiansen, S., Nelson, C., Stryker, L., Toobert, D., et al. (2004). Developing and using interactive health CD-ROMs as a complement to primary care-lessons from two research studies. *Diabetes Spectrum, 17,* 234–242.

King, W. C., & Miles, E. W. (1995). A quasi-experimental assessment of the effect of computerizing non-cognitive paper-and-pencil measurements: A test of measurement equivalence. *Journal of Applied Psychology, 80,* 643–651.

Kukafka, R., Lussier, Y. A., Eng, P., Patel, V. L., & Cimino, J. J. (2002). Web-based tailoring and its effect on self-efficacy: Results from the MI-HEART randomized controlled trial. *American Medical Informatics Association, Annual Symposium Proceedings Archive,* 410–414.

Lavoie, J. A., & Pychyl, T. A. (2001). Cyberslacking and the procrastination superhighway: A web-based survey of online procrastination, attitudes, and emotion. *Social Science Computer Review, 19,* 431–444.

Leeman-Castillo, B. A., Corbett, K. K., Aagaard, E. M., Maselli, J. H., Gonzales, R., & MacKenzie, T. D. (2007). Acceptability of a bilingual interactive computerized educational module in a poor, medically underserved patient population. *Journal of Health Communication., 12,* 77–94.

Linke, S., Murray, E., Butler, C., & Wallace, P. (2007). Internet-based interactive health intervention for the promotion of sensible drinking: Patterns of use and potential impact on members of the general public. *Journal of Medical Internet Research, 9,* e10. doi:10.2196/jmir.9.2.e10

Logan, A. G., McIsaac, W. J., Tisler, A., Irvine, M. J., Saunders, A., Dunai, A., et al. (2007). Mobile phone-based remote patient monitoring system for management of hypertension in diabetic patients. *American Journal of Hypertension, 20,* 942–948.

McCormack, L. A., Laska, M. N., Larson, N. I., & Story, M. (2010). Review of the nutritional implications of farmers' markets and community gardens: A call for evaluation and research efforts. *Journal of the American Dietetic Association, 110,* 399–408.

Noar, S. M., Clark, A., Cole, C., & Lustria, M. L. A. (2006). Review of interactive safer sex websites: Practice and potential. *Health Communication, 20*(3), 233–241.

Pequegnat, W., Rosser, B. R., Bowen, A. M., Bull, S. S., Diclemente, R. J., Bockting, W. O., et al. (2007). Conducting Internet-based HIV/STD prevention survey research: Considerations in design and evaluation. *AIDS and Behavior, 11,* 505–521.

Pew Internet & American Life Project. (2000). *The online health care revolution: How the web helps Americans take better care of themselves.* Retrieved from http://www.scribd.com/doc/219514/The-Online-Health-Care-Revolution-How-the-Web-helps-Americans-take-better-care-of-themselves

Piot, P., Bartos, M., Larson, H., Zewdie, D., & Mane, P. (2008). Coming to terms with complexity: A call to action for HIV prevention. *The Lancet, 372*(9641), 845–859.

Prochaska, J. O., DiClemente, C. C., Velicer, W. F., & Rossi, J. S. (1993). Standardized, individualized, interactive and personalized self-help programs for smoking cessation. *Health Psychology, 12,* 399–405.

Ross, M. W. (2002). The Internet as a medium for HIV prevention and counseling. *Focus, 17,* 4–6.

Rotondi, A. J., Sinkule, J., & Spring, M. (2005). An interactive Web-based intervention for persons with TBI and their families: Use and evaluation by female significant others. *Journal of Head Trauma and Rehabilitation, 20,* 173–185.

Scholes, D., McBride, C. M., Grothaus, L., Civic, D., Ichikawa, L. E., Fish, L. J., et al. (2003). A tailored minimal self-help intervention to promote condom use in young women: Results from a randomized trial. *AIDS, 17,* 1547–1556.

Smeets, T., Brug, J., & De, V. H. (2008). Effects of tailoring health messages on physical activity. *Health Education Research, 23,* 402–413.

Strecher, V. J., Kreuter, M., Den Boer, D. J., Kobrin, S., Hospers, H. J., & Skinner, C. S. (1994). The effects of computer-tailored smoking cessation messages in family practice settings. *Journal of Family Practice, 39,* 262–268.

Strecher, V. J., Shiffman, S., & West, R. (2005). Randomized controlled trial of a web-based computer-tailored smoking cessation program as a supplement to nicotine patch therapy. *Addiction, 100,* 682–688.

Taylor, C. B., Houston-Miller, N., Killen, J. D., & DeBusk, R. F. (1990). Smoking cessation after acute myocardial infarctions: Effects of a nurse-managed intervention. *Annals of Internal Medicine, 113,* 118–123.

Turner, C. F., Ku, L., Rogers, S. M., Lindberg, L. D., Pleck, J. H., & Sonenstein, F. L. (1998). Adolescent sexual behavior, drug use, and violence: Increased reporting with computer survey technology. *Science, 280,* 867–873.

Ybarra, M., & Bull, S. (2007). Current trends in Internet-based and cell-phone based HIV prevention and intervention programs. *Current HIV/AIDS Reports, 4,* 201–207.

Appendix: Technology-Based Health Promotions

INTERNET/ COMPUTER RESEARCH	Author/Year	Sample	Study Design and Target Population and Outcome	Results	Significance
Pilot Studies	Leeman-Castillo, B., Raghunath, S., Beaty, B., Steiner, J., Bull, S. 2010 (further discussed in Chapter 6)	200 self-identifying Latinos in Denver, Colorado, with diverse educational backgrounds; 70% female; 50% native Spanish speakers	Pilot: Latinos living in the Denver Metropolitan Area aged 21 and over who sought services at one of six community-based organizations (e.g., churches, schools, and social service agencies) could access a computer kiosk. They were asked to offer details on their physical activity, nutrition, and smoking habits and were offered feedback on their health and cardiovascular disease risk based on their responses. They were given an opportunity to set behavioral goals in any of these three areas. The program included Latino role models and motivational music and graphics.	Findings showed significant increases in fruit and vegetable consumption and physical activity among all participants, regardless of goal selected. No changes were observed in smoking behaviors.	The use of theoretical elements such as role models and making the program culturally relevant and appropriate with music and graphics is unique. Results are promising and need to be replicated in an RCT (randomized controlled trial).
	Cullen & Thompson, 2010	67 African American families with a 9- to 12-year-old daughter	Pilot: The Family Eats intervention (http://clinicaltrials.gov/ct2/show/) is a site that was intended to be accessed at least once a week, for 8 weeks, by a parent in each family. The families were African American with one daughter between the ages of 9 and 12 since these children are the ones at highest risk for developing obesity. The site provides healthy overviews designed to lead toward healthier habits.	Though log-on rates were low, the families that did log on consistently showed a greater likelihood of improving meal plans; adjusting their fruit, vegetable, and meat consumption; and making healthier restaurant selections. The study also found that they increased their "substitution-fat practices" (p. 46).	This pilot study leads the way for a future study on behavioral and physiological outcomes. The results show that there is a large possibility that web-based interactions may work in promoting health behavior change. Web-based interactions may also be an effective alternative when trying to reach a large population of American families.

Webber, Tate, & Quintiliani, 2008	20 women, aged 22–65 years old, all of whom were university employees: 40% with a graduate degree, 35% with a college degree, and 25% with less than a college degree	Pilot: For women who met the eligibility criteria—being between the ages of 22 and 65, having a BMI (body mass index) greater than or equal to 25 and less than 40, home access to a computer with Internet service, no orthopedic or joint problems, no psychiatric disorder within the past year, no history of anorexia or bulimia nervosa, no medical diagnosis of cancer within 5 years, no HIV, no pregnancy (current or recent), and no weight loss of over 10 lb.—the purpose of the study was to use motivational Internet-based online groups to determine whether discussions of values and motivational interviewing-based discussions produced changes in motivation and weight loss.	Weight loss was 1.5±2.2 kg in the motivational interviewing plus values group and 2.7±2.9 kg in the motivational interviewing without values group. Changes in motivation between the two groups were not different.	The use of motivational interviewing in online groups for weight loss is acceptable and produces self-motivational statements, which increases the level of motivation and weight loss.
Bull, Phibbs, Watson, & McFarlane, 2007	25 individuals between the ages of 18 and 25; 56% women, 24% White, 40% Hispanic/Latino, 16% African American, 16% mixed race/ethnic background, 4% indicating they	Focus groups: Individuals who had received service at Denver Health of Planned Parenthood and were familiar with how to access the Internet were asked to participate in focus groups. They were asked to give their supposition on attractive features of websites, including style and design considerations. In addition, they were asked to voice their opinions about how	The issues related to access that participants indicated were most often related to bandwidth and connection speed, not directly to obtaining access—as access is available at schools and libraries. In analyzing content/design, it was suggested that in order to grab attention and	The Internet can be a useful avenue to health information if attention is paid to the preference and needs of the target group. In order to gain and maintain trust with the target group, confidentiality must be ensured when dealing with health/behavior information.

(Continued)

INTERNET/ COMPUTER RESEARCH	Author/Year	Sample	Study Design and Target Population and Outcome	Results	Significance
		did not fit into any of these categories; 42% 18–20 years old, 40% 21–22 years old, 18% 23–25 years old	to best convey five theoretical constructs including risk for STD/HIV and unintended pregnancy; positive outcome expectancies related to condom use; condom use norms; self-efficacy for negotiation of condoms; and self-efficacy for condom use. Participants were shown photos of role models and asked to react through the use of those role models to convey constructs for the project.	harness the potential of the Internet for health promotion, features should be interactive and dynamic, with bold colors and unambiguous information. A key finding from the theoretical construct discussions was the expressed desire for straightforward information from a credible source and from peers. A consequence of route of access is that privacy cannot be assumed. To address this, interventions should look like content available online, and confidentiality must be protected so youth can feel secure in the online environment.	
Meta-Analysis	Noar, Black, & Pierce, 2009 (further discussed in Chapter 7)	4,639 individuals participating in original RCTs; studies published between 2002 and 2008; 10 of 12 were on heterosexually	Meta-analysis of 12 RCTs that tested the effectiveness of an intervention focused on changing sexual risk behavior(s) of people who were either HIV negative or of unknown HIV status; used condom use or unprotected sex as a dependent variable; used computer technology	Computer-based interventions have been efficacious in increasing condom use and reducing sexual activity, numbers of sexual partners, and incident STD. This method is as effective as human-delivered information	Computer technology-based interventions represent a relatively new and promising intervention type that may have great potential for dissemination of HIV prevention.

		active individuals, 2 were MSM (men who have sex with men); 6 of 12 were of mixed male/ female samples, 4 had female-only samples, 2 were male-only samples; mean age 22.52 years	in the development or delivery of intervention.	and has advantages in comparison: lower cost to deliver, greater intervention fidelity, and greater flexibility in dissemination channels. Interventions were successful with a wide range of populations.	
Methods	Curioso & Kurth, 2007	31 people living with AIDS in Peru; 3 female	In-depth interviews: report of perceptions toward use of information and communication technologies as a means to support antiretroviral medication adherence and HIV transmission risk reduction.	Positive perceptions about using the Internet, cell phones, and PDAs (personal digital assistants) for HIV health promotion; however, cell phones excited people the most to receive information about HIV, either through text messaging or prerecorded voice mails).	Suggests that cell phone use is acceptable and desirable among patients with HIV in a resource-limited setting and that it can build on existing patterns of use.
	Skinner, Rivette, & Bloomberg, 2007	8 therapeutic counselors in South Africa who are members of the community and are HIV-positive and are responsible for being advocates for antiretroviral therapy send reports back to doctors.	In-depth interviews with counselors targeted HIV-positive community members for adherence to antiretroviral therapies.	Cell phones were used to record and send data back to the health services center; interviewees claimed the phones were efficient, saved time, reduced the risk of losing patient notes, and reduced the potential breaks in confidentiality should the notes be lost.	Use of cell phones assisted communication between health care staff and community counselors; counselors thought the use of cell phones could contribute to the management of antiretroviral therapies in South Africa.

(Continued)

INTERNET/ COMPUTER RESEARCH	Author/Year	Sample	Study Design and Target Population and Outcome	Results	Significance
	Kirk et al., 2007	180 people (no indication of how many men/ women or race) with a BMI greater than 30 kg/m^2. They must be 18–65 years old and able to access the Internet at least once a week.	Participants will be split into either an intervention group (via the Internet) or a "usual care group" (control). The purpose of the study is to test the promising effects of an Internet-based intervention of weight loss in comparison to a standard, usual form of care.	Projected outcomes are more changes in lifestyle and more participation in managing health care for online users. The cost of an online health service will also be estimated.	If the experiment succeeds, then there will be more options available for handling the problem of obesity. If it fails, then there will at least be confirmation that other strategies will be needed.
Surveillance	Kainth et al., 2004	11 studies: 1 examining one-to-one education, 2 RCTs, 1 controlled trial, and 8 before-and-after studies. Studies were aimed at reducing patient and/or prehospital delay.	Surveillance: Study targets studies conducted on cardiac care. Purpose of the study is to evaluate the effectiveness of interventions aimed at reducing the time from onset for the symptoms of an acute myocardial infarction to seeking medical help at a hospital.	Of the 8 before-and-after studies, 3 reported a significant reduction in delay after intervention, 2 found no statistically significant difference in the people seeking help, 1 found a statistically significant reduction in median delay, 1 reported an increase in the percentage of persons delaying treatment 2 hours or less, and 1 reported mortality rates and found no significant effects of intervention. Neither RCT reported significant effects due to the intervention.	Little evidence supports the idea that community-wide media-based or educational interventions are successful at reducing delay time for treatment in patients with suspected heart attack.

| Interventions | Grimley & Hook, 2009 | 430 individuals: 88% Black, 54.5% women, mean age 24.5 years | RCT: Participants were randomly assigned to the intervention or comparison group. Baseline data were collected including sexual risk behaviors and number of partners. They were also required to submit biological samples to test for Neisseria gonorrhoeae and Chlamydia trachomatis. The intervention was delivered via an audio, multimedia, computerized application. Intervention was individualized based on answers to risk behavior questions. The comparison group was asked questions on many different health risk behaviors with no intervention. The study evaluated the effectiveness of a 15-minute intervention measured by condom use and change of infection for two STDs. Follow-up data were collected after a 6-month time lapse. | Increased condom use and decreased prevalence of Neisseria gonorrhoeae and Chlamydia trachomatis were reported in the intervention group. | Brief, interactive, computer-delivered interventions provided at the evaluation visit increase condom use and reduce STDs without putting an additional burden on clinicians or staff. |
| | Bowen, Williams, Daniel, & Clayton, 2008 | 475 MSM residing in rural areas | RCT: online recruiting, three intervention modules each with two sessions, and online questionnaires. The purpose of the study is to assess the effectiveness of reducing risky sexual behavior in rural MSM through presentation of content via the Internet. | Knowledge of risk, self-efficacy, outcome expectancies, and motivation increase in a dose-response fashion. Postintervention behavior changes included reduced anal sex and significant increases in condom use. | The results of the study provide support for the efficacy of Internet-based interventions to reduce risk of HIV infection. |

INTERNET/ COMPUTER RESEARCH	Author/Year	Sample	Study Design and Target Population and Outcome	Results	Significance
	Gilbert et al., 2008	471 individuals who were English speaking, were HIV positive for at least 3 months, and reported substance use or sexual risk recruited from five San Francisco outpatient HIV clinics; majority male	RCT: face-to-face recruitment, individuals reporting 1+ risky behaviors were stratified by risk combination and then randomized. All participants completed a baseline survey. The intervention group received personalized counseling for risk reduction from a "Video Doctor" by laptop and through a printed educational worksheet together known as Positive Choice.	Intervention participants reported fewer average days of ongoing illicit drug use than the control participants and had fewer casual sex partners.	The Positive Choice intervention was able to attain cessation of illicit drug use and number of casual sex partners in comparison to the control group both at the group level and individually and functions as a complement to education received in the outpatient clinic.
	Rosser et al., 2009	1,026 high-risk Latino MSM	Survey design: Study targets MSM as an HIV risk. Purpose of the study is to describe the sexual risk behavior of an Internet-based sample of Latino MSM, investigate the relationship between the Internet as a risk environment and unsafe sex, and assess the ability to conduct online survey research of Latino MSM.	99% of the participants reported having used the Internet to seek sex with another man. Two thirds had unprotected anal sex in the last year, 57% of these with multiple partners.	Study confirms the use of the Internet in conducting online research with Latino MSM. A large number of high-risk Latino MSM were recruited for this study. The primary factor that contributes to the sexual risk behavior in online sexual liaisons is the high rate of unprotected sex due to the Internet enhancing the efficiency of initiating sexual behavior.

De Bourdeaudhuij, Stevens, Vandelanotte, & Brug, 2007	337 participants from six different Belgian companies assigned to either a computer-tailored intervention, a generic intervention, or no intervention (control group); no gender specified	RCT: Six companies were randomly assigned to one of two intervention groups, or a control group, to test benefits of a tailored Internet education.	The computer-tailored intervention group proved to be more effective in regulating/reducing total fat intake than the generic or control group.	Since this computer-tailored intervention proved to be effective, it might prove beneficial to apply this study to other forms of health promotions.
Hurling et al., 2007	77 healthy adults (control = 30, randomized to intervention = 47)	RCT: average adults to increase self-efficacy and motivation to become more physically active	Self-efficacy of test group (Internet technology to deliver automated physical activity program) was higher than that of the control group (no support), but motivation to increase duration/ amount of physical activity was not.	A fully automated Internet-based motivation and action support system can significantly increase and maintain the level of physical activity in healthy adults.
Jacobi et al., 2007	100 healthy females, 18- to 19-year-old university students	RCT: Out of 100 females, 50 were randomly assigned to an intervention (Internet) group, and 50 were assigned to a control (wait list) group to measure the effectiveness of an Internet-based prevention on lowering the possibility of developing eating disorders.	The intervention-based group proved to have more knowledge about eating disorders, exercise, and healthy eating based on the WCR questionnaire. They were also found to be less concerned about being thin.	The results show how an Internet-based prevention is effective and how it could potentially apply "across cultures and languages" (p. 118).

(Continued)

(Continued)

	Author/Year	Sample	Study Design and Target Population and Outcome	Results	Significance
INTERNET/ COMPUTER RESEARCH	Murray et al., 2007	Users who have found the "Down Your Drink" website and are aged 18 or over with a score of 5 or above on the AUDIT-C (Alcohol Use Disorders Identification Test)	RCT: online intervention with two different groups. The first group is an interactive, psychologically enhanced website with components known to be effective in alcohol interventions. The control is a text-based site only giving health information and by itself is unlikely to be effective. The purpose of the study is to determine the effectiveness and cost-effectiveness of an online, psychologically enhanced, interactive computer-based intervention in reducing alcohol consumption.	Primary outcomes will be a difference in the two groups used in the study and will provide valuable information about whether an online trial will be effective.	Given the rapid rise in health-related websites and their increasing use by health professionals and public members, this study will determine whether website interactivity adds to the potential impact on the users' health.
	Paxton, McLean, Gollings, Faulkner, & Wertheim, 2006	116 women aged 18–35 years (42 in the face-to-face [FF] group, 37 in the Internet [INT] group, and 37 in the delayed treatment control [DTC] group).	RCT: women aged 18–35 years, with access to and ability to use the Internet, a Body Shape questionnaire score of greater than or equal to 100 or a combined bulimia test score of above 104. Purpose of the study is to compare body image, eating behavior, and psychological outcomes in adult women in the following treatment groups: face-to-face, online synchronous Internet, and delayed treatment control group. Expected result is both intervention groups will show improvement, and delayed treatment control group will show no to little improvement.	ITT analyses for Time 1 showed no clear differences, typical of women seeking body image therapy. From Time 1 to Time 2, the FF and INT groups compared to the DTC group showed improvements in body dissatisfaction, body attitudes, eating attitudes and behaviors, psychopathology, and session attendance (see Table 1, pp. 696 and 698. and Figure 2, p. 696). Improves from Time 2 to Time 3 for all measures.	Gains at the end of treatment in the FF approach were larger than in the INT approach. Six-month follow-up for the INT group indicates that the effects of the program were equivalent in both delivery modes, so although initial gains were apparent, after the 6-month follow-up, both groups were no longer clearly different from each other.

Polzien, Jakicic, Tate, & Otto, 2007	58 individuals: 57 females and 1 male with a BMI of 25 to 39, an age of 18–55 years, and a sedentary lifestyle	RCT: Participants received a 12-week weight loss intervention. They were randomized to one of three groups; SBWP (standard in-person behavioral weight control program), INT-TECH (intermittent technology-based behavioral weight control program), or CON-TECH (continuous technology-based behavioral weight control program). Purpose was to examine the efficacy of adding a technology-based program to a weight loss program and to evaluate the differences between a continuous and a noncontinuous program.	Weight loss for each group: CON-TECH = 6.2 ± 4.0 kg, INT-TECH = 3.4 ± 3.4 kg, SBWP = 4.1 ± 2.8 kg. Results show that weight loss is significantly greater when the two programs are used continuously.	Use of a continuous technology-based system for weight loss results in an increased amount of weight loss. Interventions not using technology and that are not continuous are not as effective.
Winett, Anderson, Wojcik, Winett, & Bowden, 2007	1,071 participants: 33% male, 23% African American, 57% overweight or obese, 60% sedentary	RCT: Study targets churches because socially mediated interventions are most effective when delivered within social networks. Purpose of the study is to assess the impact of an Internet program (GTH) to improve the nutrition and physical activity of adults.	GTH-plus and GTH-only increased fiber intake by 3.0 g/day, increased F&V intake by 1.5 servings a day. GTH-plus decreased fat intake by 0.6%, and no differences were observed for GTH-only. GTH-plus increased the number of steps (physical activity) by 1,500 steps a day and GTH-only by 1,400 steps a day.	Participants in the GTH-plus and GTH-only groups made much greater changes in their nutrition self-regulation behaviors. The results suggest supports in socially mediated intervention play a role in behavior change.
Bensley et al., 2006	39,541 clients who completed the learning module session; 94.8% were parents of a WIC	Survey design: WIC participants who were not considered high risk for nutritional issues. The purpose of the study was to determine the usefulness of Internet-based intervention and	46.5% of users who began in the precontemplation stage advanced to the action stage by the end of the study. 77% of users who	Wichealth.org is useful and helpful in impacting positive stage advancement with parent–child feeding issues.

(Continued)

(Continued)

	Author/Year	Sample	Study Design and Target Population and Outcome	Results	Significance
INTERNET/ COMPUTER RESEARCH			the movement in stage of change associated with WIC nutrition issues.	entered during the preparation stage advanced to the contemplation stage. 98.4% of users who entered in the preparation stage advanced to the action stage.	
	Christensen, Griffiths, Mackinnon, & Brittliffe, 2006	2,794 participants: 1,846 women and 948 men; 61.7% logged in from Australia, 12.6% from the United Kingdom, 10% from the United States, 4.5% from Canada, and 2.5% from New Zealand	RCT: Study targets participants with elevated scores on the Goldberg Depression Scale of 5.96. Purpose of the study was to investigate whether CBT (cognitive behavior therapy) was effective as an extended version or whether add-on components contributed to positive outcomes.	20.4% of participants completed the intervention. CBT was not effective in reducing depression symptoms. Extended CBT with or without additional components was effective at reducing depression.	Short CBT programs are not effective interventions for decreasing depression. Longer programs are much more effective but are associated with higher dropout rates.
	Huang et al., 2007	120 women	Quasi-experimental: Study targets women at 29–36 weeks using the Internet on a regular	Women receiving web education on breast-feeding had high	Results suggest web-based breast-feeding education may

		basis. Purpose of the study is to examine the effects of an online breast-feeding education program in Taiwan. The study aims to increase breast-feeding knowledge and to increase its behavior.	knowledge of the subject and a more positive attitude toward breast-feeding.	contribute to high knowledge about, positive attitude toward, and high rate of breast-feeding.
Japuntich et al., 2006	284 smokers, roughly 55% female and 45% male, 79.1% of whom are White, who smoke approximately 40.8 cigarettes per day	RTC: 140 were randomly placed in the treatment group (Internet-CHESS SCRP website), and 144 were randomly placed in the control group. The purpose was to determine the effectiveness of smoking interventions via the Internet.	63 patients withdrew (21 CHESS SCRP, 32 control). After 3 months postquit, 22.9% in CHESS SCRP and 20.8% of control were abstinent. After 6 months, 15% of CHESS SCRP and 11.8% were abstinent. No significant results have occurred. There was no relationship between the amount of Internet usage and "ethnicity, gender, or education level" (p. S65).	This study shows the limits of generalizability. Internet intervention might show a benefit if it is used on a wide-scale population size. If the project was made into a longer intervention, possible build-up effects might be seen.
Vildrine, Arduino, & Gritz, 2006	95 participants from an inner-city HIV/AIDS clinic in Texas (control = 47, randomized to intervention = 48); 71.6% African American, 18.9% White, 8.4% Hispanic	RCT: For HIV-positive adults who smoke, cell phone counseling sessions (8 total) will help smoking cessation.	Intervention group experienced significantly greater reductions in anxiety and depression and significantly greater increases in self-efficacy. Patients in the intervention group were 5 times more likely to abstain from smoking at the first follow-up assessment (3 months).	Cell phones can be effective in addressing some factors for smoking cessation in people living with AIDS (increasing self-efficacy, decreasing depression and anxiety), which could also impact medical adherence.

(Continued)

(Continued)

INTERNET/ COMPUTER RESEARCH	Author/Year	Sample	Study Design and Target Population and Outcome	Results	Significance
	van Wier et al., 2006	1,386 eligible Dutch employees (no gender specified) from seven different companies. For the two intervention groups, 462 were put in a phone group, and 464 were placed in an Internet group, while 460 were placed in the control group.	RCT: Targeted individuals were assigned to a phone intervention group, an Internet intervention group, or a control group to evaluate betterment of BMI, physical activity, diet, and so forth.	So far, the study is projected to show that distance counseling programs via Internet and phone should be more cost efficient, more time saving, and more effective. Results are not complete. There will be a 2-year follow-up of the study.	After the follow-up, the study should be the first to assess "economic evaluations from the societal perspective of weight control intervention" (p. 10), which are grounded upon actual costs and results of the study.
	Clarke et al., 2005	255 adults with depression (no gender preference)	RCT: Of the 255 adults, 100 were assigned to a control group (no access to Overcoming Depression on the Internet [ODIN] site), 75 were assigned to postcard reminders, and 80 were assigned to the ODIN program reminders. The purpose is to see whether a self-help method to treating depression is feasible online.	The randomized trial found that those involved in the ODIN program had a lower prevalence of depression indicators and a moderate increase in their overall health. Follow-up rates, however, were shown to be fairly low. This made the follow-up brief.	It was suggested that online intervention programs such as ODIN are very efficient and cost-effective. Over time, they may prove beneficial when trying to access a widespread population.
	Kim, Yoo, & Shim, 2005	51 subjects (no specific number of men and women), all with a history of diabetes	Quasi-experimental design: 25 subjects were designated toward the intervention (web-based or cellular communication), and 26 were designated toward the control (face-to-face interaction).		

	Sample	Methodology	Findings	Implications
		Both the intervention and control groups were then split into two groups based on their "glycosylated haemoglobin at baseline with type 2 diabetes" (p. 11361). From there, they test which group will maintain the best blood glucose levels.		
Papadaki & Scott, 2005	72 healthy women, ages 25–55 with Internet/e-mail access participated; 53 were part of the intervention group that came from University of Glasgow—19 were the control group that came from Glasgow Caledonian University.	Quasi-experimental design: The two groups were designated toward either a feedback/brochure method (control) or an Internet method (intervention) by the researchers to promote the Mediterranean diet.	The Internet-based intervention group proved to be more effective in regulating a Mediterranean diet (and with healthier outcomes), than the control group (brochures and feedback).	An Internet-based reach appears to be more engaging than the traditional "feedback and brochures" method. This study shows how a Mediterranean diet can be extended to promote health (through diet) via the Internet.
Verheijden et al., 2004	146 randomized Canadian patients at risk for cardiovascular disease (no gender amount specified)	RCT: 73 patients were placed in the web-based intervention group, and 73 were placed in the control group (standard counseling) to assess whether an online "nutrition counselling site and social support measures" (p. 1) would benefit the health of those at risk for cardiovascular disease.		

(Continued)

(Continued)

INTERNET/COMPUTER RESEARCH	Author/Year	Sample	Study Design and Target Population and Outcome	Results	Significance
	Glasgow, Boles, McKay, Feil, & Barrera, 2003 (further discussed in Chapters 3 and 7)	320 patients with type II diabetes; average age 59, equally divided between men and women	RCT: All participants received a computer for use at home to access a user-friendly diabetes self-management website. The intervention group had, in addition, access to a tailored self-management tool and a peer support group online.	All conditions were significantly improved from baseline on behavioral, psychosocial, and some biological outcomes, and there were few differences between conditions. Results were robust across online coaches, patient characteristics, and participating clinics.	One of the only strongly theoretically focused interventions. The authors used largely a Web 1.0 framework but also added peer support. Showed no additional benefits with tailored information or peer support.
CELL PHONE RESEARCH					
Pilot Studies	Patrick et al., 2009	65 participants who agreed to participate in a weight control study: mean age 44.9 years, mean weight 89 kg, mean BMI 33.2 kg/m^2. 80% of participants were women, and 75% of participants were White while 17% were African American.	RCT: Participants were randomly assigned to one of the two groups: intervention-receiving personalized text and picture messages sent 2–5 times daily, printed materials, and brief monthly phone calls from a health counselor or comparison/control receiving monthly printed materials on weight control. Assessments were completed at baseline, 2 months, and 4 months. The objective of the study was to evaluate a mobile phone-based application designed as an assessment and intervention tool	At the end of 4 months, the intervention group lost more weight than the comparison after adjusting for time, sex, and mean age (1.97 kg more).	Text messages might prove to be a productive channel of communication to promote behaviors that support weight loss in overweight adults. Further studies are needed with a larger sample size and a longer intervention period.

Citation	Sample	Design/Method	Results	Conclusions
		to improve dietary behaviors and reduce weight with primary outcome determined by weight in kilograms as measured by calibrated scales in research offices. Results were adjusted for age and gender.		
Cornelius & St. Lawrence, 2009	14 adolescents primarily 14 and 16 years of age (within the age range 13–17) and in high school: 7 males, 7 females	Focus groups: Participants were first given a survey about mobile phone use. Adolescents were asked what they could tell us about how they used text messaging (TM), what they knew about HIV, what they thought about TM HIV-prevention messages to adolescents their age, and how the curriculum could be modified for TM delivery	Adolescents in the study reported readily having access to a cell phone with TM capabilities, and reported consistent use of such a device. Not all of the adolescents were knowledgeable about modes of HIV/AIDS transmission and prevention. The participants were open to the idea of receiving text messages as a supplement to other curriculum.	Teens are open to receiving sexual health information through text messages: 1–3 daily as a supplement to traditional education methods.
Logan et al., 2007 (further discussed in Chapter 8)	33 type 2 diabetic patients with uncontrolled ambulatory BP (blood pressure) recruited from family practice physicians to use a home BP tele-management system	Pilot: Diabetic patients with BP problems in order to help control BP issues	24-hour ambulatory BP fell, and BP control improved significantly; patients perceived the system as acceptable and effective.	Believe results are encouraging for a home BP tele-management system to improve BP control in the community among patients with uncontrolled hypertension.

(Continued)

INTERNET/ COMPUTER RESEARCH	Author/Year	Sample	Study Design and Target Population and Outcome	Results	Significance
	Puccio et al., 2006	8 patients ages 16–24; half history of substance use; 1 female, 1 White, 2 African American, 5 Latino	Pilot: HIV-positive youth to receive cell phone reminder calls in order to increase adherence in ARVs	5 in 8 achieved a viral load of <=50 at week 12 (all 8 experienced a significant rise after intervention period at week 24); 4 in 8 left study before 12 weeks because of lost phone access; one patient never took HAART despite receiving phone calls.	Authors judged the phones useful although study design did not include a control group so effect is difficult to measure; 7 in 8 went over the time limit, and 4 in 8 lost phones.
Meta-Analysis	Fjeldsoe, Marshall, & Miller, 2009 (further discussed in Chapter 2)	14 articles published between January 1990 and March 2008 using an intervention to promote healthy behavior through SMS (text messaging)	Meta-analysis of articles that evaluated an intervention delivered primarily in SMS, assessed a change in health behavior using pre- and postassessment, and were published in English in a peer-reviewed scientific journal to examine current literature strengths and weaknesses in bringing about behavior change	Most studies analyzed using SMS as a reminder to increase adherence to treatment programs among sick individuals. Fewer studies have focused on promoting preventive health behaviors to healthy individuals through SMS. Of the 14 studies analyzed, 13 showed positive behavior changes, although some studies were statistically underpowered. In the future studies should use adequate sample sizes and sufficient statistical power, and include an assessment of the maintenance of	Research on the effects of specific SMS characteristics is now required to better understand the potential of this medium.

				behavioral changes after the intervention period. Further investigation is needed into the effectiveness of various elements in behavior changes such as intervention initiation, initiation of SMS dialogue, tailoring of SMS content, and the opportunity for SMS interaction between participants and researchers to optimize and enhance intervention effectiveness.	
Meta-analysis	Krishna, Boren, & Balas, 2009	25 articles that evaluated cell phone voice and text messaging interventions: 20 were RCTs, 5 were controlled studies, 19 studies assessed outcomes of care, and 6 assessed processes of care. Selected studies included 38,060 participants with 10,374 adults and 27,686 children. Studies took place in 13 countries.	Meta-analysis to evaluate the empirical evidence related to the role of cell phones and text messaging interventions in improving health outcomes and processes of care	Message delivery ranged from 5 times per day for diabetes and smoking cessation support to once a week for advice on how to overcome barriers and maintain regular physical activity. Duration of studies ranged from 3 to 12 months. Overall, the studies found improvement in both process of care and outcomes of care, which includes behavior change, clinical improvement, and social functioning.	Health care can be improved through the use of wireless mobile technology. It has the potential to reach diverse and hard-to-reach populations and reduce health disparities. Further studies are needed to analyze effectiveness with larger sample sizes and to investigate the cost-effectiveness of adoption in clinical settings.

(Continued)

INTERNET/ COMPUTER RESEARCH	Author/Year	Sample	Study Design and Target Population and Outcome	Results	Significance
Meta-analysis	Lim, Hocking, Hellard, & Aitken, 2008	9 articles on the use of text messaging in the promotion of sexual health	Meta-analysis to investigate the evidence base for the use of SMS in clinical management, sexual health services, and health promotion	SMS has the capacity to improve services and increase knowledge and understanding of the condition on interest, and since it is of low cost, easy and convenient to use, highly accessible, and popular it has been used in a variety of ways to improve sexual health: SMS has been employed to deliver STI test results, to remind patients of appointments, as a condom request service, as a reminder to take birth control, as a reminder of the best time of the cycle to try to conceive, and finally in general health promotion.	Evaluation of SMS benefits and effectiveness is important. Because of SMS's low cost and its capability to reach a large number of people, it has the potential to be an important tool in sexual health. In order to utilize it as such, we must ensure that messages are clear, have resonance with the group at risk, and are reaching their target population.
Methods	Levine, McCright, Dobkin, Woodruff, & Klausner, 2008	4 focus groups of youth; 4,500 message inquiries to SexInfo Campaign; surveys from 322 patients from 3 San Francisco clinics aged	Focus groups: to assess the possibility of using text messages to communicate sexual health information including referrals to services, to develop content and marketing. Survey design: The SexInfo Campaign was developed including a text message tree, and a corresponding website was	Marketing took place by running banner ads on Yahoo! and distributing palm cards in schools and neighborhoods with targeted demographics as well as through media news coverage. In the first 25 weeks, there were more than 4,500	Text messaging is a reasonable and culturally acceptable way to communicate sexual health information. Results show success in reaching the highest-risk individuals based on demographic and

(Continued)

				geographic risk factors as demonstrated by campaign awareness.
	12–24 years; additional 214 patients from 10 San Francisco clinics aged 12–24 years surveyed	designed. The program was participant initiated; upon exposure to marketing individuals texted a phone number to receive general sexual health information and referrals to resources. Surveys were given face-to-face in clinics to assess demographics and awareness of campaign.	inquiries; 2,500 of those inquiries led to access to more information and referrals. The most common messages for information were (a) what 2 do if ur condom broke, (b) 2 find out about STDs, and (c) if u think ur pregnant. In survey analysis, positive correlations were found between demographic risk factors for STIs and campaign awareness. African Americans were more likely than any other race to be aware of the program. Additionally, youth living in target areas, younger participants (ages 12–18 years), and youth with the least expensive cell phone providers were more likely to be aware of the program than their counterparts.	
Curioso & Kurth, 2007	31 people living with AIDS in Peru; 3 female	In-depth interviews: report of perceptions toward use of information and communication technologies as a means to support antiretroviral medication adherence and HIV transmission risk reduction	Positive perceptions about using the Internet, cell phones, and PDAs for HIV health promotion; however, cell phones excited people the most to receive information about HIV, either through text messaging or prerecorded voice mails.	Suggests that cell phone use is acceptable and desirable among patients with HIV in a resource-limited setting and that it can build on existing patterns of use.

INTERNET/ COMPUTER RESEARCH	Author/Year	Sample	Study Design and Target Population and Outcome	Results	Significance
	Skinner, Rivette, & Bloomberg, 2007	8 therapeutic counselors in South Africa who are members of the community, are HIV-positive, and are responsible for being advocates for antiretroviral therapy; send reports back to doctors	In-depth interviews with counselors: targeted HIV-positive community members for adherence to ARVs	Cell phones were used to record and send data back to the health services center; interviewees claimed the phones were efficient, saved time, reduced the risk of losing patient notes, and reduced the potential breaks in confidentiality should the notes be lost.	Use of cell phones assisted communication between health care staff and community counselors; counselors thought the use of cell phones could contribute to the management of ARVs in South Africa.
	McKee, Picciano, Roffman, Swanson, & Kalichman, 2006	1,196 callers who were screened for eligibility to participate in an HIV prevention study	Survey design: Participants who initiated contact to participate in an HIV prevention study were screened by telephone to determine eligibility. Those who were eligible and wished to enroll were asked to complete a two-part, pretreatment baseline assessment composed of a telephone interview and a mailed self-administered questionnaire. During the intake interview, callers were asked how they heard of Sex Check (the study). Other information collected included demographic information, HIV status, sexual identity, closetedness, and	The use of recruiters at gay events and venues was important to marketing success. Encouraging enrolled individuals to help publicize the study within their social group cost nothing but had a substantial effect on enrollment. Paid advertisements in widely read alternative newspapers reached a large number of individuals. Paid media (nongay) was most effective in recruiting	Marketing HIV prevention counseling services requires a multicomponent strategy that must be creative to reach men at risk. Nongay media resources may be more effective than gay media resources at successfully reaching bisexual and more closeted MSM— due to the mainstreaming of gay and bisexual cultures. Each marketing channel worked well within specific subgroups, so a

		sexual behavior. Current motivation to adopt safer sex behaviors was assessed with a 5-point item and stage of change—the degree to which they do or do not plan to change or maintain their behavior. The objective of the paper was to find the relative effectiveness of an array of marketing and service strategies to enroll participants in an HIV prevention counseling trial designed to reduce enrollment barriers including logistical burdens, stigma, culture (i.e., insensitivity and mistrust in research), and motivation (i.e., HIV prevention fatigue, ambivalent attitude toward sexual behavior).	Those with less education, bisexuals, closeted men, individuals who had recently had sex with women, and those who more frequently engaged in sex while using drugs. Recruiters were most effective at reaching younger MSM and individuals who frequently engaged in sex while consuming alcohol. Posters/brochures/flyers/matchbooks reached Latinos and HIV-positive MSM and men with less motivation to be sexually safer. Referrals by professionals reached HIV-positive MSM, and referrals by friends and family more successfully reached MSM at an earlier stage of readiness for change and IDUs (injection drug users).	successful marketing campaign depends on being consciously creative throughout the project's duration as to decision making concerning the use of specific channels when recruiting specific subgroups.
Interventions	Haug, Meyer, Schorr, Bauer, & John, 2009	174 participants recruited from the cafeteria of University of Greifswald	RCT: Participants were assigned to one of the three groups: control group without intervention, intervention with one weekly SMS feedback, or intervention with three weekly SMS feedbacks. SMS messages were personalized based on information obtained from a baseline survey. Intervention lasted 3 months. The objective of	Acceptance of the program did not vary between the intervention groups. No significant differences between the three study groups were found based on smoking variables.	High participation and retention rates suggested that SMS-based smoking cessation interventions are attractive for young adults. The effectiveness of text messaging in causing the desired behavior change needs to be further investigated.

(Continued)

(Continued)

INTERNET/COMPUTER RESEARCH	Author/Year	Sample	Study Design and Target Population and Outcome	Results	Significance
			the study was to test the feasibility and acceptance of an intervention using text messaging for continuous individual support of smoking cessation in young adults. Optimal feedback intensity was investigated.		
	Reynolds et al., 2008	109 antiretroviral therapy subjects (control = 55, randomized to intervention = 54)	RCT: targeted ART subjects who received standard clinic-based patient education or that plus structured telephone calls to improve ART adherence	Adherence for trial group (standard education plus phone calls for 16 weeks from trained RN) higher than that of control group (standard care only)	Customized, proactive phone calls have good potential to improve long-term adherence to ART.
	Vildrine, Arduino, & Gritz, 2006	95 participants from an inner-city AIDS clinic in Texas (control = 47, randomized to intervention = 48); 71.6% African American, 18.9% White, 8.4% Hispanic; 35% history of substance use	RCT: HIV-positive adults who smoke; cell phone counseling sessions (8 total) will help smoking cessation for these adults.	Intervention group experienced significantly greater reductions in anxiety and depression and significantly greater increases in self-efficacy. Patients in the intervention group were 5 times more likely to abstain from smoking at the first follow-up assessment (3 months).	Cell phones can be effective in addressing some factors for smoking cessation in people living with AIDS (increasing self-efficacy, decreasing depression and anxiety), which could also impact medical adherence.

van Wier et al., 2006	1,386 eligible employees from 7 different companies. For the two intervention groups, 462 were put in a phone group, and 464 were placed in an Internet group. 460 were placed in the control group.	RCT: Targeted individuals were assigned to a phone intervention group, an Internet intervention group, or a control group to evaluate betterment of BMI, physical activity, diet, and so forth.	So far, the study is projected to show that distance counseling programs via Internet and phone should be more cost efficient, more time saving, and more effective. Results are not complete. There will be a 2 year follow-up of the study.	After the follow-up, the study should be the first to assess "economic evaluations from the societal perspective of weight control intervention" (p. 10), which are grounded upon actual costs and results of the study.
Downer, Meara, & Da Costa, 2005	2,151 patients who had a scheduled appointment at the hospital (control = 769, randomized to intervention = 1,382)	RCT: targeted patients who had appointments who gave their cell phone numbers in order to increase attendance rates for appointments.	The failure-to-attend (FTA) rate was significantly lower in the trial group than in the control group (14.2% vs. 23.4%).	The ease with which large numbers of messages can be customized and sent by text messaging, along with its availability and low cost, suggest it may be a suitable means of improving patient attendance.
Kim et al., 2005	51 subjects (men and women), all with a history of diabetes	Quasi-experimental design: 25 subjects were designated toward the intervention (web-based or cellular communication), and 26 were designated toward the control (face-to-face interaction). Both the intervention and control groups were then split into 2 groups based on their "glycosylated haemoglobin at baseline with type 2 diabetes" (p. 11361). From there, they test which group will maintain the best blood glucose levels.	Patients in the intervention (Internet/cell phone) group were significantly able to maintain better control of their baseline hemoglobin and also improved in their control of HbA1c and Pg levels.	Results show how an Internet/cellular-based approach to patient contact can influence a patient's health outcome better than standard checkups. In the future, other nurses could utilize these forms of communication to have effective results of maintaining/controlling HbA1c or Pg levels.

(Continued)

(Continued)

INTERNET/ COMPUTER RESEARCH	Author/Year	Sample	Study Design and Target Population and Outcome	Results	Significance
	Rodgers et al., 2005	1,705 smokers from throughout New Zealand who wanted to quit, were over 15 years of age, and owned a mobile phone	RCT: Participants were randomly assigned to either the control group or the intervention group. Intervention group received personalized text messages to provide smoking cessation advice, support, and distraction. Follow-up was conducted at 6 weeks and 6 months. The objective of this study was to investigate the effectiveness of using text messages to aid smoking cessation.	More participants had quit at 6 weeks in the intervention in comparison to the control group (28% vs. 13%). Reported quit rates remained high at 6 months, but there was uncertainty between groups because of incomplete follow-up.	Use of text messages to assist in smoking cessation potentially offers a new way to help young smokers quit, being affordable, personalized, age appropriate, and not location dependent.
Broad-Based Technology Focus					
Review Report	VW Consulting, 2009	51 studies relating to the use of some form of technology to present health-related information	Review: Most of the studies were targeting populations in rural and underserved areas, focusing on illness and disease including HIV/AIDS, avian flu, SARS, tuberculosis, diabetes, cardiovascular disease, and others. Some studies conveyed information directly to patients while others provided training and resources to health care providers. Overall, the review investigated the effectiveness of mHealth in its documented applications.	Studies examined showed that mHealth applications have the proven potential to (a) make health care more accessible for people living in underserved areas; (b) improve the ability of health care officials to diagnose and track disease; (c) collect and act on information quicker, such as knowledge of a cluster of people with a communicable disease;	Many mHealth studies have proven the application effective by improving efficiency of health care delivery resulting in more positive health care outcomes. In the future we will see the scope of mHealth increase. In the future, the report notes that studies should run longer to prove the effectiveness, and that there is a need

			and (d) provide health care workers with continuing education and training. They have done so by using a variety of approaches: (a) providing education and promoting awareness, (b) using remote data collection, (c) using remote monitoring of patients, (d) providing communication and training for health care workers, (e) monitoring and tracking disease and epidemic outbreak, and finally (f) providing diagnostic and treatment support. Aspects of mHealth applications that are effective include finding partners in research that contribute to the goals of the study, keeping the user in mind in approach and presentation, finding long-term funding, and setting goals that can be assessed to measure effectiveness		for a global facilitation body to examine gaps in mHealth presentation. There is also the need for multigroup collaboration.
Other					
Meta-analysis	Baranowski, Buday, Thompson, & Baranowski, 2008	27 articles were identified on 25 video games that promoted health-related behavior change through December 2006	Meta-analysis of articles on video games that promoted health-related behavior	Most of the articles demonstrated positive health-related changes through the use of fantasy, attention-maintaining properties of stories, fantasy, interactivity, and behavior change technology.	Further research is needed to investigate the optimal use of game-based intervention in promotion of health-related behavior change.

INTERNET/ COMPUTER RESEARCH	Author/Year	Sample	Study Design and Target Population and Outcome	Results	Significance
Interventions	Andrade et al., 2005	64 subjects who were HIV-positive and over the age of 18 with the ability to self-administer their medication, results from 58 subjects who completed the entire study. There was a majority of African Americans among study participants and a slight majority of male participants in relation to other demographic qualities.	RCT: The intervention group used a disease management assistance system (DMAS) device programmed with verbal reminders at dosing times for all HAART medication. Adherence to HAART regimen was measured through the use of electronic drug exposure monitor (eDEM) caps on specific medications within the HAART regimen. Both the control and intervention groups received monthly drug adherence counseling and were subjected to a biological test for plasma HIV RNA loads and CD4 cell counts. Follow-up evaluations after 24 weeks assessed adherence, neuropsychological status, and mood disorder and substance use.	An electronic verbal prompting device can improve adherence to HAART by HIV-infected subjects who have memory impairment. The effect of the DMAS device at 24 weeks was only evident in the memory-impaired group, resulting in a 20% increase in the adherence rate, compared with 6% for the memory-intact patients. (Memory assessed under "neuropsychological status.")	Poor adherence to HAART may be explained in part by HIV-associated memory deficits. Patients' adherence to treatment may improve with the use of a memory-prompting device.

SOURCES

Andrade, A. S. A., McGruder, H. F., Wu, A. W., Celano, S. A., Skolasky, R. L., Jr., Selnes, O. A., et al. (2005). A programmable prompting device improves adherence to highly active antiretroviral therapy in HIV-infected subjects with memory impairment. *Clinical Infectious Diseases, 41,* 875–882.

Baranowski, T., Buday, R., Thompson, D. I., & Baranowski, J. (2008). Playing for Real: Video games and stories for health-related behavior change. *American Journal of Preventive Medicine, 34,* 74–82.

Bensley, R., Brusk, J., Anderson, J., Mercer, N. F., Rivas, J. F., & Broadbent, L. (2006). Impact of a stages of change-based Internet nutrition education program. *Journal of Nutrition Education and Behavior, 38*(4), 222–229.

Bowen, A. M., Williams, M. L., Daniel, C. M., & Clayton, S. (2008). Internet based HIV prevention research targeting rural MSM: Feasibility, acceptability, and preliminary efficacy. *Journal of Behavioral Medicine, 31*(6), 463–477.

Bull, S. S., Phibbs, S., Watson, S., & McFarlane, M. (2007). What do young adults expect when they go online? Lessons for development of an STD/HIV and pregnancy prevention website. *Journal of Medical Systems, 31,* 149–158.

Christensen, H., Griffiths, K. M., Mackinnon, A. J., & Brittliffe, K. Y. (2006). Online randomized controlled trial of brief and full cognitive behaviour therapy for depression. *Psychological Medicine, 36,* 1737–1746.

Clarke, G. F., Eubanks, D. F., Reid, E., Kelleher, C. F., O'Connor, E., DeBar, L. L., et al. (2005). Overcoming Depression on the Internet (ODIN) (2): A randomized trial of a self-help depression skills program with reminders. *Journal of Medical Internet Research, 7*(2), e16.

Cornelius, J. B., & St. Lawrence, J. S. (2009). Receptivity of African American adolescents to an HIV-prevention curriculum enhanced by text messaging. *Journal for Specialists in Pediatric Nursing, 14,* 123–131.

Cullen, K. W., & Thompson, D. (2010). Feasibility of an 8-week African American web-based pilot program promoting healthy eating behaviors: Family Eats. *American Journal of Health Behavior, 3*(1), 40–51.

Curioso, W. H., & Kurth, A. (2007). Access, use and perceptions regarding Internet, cell phones and PDAs as a means for health promotion for people living with HIV in Peru. *BMC Medical Informatics and Decision Making, 7,* 24.

De Bourdeaudhuij, I., Stevens, V., Vandelanotte, C., & Brug, J. (2007). Evaluation of an interactive computer-tailored nutrition intervention in a real-life setting. *Annals of Behavioral Medicine, 33,* 39–48.

Downer, S. R., Meara, J. G., & Da Costa, A. C. (2005). Use of SMS text messaging to improve outpatient attendance. *Medical Journal of Australia 18*(7), 366–368.

Fjeldsoe, B. S., Marshall, A. L., & Miller, Y. D. (2009). Behavior change interventions delivered by mobile telephone short-message service. *American Journal of Preventive Medicine, 36,* 165–173.

Gilbert, P., Ciccarone, D., Gansky, S. A., Bangsberg, D. R., Clanon, K., McPhee, S. J., et al. (2008). Interactive "Video Doctor" counseling reduces drug and sexual risk behaviors among HIV-positive patients in diverse outpatient settings. *Public Library of Science ONE, 3,* 1–10.

Glasgow, R. E., Boles, S. M., McKay, H. G., Feil, E. G., & Barrera, M., Jr. (2003). The D-Net diabetes self-management program: Long-term implementation, outcomes, and generalization results. *Preventive Medicine, 36,* 410–419.

Grimley, D. M., & Hook, E. W. I. (2009). A 15-minute interactive, computerized condom use intervention with biological endpoints. *Sexually Transmitted Diseases, 36,* 73–78.

Haug, S., Meyer, C., Schorr, G., Bauer, S., & John, U. (2009). Continuous individual support of smoking cessation using text messaging: A pilot experimental study. *Nicotine and Tobacco Research, 11,* 915–923.

Huang, M. Z., Kao, S. C., Avery, M. D., Chen, W., Lin, K., & Gau, M.(2007). Evaluating effects of a prenatal web-based breastfeeding education programme in Taiwan. *Journal of Clinical Nursing 16*(8), 1571–1679.

Hurling, R., Catt, M., De Boni, M., Fairley, B. W., Hurst, T., Murray, P., et al. (2007). Using Internet and mobile phone technology to deliver an automated physical activity program: Randomized controlled trial. *Journal of Medical Internet Research, 9*(2), e7.

Jacobi, C. F., Morris, L. F., Beckers, C. F., Bronisch-Holtze, J. F., Winter, J. F., Winzelberg, A. J., et al. (2007). Maintenance of internet-based prevention: a randomized controlled trial. *International Journal of Eating Disorders, 40*(2), 114–119.

Japuntich, S. J., Zehner, M. E., Smith, S. S., Jorenby, D. E., Valdez, J. A., Fiore, M. C., et al. (2006). Smoking cessation via the Internet: A randomized clinical trial of an Internet intervention as adjuvant treatment in a smoking cessation intervention. *Nicotine Tobacco Research, 8,* S59-S67.

Kainth, A., Hewitt, A., Pattenden, J., Sowden, A., Duffy, S., Watt, I., et al. (2004). Systematic review of interventions to reduce delay in patients with suspected heart attack. *Heart, 90,* 1161.

Kim, H. S., Yoo, Y. S., & Shim, H. S. (2005). Effects of an Internet-based intervention on plasma glucose levels in patients with type 2 diabetes. *Journal of Nursing Care Quality, 20,* 335–340.

Kirk, S. F., Harvey, E., McConnon, A. F., Pollard J. E., Greenwood, D., Thomas, J., Ransley, J., et al. (2007). A randomised trial of an Internet weight control resource: The UK Weight Control Trial. *BMC Health Services Research, 7,* 206.

Krishna, S., Boren, S. A., & Balas, E. A. (2009). Healthcare via cell phones: A systematic review. *Telemedicine and e-Health, 15,* 231–240.

Leeman-Castillo, B., Raghunath, S., Beaty, B., Steiner, J., Bull, S. (2010). LUCHAR: Battling heart disease with computer technology for Latinos. *American Journal of Public Health, 100*(2), 272–275.

Levine, D., McCright, J., Dobkin, L., Woodruff, A. J., & Klausner, J. D. (2008). SEXINFO: A sexual health text messaging service for San Francisco youth. *American Journal of Public Health, 98,* 393–395.

Lim, M. S. C., Hocking, J. S., Hellard, M. E., & Aitken, C. K. (2008). SMS STI: A review of the uses of mobile phone text messaging in sexual health. *International Journal of STD & AIDS, 19,* 287–290.

Logan, A. G., McIsaac, W. J., Tisler, A., Irvine, M. J., Saunders, A., Dunai, A., et al. (2007). Mobile phone-based remote patient monitoring system for management of hypertension in diabetic patients. *American Journal of Hypertension 20,* 942–948.

McKee, M. B., Picciano, J. F., Roffman, R. A., Swanson, F., & Kalichman, S. C. (2006). Marketing the "Sex Check": Evaluating recruitment strategies for a telephone-based HIV prevention project for gay and bisexual men. *AIDS Education and Prevention, 18,* 116–131.

Murray, E., McCambridge, J., Khadjesari, Z. F., White, I. R., Thompson, S., Godfrey, C. F., et al. (2007). The DYD-RCT protocol: An on-line randomised controlled trial of an interactive computer-based intervention compared with a standard information website to reduce alcohol consumption among hazardous drinkers. *BMC Public Health, 7,* 307.

Noar, S., Black, H., & Pierce, L. (2009). Efficacy of computer technology-based HIV prevention interventions: A meta-analysis. *AIDS, 23,* 107–115.

Papadaki, A., & Scott, J. A. (2005). The Mediterranean Eating in Scotland Experience project: Evaluation of an Internet-based intervention promoting the Mediterranean diet. *British Journal of Nutrition, 94,* 290–298.

Patrick, K., Raab, F., Adams, M. A., Dillon, L., Zabinski, M., Rock, C. L., et al. (2009). A text message-based intervention for weight loss: Randomized controlled trial. *Journal of Medical Internet Research, 11,* e1.

Paxton, S. J., McLean, S., Gollings, E. K., Faulkner, C., & Wertheim, E. H. (2006). *How effective are synchronous online interventions for body dissatisfaction in adult women and adolescent girls?* Paper presentation at Eating Disorders Research Society Conference, Port Douglas, Australia.

Polzien, K. M., Jakicic, J. M., Tate, D. F., & Otto, A. D. (2007). The efficacy of a technology-based system in a short-term behavioral weight loss intervention. *Obesity, 15,* 825–830.

Puccio, J. A., Belzer, M., Olson, J., Martinez, M., Salata, C., Tucker, D., et al. (2006). The use of cell phone reminder calls for assisting HIV-infected adolescents and young adults to adhere to highly active antiretroviral therapy: A pilot study. *AIDS Patient Care and STDs, 2*(6), 438–444.

Reynolds, N. R., Testa, M. A., Su, M., Chesney, M. A., Neidig, J. L., Frank, I., et al. (2008). Telephone support to improve antiretroviral medication adherence. *Journal of Acquired Immune Deficiency Syndrome, 4*(7), 62–68.

Rodgers, A., Corbett, T., Bramley, D., Riddell, T., Wills, M., Lin, R. B, et al. (2005). Do u smoke after txt? Results of a randomised trial of smoking cessation using mobile phone text messaging. *Tobacco Control, 14,* 255–261.

Rosser, B., Miner, M., Bockting, W., Ross, M., Konstan, J., Gurak, L., et al. (2009). HIV risk and the Internet: Results of the Men's Internet Sex (MINTS) Study. *AIDS and Behavior, 13,* 746–756.

Skinner, D., Rivette, U., & Bloomberg, C. (2007). Evaluation use of cellphones to aid compliance with drug therapy for HIV patients. *AIDS Care, 19*(5), 605–607.

van Wier, M., Ariens, G., Dekkers, J., Hendriksen, I., Pronk, N., Smid, T., et al. (2006). ALIFE@Work: A randomised controlled trial of a distance counselling lifestyle programme for weight control among an overweight working population. *BMC Public Health, 6,* 140.

Verheijden, M., Bakx, J. C., Akkermans, R., van den Hoogen, H., Godwin, N. M., Rosser, W., et al. (2004). Web-based targeted nutrition counselling and social support for patients at increased cardiovascular risk in general practice: Randomized controlled trial. *Journal of Medical Internet Research, 6,* e44.

Vildrine, D. J., Arduino, R. C., & Gritz, E. (2006). Impact of a cell phone intervention on mediating mechanisms of smoking cessation in individuals living with HIV/AIDS. *Nicotine and Tobacco Research, 8*(1), S103–S108.

VW Consulting. (2009). *mHealth for development: The opportunity of mobile technology for healthcare in the developing world.* Washington, DC, and Berkshire, UK: United Nations.

Webber, K. H., Tate, D. F., & Quintiliani, L. M. (2008). Motivational interviewing in Internet groups: A pilot study for weight loss. *Journal of the American Dietetic Association, 108,* 1029–1032.

Winett, R., Anderson, E., Wojcik, J., Winett, S., & Bowden, T. (2007). Guide to health: Nutrition and physical activity outcomes of a group-randomized trial of an Internet-based intervention in churches. *Annals of Behavioral Medicine, 33,* 251–261.

Name Index

Subject Index

Note: Page numbers with *t* are tables, *f* are figures, and *b* are boxes.

implementation of, 46–47
mobile phones and, 102
purpose of, 52*t*
Health Promotion Practice, 110
Health-e-Solutions project,
104, 176
Healthy People 2010, 75
Hepatitis B virus (HBV), 80
Hierarchical linear modeling
(HLM), 125–126
HIPAA. *See* Health Insurance
Portability and
Accountability Act (HIPAA)
HIV Connect, 130
HIV/AID prevention programs
enrollment challenges of,
76–77
Project LIGHT, 167, 169–174
WRAPP, 184–192
HIV/AIDS
behavior risk profiles, 22–23
bug chaser/gift giver and, 12–14
prevention programs, 95
HLM. *See* Hierarchical linear
modeling (HLM)
Howard Brown Health Center,
98–99
HTML, 78, 82–83*t*
Hybrid programs
evolution of, 80–81
observational studies, 20–21
potential of, 230–233
surveillance facilitation, 22–23

Identification. *See* User
identification
Incentives, 155*t*, 192
Infectious diseases, 76–77, 192
Infomediary
decision-making with, 94*b*
defined, 89
disadvantages of, 93
skills/competencies for, 93*b*
technical difficulties and, 104
use of, 92–95
Information
standardizing, 8–9
tailoring of, 9
technology experts, 71, 74
Informed consent, 44–46

Instant messages, 112*t*
Institutional review boards (IRBs)
defined, 17
steps for, 44*f*
working with, 43–44
Interactive voice response (IVR)
advantages of, 122
defined, 121
development of, 141–143*f*
programs, 140
Interactivity, 5*b*, 9–10
International mobile
telecommunications, 219*t*
Internet and computer research
ACASI in, 130, 140
beneficence in, 38–39
broad-based focus, 260*t*–261*t*
confidentiality in, 40, 128
database development, 68–69
digital divide, 97
equity in, 40
evaluation design, 119–120
generalizability, 12–14
GIS in, 148–149
informed consent in, 44–45
interventions, 80,
241*t*–250*t*, 262*t*
issues facing, 17–19
meta-analysis, 252*t*–254*t*, 261*t*
methods, 239*t*–240*t*, 254*t*–257*t*
mobile phone, 250*t*–252*t*
pilot studies, 236*t*–238*t*
process of, 66
privacy and, 10
public health impact, 8
security issues, 46–49
social networks and, 25–27,
151, 194–200
statistical analysis of, 119–120
surveillance, 240*t*
tailoring and, 9
transparency in, 36
Internet protocol address, 101
Internet service provider
(ISP), 98
Internet-based programs
advantages of, 60
applications, security of, 48
attention spans and, 15
best practices by, 192–194

considerations for, 63–64*b*
D-NET, 184–192
data collection for, 121
disadvantages of, 61–62
evaluation designed for, 20
health promotion reach and, 3
number of sessions for, 193
participant retention
by, 192–192
popularity of, 25
resources for, 202
social networking sites and,
194–200
summary of, 200–201
technical difficulties with, 104
updates for, 193–19
user identification and, 14
Web 2.0 elements, 194
WRAPP, 184–189, 184–192
Intervention programs
additional resources for, 30
behavior change and, 18–19
at individual level, 18–19
stand-alone, 24–25
targeted, 80
3-minute, 80
types of, 18
research example,
241*t*–250*t*, 262*t*
Interviews, self, 10
iPhones, 216
IRBs. *See* Institutional review
boards (IRBs)
IVR. *See* Interactive voice
response (IVR)

Java virtual machine, 219*t*

Kiosks. *See* Computer kiosks

Laptops, 47
Latinos
cardiovascular risk to, 162–163
digital divide and, 76, 92
health disparities of, 75
mobile phone use by, 215
LinkedIn
defined, 195
page, example of, 199*t*
purpose of, 198

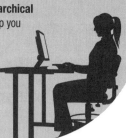
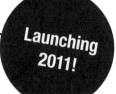
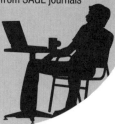
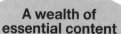